Xenobiotic Metabolism: Nutritional Effects

Xenobiotic Metabolism: Nutritional Effects

John W. Finley, EDITOR
Nabisco Brands, Inc.

Daniel E. Schwass, EDITOR
Oregon Health Sciences University

Based on a symposium sponsored by
the Division of Agricultural and Food Chemistry
at the 187th Meeting
of the American Chemical Society,
St. Louis, Missouri,
April 8–13, 1984

American Chemical Society, Washington, D.C. 1985

Library of Congress Cataloging in Publication Data

Xenobiotic metabolism.
  (ACS symposium series, ISSN 0097-6156; 277)

  "Based on a symposium sponsored by the Division of
Agricultural and Food Chemistry at the 187th meeting
of the American Chemical Society, St. Louis, Missouri,
April 8–13, 1984."

  Includes bibliographies and indexes.

  1. Xenobiotics—Metabolism—Nutritional aspects—
Congresses.

  I. Finley, John W., 1942–   . II. Schwass, Daniel
E., 1951–   . III. American Chemical Society.
Division of Agricultural and Food Chemistry.
IV. American Chemical Society. Meeting (187th: 1984:
St. Louis, Mo.) V. Series.

QP529.X46   1985   612'.39   85-6191
ISBN 0–8412–0912–X

ACS Symposium Series

M. Joan Comstock, *Series Editor*

FOREWORD

The ACS SYMPOSIUM SERIES was founded in 1974 to provide a medium for publishing symposia quickly in book form. The format of the Series parallels that of the continuing ADVANCES IN CHEMISTRY SERIES except that, in order to save time, the papers are not typeset but are reproduced as they are submitted by the authors in camera-ready form. Papers are reviewed under the supervision of the Editors with the assistance of the Series Advisory Board and are selected to maintain the integrity of the symposia; however, verbatim reproductions of previously published papers are not accepted. Both reviews and reports of research are acceptable, because symposia may embrace both types of presentation.

CONTENTS

vii

viii

PREFACE

OUR ENVIRONMENT exposes us daily to a wide variety of xenobiotics: in our food, in the air we breathe, or as a result of industrial exposure and toxic wastes. However, despite this exposure, most of us are living long, healthy lives. Certainly individual variation could account for some of the variability in resistance to disease, but other factors are undoubtedly involved. According to a growing body of evidence, diet may be extremely important in increasing resistance to chronic disease. One is tempted to speculate, or hope, that improved dietary habits could improve individual resistance to chemically induced chronic disease.

In this volume, we have focused on how xenobiotics are metabolized in higher animals and how this metabolism is mediated by the nutritional status of the target animal. Emphasis has been placed on the toxic, mutagenic, carcinogenic and potentially mutagenic or carcinogenic compounds. The topic is a natural follow-up and expansion of "Xenobiotics in Foods and Feeds" (ACS Symposium Series No. 234, Finley and Schwass, Eds.) in which sources of xenobiotics were identified and discussed at length. The authors in this volume discuss how and why these xenobiotics are toxic and how nutritional intervention can mediate some of the toxicities.

Current nutritional awareness in the western world is probably unparalleled in the history of man. One need only look in health food stores and supermarkets to see the results of this awareness. Many food companies now place major emphasis on the natural, pure, low-calorie, additive-free, health- and fitness-oriented ingredients in their products. Nutritionists have established requirements for normal individuals, and additional data are being acquired rapidly on diets designed especially for individuals who experience high stress due either to illness or life style.

This volume presents a state-of-the-art assessment of how diet can intervene and aid in the prevention of chronic disease. The editors hope this effort will stimulate further research in this important area of food biochemistry and nutrition.

The authors wish to express their sincere gratitude to Miles Laboratories, Stroh Brewing Co., Nabisco Brands, Cutter Laboratories, Best Foods, General Mills, Inc., Warner Jenkinson, McCormick and Co., H. J. Heinz, and Lipton, Inc. for their generous support in helping many of the authors attend the symposium upon which this volume is based.

JOHN W. FINLEY
Nabisco Brands, Inc.
Fair Lawn, New Jersey

September 21, 1984

DANIEL E. SCHWASS
Oregon Health Sciences University
Portland, Oregon

The editors would like to dedicate this volume to the memory of Morris N. Joselow whose untimely death in 1983 was a loss to all, particularly those in the area of preventative medicine. Dr. Joselow was Professor of Preventative Medicine and Community Health at the College of Medicine and Dentistry in Newark, New Jersey. One of his last published works, "Systematic Toxicity Testing for Xenobiotics in Foods," appeared in "Xenobiotics in Foods and Feeds" (ACS Symposium Series No. 234). In addition to his other duties, he was organizer and principal lecturer in the American Chemical Society Toxicology Short Course. Dr. Joselow's research interests included environmental sciences, industrial hygiene and safety, toxicology, trace metals, and biochemical monitoring. During his career he published more than 100 papers. Dr. Joselow will be missed as a friend, a coworker, and a scientist.

Overview: The Influence of Nutrition on Xenobiotic Metabolism

D. E. SCHWASS[1,3] and J. W. FINLEY[2]

[1]U.S. Department of Agriculture, Western Regional Research Center, Berkeley, CA 94610
[2]Nabisco Brands, Inc., Fair Lawn, NJ 07410

In the course of living in the modern world it is inevitable that man and animals will be exposed to compounds in the environment which are not essential for life or even "normal" from the standpoint of the evolution of the species. The term "xenobiotic" (from the Greek "xenos" and "bios", meaning stranger to life) was coined by Mason, et al [1] to describe the myriad of compounds including carbohydrates, lipids, proteins, alkaloids, natural and synthetic drugs, flavorings, pigments, preservatives, polycyclic hydrocarbons, flavonoids, terpenoids, etc., which may enter the organism as non-essential or non-functional materials. The assumption inherent in the use of the term is that one is speaking relative to an organism of reference. For example, the drug quinine is a xenobiotic relative to man but not to the South American tree, Chinchona officinalis, in which quinine is a major constituent of the bark. Xenobiotics which enter the biosphere of the organism are not necessarily toxic. In fact, based on the Mason definition, non-essential amino acids could be referred to as xenobiotics. For the purpose of this symposium, however, xenobiotic does not include non-essential nutrients which occur in the diet, but will be restricted to environmental compounds which are acutely toxic, potentially toxic requiring activation, or which exhibit long term effects, such as mutagens, carcinogens or teratogens. In general, the discussions in this symposium are relative to man and/or animals. It is important to remember that xenobiotics range from the inocuous (i.e. vanillin) through the chronically toxic (i.e. ethanol) to the acutely toxic (i.e. curare). Some xenobiotics, although not toxic in and of themselves, are metabolically converted to toxic substances. The metabolic conversion of xenobiotics to toxic substances can be dramatically influenced by the nutritional status of the organism.

Smoking, drugs, industrial chemicals and foods, represent the major sources of exposure to xenobiotics for modern man. Because diet furnishes the most variable and continuous array of xenobiotic exposure, the emphasis of this symposium is the

[3]Current address: Oregon Health Sciences University, Portland, OR 97201

0097-6156/85/0277-0001$06.00/0
© 1985 American Chemical Society

influence of food-borne xenobiotics and how diet can mediate the
metabolism of these compounds. Food borne xenobiotics can be
endogenous to the foodstuff (flavinoids in tea), can result from
processing and storage (lipid oxidation or non-enzymatic
browning) or can be the result of deliberate addition (the
antioxidant, butylated hydroxyanisole).

Exposure to xenobiotics is inevitable and although the degree
of exposure can be controlled, it is impossible to prevent
exposure altogether. Fortunately, the healthy, well-nourished
individual or animal under normal circumstances can resist long-
term effects of many of these compounds by metabolizing them and
excreting them as metabolites or conjugates of metabolites.

A major source of exposure to xenobiotics is tobacco smoke.
Cigarette smoke consists of a large variety of compounds
including oxidants, free radicals, benzo-(a)-pyrene and carbon
monoxide. Long term exposure to cigarette smoke entails exposure
to both acutely toxic materials and chronically toxic materials.
We are all exposed to smoke in various degrees both from tobacco
and from the environment through the burning of fuels and from
cooking. Exposure to industrial sources of xenobiotics can come
via the air or through exposure and absorption by the skin.
Although major industrial exposure receives much publicity when
it occurs. This type of event usually accounts for exposure to
relatively few compounds over a prolonged period of time.
Fortunately, chemical companies have made great strides in
reducing the incidence of such exposure, although it is likely
that some exposure will continue to occur either through
accidents or lack of knowledge. Industrial pollution in the form
of toxic waste should be reduced significantly in the next
several years as efforts continue to correct this problem.
Exposure from toxic waste dumps is likely to continue but at
lower levels. Pharmaceutical drugs can be considered xenobiotics
and in the western world an individual might expect to be exposed
significantly to two-to-three dozen compounds in a lifetime under
normal circumstances. Frequently these exposures are over
relatively short periods of time.

Food represents a large and continuous exposure to a vast
array of xenobiotics. Xenobiotics from food can range from the
inocuous to the extremely dangerous. Plants frequently produce a
variety of xenobiotics which subsequently are consumed by man or
animals. In addition, during storage and processing of foods,
(including home cooking), xenobiotics can be produced. A recent
symposium (Finley and Schwass) (2) reviewed many of these
sources of xenobiotics in the diet.

Historically, the impact of diet on health has been a concern
of man. In recent years we have seen greater emphasis on how
nutrition relates to health and the prevention of chronic
afflictions such as coronary heart disease, hypertension,
obesity, and cancer. Consequently, several health organizations
have proposed guidelines to promote better health and reduce risk

of chronic disease. The National Research Council $(\underline{3})$
published an extensive study and guidelines regarding nutritional
means to reduce the risk of cancer. In this volume, Palmer $(\underline{4})$
discusses these guidelines in terms of current evidence. One of
the problem areas discussed is dietary fat and its relationship
to cancer as well as previously established relationships to
coronary heart disease and obesity.

Throughout this symposium one observes a common thread in
many of the papers: the many problems associated with lipids in
the diet. It is important to note however, that the problems may
not be due simply to fat but more likely to oxidized lipid
products. Pryor $(\underline{5})$ reviews the mechanisms of lipid oxidation
and discusses the chemical basis for a relationship between lipid
oxidation and chronic disease. It would seem from this and other
evidence $(\underline{6})$ $(\underline{7})$ $(\underline{8})$ that peroxidizing lipids could be a major
dietary concern in the development of certain types of cancers.
If one considers the early stages of tumor development to be
initiation followed by promotion, one could speculate a number of
roles for peroxidizing lipids. Initiation for the purpose of
this discussion will be considered the initial chemical change in
the DNA of a cell which has the potential to lead to the
development of a tumor. In the promotion stage, the damaged cell
begins to multiply as a result of chemical insult and tumor
development proceeds. The initial damage or initiation can be
caused by a variety of compounds, many of which are used as model
compounds for the study of carcinogenesis. One might speculate
that these compounds (i.e., DMBA, benzo-(a)-pyrene) could act as
initiators and the oxidizing lipids as promoters. Indeed, much
of the evidence in the present symposium will support this
speculation. If one then considers the protective role against
tumor development of retenoids, BHT, ascorbic acid and
tocopherol, all of which are antioxidants, the argument is
strengthened (Chow, $(\underline{5})$ $(\underline{8})$; King, $(\underline{9})$; Newberne, $(\underline{10})$
C. Reddy, $(\underline{11})$; Anderson, $(\underline{12})$; Seifter et al $(\underline{13})$; Baird,
$(\underline{14})$. The issue is certainly more complicated than simple
control of oxidation, but the evidence does suggest an important
correlation. In addition, peroxidizing lipids represent a group
of xenobiotics which can be controlled in the diet. Oxidized
lipids are important in the development of certain flavors in
foods such as frying and in the flavor profiles of certain
meats. Through reduced consumption of meats and fried foods, as
suggested in the NRC Guidelines $(\underline{3})$, exposure to oxidized
lipids can be reduced. Assuming that the oxidation products or
intermediates act as promoters or modify the ability of the cell
to metabolize the initiating carcinogen in a harmless way,
reducing the level of these xenobiotics in the diet could
significantly reduce the risk of tumor development.

The impact of xenobiotics on health can occur in a number of
ways. As we have noted, the xenobiotic can be a carcinogen, be
metabolized to a carcinogen, inhibit the detoxification of

another xenobiotic, act as a tumor promoter or act as an acute
toxin. Clearly we are and will continue to be exposed to
compounds which are both acutely toxic and those which exhibit a
long term effect such as carcinogens. Acute toxins are usually
detectable and can be controlled in diet. On the other hand,
chronic xenobiotics can occur at extremely low levels in the diet
over several years before any clinical manifestations are
observed, and because of the extremely low levels and wide
variety of candidate materials, chemical detection is difficult.
Complete analysis for and subsequent control of these compounds
is unlikely. Furthermore, these materials can result from
processing, storage and home preparation, making control even
more difficult. Dietary restraint and assuring that the
detoxification system is functioning correctly would appear to be
the best current means of preventing chronic disease.

In the process of attempting to detoxify materials, the
animal of man frequently converts them to carcinogens in the
process. One of the principle means of detoxification in higher
animals is the microsomal mixed function oxidases (MFO).
Xenobiotics including polycyclic hydrocarbons which appear in
food cooked using hish temperatures, smoke, drugs, or chemical
processes are frequently metabolized by the MFO system. These
cytochrome P-450-linked systems, when coupled with other
metabolically juxtaposed adjacent enzymes, provide cells with an
important pathway whereby the various xenobiotics can be
converted to metabolites that are water soluble, allowing them to
be safely excreted. These systems are clearly beneficial and
indeed essential to the organism. Unfortunately, these same
systems can also convert xenobiotics to metabolites which are
toxic, mutagenic, teratogenic and carcinogenic. A typical
example of this type of enzyme is the aryl hydrocarbon
hydroxylase (AHH) which oxygenates polycyclic aromatic
hydrocarbons. This enzyme is nearly ubiquitous in animal
tissues. It is a multicomponent system consisting of a
cytochrome P-450, NADPH cytochrome P-450 reductase, and a
phospholipid cofactor. The enzyme system is induced when the
system is exposed to polycyclic aromatic hydrocarbons, or various
drugs or hydrocarbons, with the activity increasing as much as
one hundred fold. The ability of the organism to respond in this
way is important for it to respond to normal exposures to
xenobiotics. Typically, benzo-(a)-pyrene can be used to measure
the activity of the enzyme so the phenolic procuts can be easily
measured. The products also represent an excellent example of
possible benefits and dangers of the enzyme system. Figure 1
shows that partial oxidation products can bind DNA, while a more
favored route would be the formation of conjugates with
glutathione. The activation of the enzyme and the levels of
glutathione are factors that could be dramatically affected by
the nutritional status of the organism. Also, one could
speculate that other compounds in the cell could compete for

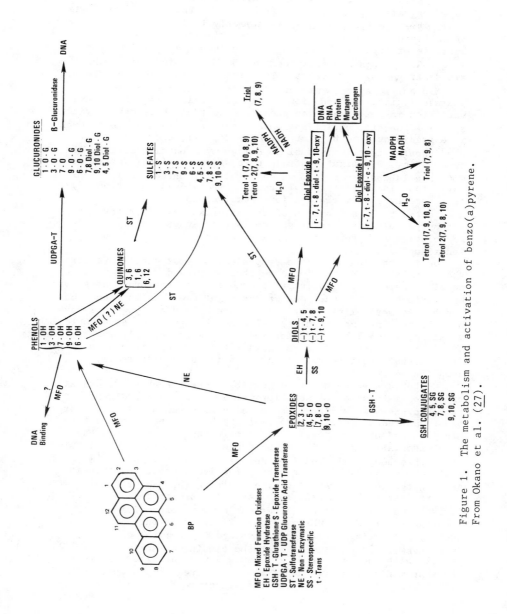

Figure 1.   The metabolism and activation of benzo(a)pyrene.
From Okano et al. (27).

glutathione conjugation and therefore increase the chance of DNA binding by the epoxide intermediates.

Examples of how variation in dietary status can influence drug metabolism in humans are discussed by Vesell [15] and Carr [16]. Both report that diet can greatly influence the effectiveness of drugs. Dietary manipulations that would activate or depress the MFO system influence activity of the drug. Some drugs are activated by the MFO system while others are destroyed by the system. Therefore, diets which influence the MFO enzyme systems are of significant concern to the pharmacologist. In addition to dietary variations, individual variation may exert an even greater effect on these detoxifying systems. Genetic variation could cause an individual to be much more predisposed to high or low MFO activity, thereby predisposing that individual to damage by a particular type of xenobiotic. One might contrast this wide individual variation with the laboratory animal which is highly inbred. All variations in diet are complicated by individual variation and environment. The variation in effectiveness of drugs can be considered to be a function of these variables. Therefore it is not unreasonable to expect variability in suseptibility to xenobiotics from food, industrial exposure, or smoking in individuals.

During the course of the symposium, several dietary factors that can influence xenobiotic metabolism were discussed in detail. Here we will attempt to summarize in the broadest terms how various classic nutrient groups might exert an influence on xenobiotic metabolism. For convenience, the dietary groups have been broken into carbohydrates, lipids, proteins, water-soluble vitamins, fat-soluble vitamins and trace elements. It is difficult to take any one group individually, and it must be kept in mind that the interactions are continuous and extremely complicated.

Carbohydrates which are digestible appear to have no dramatic effect on metabolism of xenobiotics; however, the nondigestible carbohydrates can mediate the toxicity of a xenobiotic. Dietary fiber can reduce nutrient availability by absorbtion of certain minerals and/or vitamins. Inclusion in the diet of fiber has been associated with a lower incidence of colon cancer, and this effect has been explained in a number of ways (B. Reddy, [17]; Kritchevsky, [18]. Fiber can be effective in reducing transit time in the gut, thereby lowering the time for bacteria to convert intestinal content into toxic or carcinogenic derivatives. In addition, fiber can be very effective as an absorbant to bind and carry certain xenobiotics through the system, preventing their absorption and any harmful effect. Kritchevsky [18] points out that the binding capacity varies greatly with the type of fiber; hence different fibers protect the system differently. As in may other areas, much more work will be necessary to establish the structure function

relationship for these phenomena. Variations in dietary fiber
also alter the nature of the gut flora. Inclusion of fermentable
fiber such as pectin in the diet, results in a higher
concentration of cecal bacteria, hence greater metabolism of 2,
6-dinitrotoluene or nitrobenzene. The result of the greater
bacterial fermentation appears to be greater absorption and
hepatic binding of the aromatics. The results suggest that
non-fermentable fiber may offer the advantage that the bound
xenobiotics would not be released and subsequently abosrbed.

High levels of dietary fat have been associated with
increased risk of colon, (B. Reddy, [17]), prostrate, uterus,
ovary and mammary cancers (Carroll, [19] in humans. It is
important to recognize that diets higher in polyunsaturated fatty
acids exhibit higher incidence of colon cancer than diets high in
saturated or monounsaturated fatty acids (B. Reddy, [17]. The
polyunsaturated fatty acids appear to act at the promotion state
of tumorogenesis rather than as initiators. Because diets
containing polyunsaturated fatty acids are susceptible to
oxidation, the question of the importance of lipid oxidation or
lipid oxidation products in the initiation or promotion of tumor
development becomes very important. Pryor [5] reports that the
free radicals from the oxidation reactions can bind
macromolecules and that the free radicals can themselves by
involved in tumor promotion. Rahimtula et al [7] demonstrated
that lipid peroxidation is involved in chemical carcinogenesis
initiated by benzo-(a)-pyrene, aminofluorene, benzidine and
methylaminobenzene. The products were shown to be bound
irreversibly to protein and DNA. Wheeler, et al [20]
demonstrated that varying the oxidation state of sulfur amino
acids in the diet caused variation in the forms of MFO in the
liver and therefore affected the nature of metabolites of
benzo-(a)-pyrene formed. The results suggest again that
oxidation state may be important. The various oxidation states
of sulfur amino acids can be a secondary effect of lipid
oxidation. As lipid oxidation proceeds, increased levels of
oxidized sulfur amino acids would be expected in the diet.

The nature of protein in the diet also appears to alter
xenobiotic metabolism. Clinton and Visek [6] and Clinton and
Visek [21] observed that protein alters carcinogen metabolism
and that fat level in the diet alters the absorption and
distribution of DMBA in the tissue. The effects of protein
nutriture also are observed when 1, 2-dimethylhydrazine is
included in the diet. It appears that inadequate protein in the
diet causes a significant decrease in hepatic MFO activity.
Hayes [22] observed that in protein-deficient animals,
aflatoxin B^1 was more acutely toxic and not as carcinogenic.
This was explained by lower MFO activity in the liver. Animals
with the decreased MFO activity were unable to detoxify the
aflatoxin B^1, thus it was acutely toxic. Because the aflatoxin
was not hydroxylated by the MFO, it was not converted to the

carcinogenic derivative. It appears that the state of the sulfur amino acids and the quantity of protein both influence the ability of the organism to metabolize xenobiotics.

Water-soluble vitamins and co-factors also appear to elicit an effect on xenobiotic metabolism. Ascorbic acid has been shown to inhibit chemically induced chemical carcinogenesis in test systems (Shamberger, [8]. When diets are deficient in choline, the animals appear to become much more susceptible to chemically-induced carcinogenesis (Shinozuka, et al, [23]. It was observed in this work that there was more lipid peroxidation in the livers of the choline-deficient animals. This may be important in relation to the tumor-promoting effects of lipid peroxides. Herbert [24] observed that chemically-induced tumors of the liver, colon and esophagus may be enhanced by diets deficient in folic acid, vitamin B^{12}, choline and methionine. Conversely, he observed that vitamin B^{12} may serve to enhance the carcinogenic effect of p-dimethylaminoazobenzene in rats fed a methionine-deficient diet. It is important to note, however, that this was only true in rats on a methionine-deficient diet.

Fat-soluble vitamins, in addition to their antioxidative effects on lipids, appear to exert a general protective effect in animals. Vitamin A and beta-carotenes protect lab animals from toxicity of citral, cyclophosphamide and some hydrocarbons (Seifter et al, [13]. In related but independent studies, it was observed that high levels of vitamin A inhibit tumorogenesis and that low levels of vitamin A appear to enhance tumorogenesis (Baird, [14]. Vitamin E inhibited chemically-induced carcinogenesis in test systems (Shamberger, [8] and also reduced the susceptibility of rats to cigarette smoke (Chow, [25]. These observations support the NRC guidelines urging increased consumption of fruits and vegetables which are rich in these vitamins.

Selenium levels in the diet and blood have been shown to be inversely correlated with human cancer mortality (Shamnberger, [8]. Also, selenium-dependent glutathione peroxidase activity has been shown to be reduced in selenium-deficient rats (C. Reddy, [11]. Selenium appears to inhibit both the initiation and promotion phases of carcinogenesis (Milner, [26]. These results suggest that selenium is critical for glutathione peroxidase activity, but apparently functions in other ways as well to inhibit carcinogenesis.

In summary, it is clear that a multitude of dietary factors can influence the metabolism of xenobiotics, particularly those that can be involved in carcinogenesis. We are and will continue to be exposed to xenobiotics of various types from our food, industrial sources, toxic wastes, drugs, and smoke. The well nourished animal or man appears, within the limits of individual variation, to be able to metabolize and excrete most of these xenobiotics harmlessly. It is important that we use the best diet possible to reduce fat in the diet, particularly where lipid

oxidation is present, and adhering to the proposed NRC
guidelines. Following these guidelines will, in effect, assure
adequate levels of vitamins, selenium, protein and fiber.

Literature Cited

1. Mason, H. S., North J. C. and Vanneste, M. (1965) Fed. Proc.
   24, 1172.
2. Finley, J. W. and Schwass, E.E., Xenobiotics in Foods and
   Feeds. ACS Symposium Series #234 American Chemical Society
   Washington, DC 1983.
3. National Research Council (1982) Diet, Nutrition, and
   Cancer. Committee on Diet, Nutrition and Cancer, Commission
   on Life Sciences, National Academy Press, Washington, DC.
   496pp.
4. Palmer, S. (1985) Interim Dietary Guidelines to Lower the
   Risk of Cancer. This Volume.
5. Pryor, W.A. (1985) Free Radical Reactions in Autoxidation,
   Cancer, Heart and Blood Vessel Diseases and Aging. This
   Volume.
6. Clinton, S.K. and Visek, W.J. (1985) The Interactions of
   Dietary Fat and Protein on Breast Cancer. This Volume.
7. Rahimtula, M., Washington, W., Gregory, B. and O'Brien, P.J.
   (1985). Xenobiotic Adduct Formation with DNA or GSH
   Following Oxidation by Lipid Peroxide or H2O2-Peroxidase.
   This Volume.
8. Shamberger, R.J. (1985) Antioxidants and Malonaldehyde in
   Cancer. This Volume.
9. King, M.M. (1985) Modulation of Mammary Tumor Incidence by
   Dietary Fat and Antioxidants - A Mechanistic Approach. This
   Volume.
10. Newberne, P.M. (1985) Dietary Factors Affecting Biological
    Responses to Chemicals. This Volume.
11. Reddy, C.C. (1985) Effects of Inadequate Vitamin E and/or
    Selenium nutrition on enzymes associated with Hydroperoxide
    Metabolism. This Volume.
12. Anderson, M.W. (1985) Inhibition in Vivo of the Binding of
    Benzo-a-pyrene Metabolites to DNA in Target Tissues by
    Butylated Hydroxyanisole. This Volume.
13. Seifter, E., Demetriou, A.A., Levenson, S.M. and Rettura, G
    (1985) The Anti-Toxic Properties of Vitamin A. This Volume.
14. Baird, M.B. (1985) Modulation of Chemical Mutagenesis in a
    Salmonella/Mamalian Tissue Bioassay by Vitamin A and Other
    Retinoids. This Volume.
15. Vesell, E.S. (1985) To What Extent do Dietary Factors
    Account for Interindividual Variation of Normal Human
    Subjects in Drug Disposition. This Volume.
16. Carr, C.J. (1985) Food and Drug Interactions. This Volume.
17. Reddy, B. (1985) Influence of Types and Levels of Dietary
    Fat on Colon Cancer. This Volume.

18. Kritchevsky, D. (1985) Influence of Dietary Fiber on
    Xenobiotics. This Volume.
19. Carroll, K.K. (1985) Influence of Diet on Hormone-Dependent
    Cancers. This Volume.
20. Wheeler, E.L., Schwass, D.E., and Berry, D.L. Modulation of
    Benzo-a-pyrene Metabolism by Dietary Sulfur Amino Acids.
    This Volume.
21. Visek, W.J. and Clinton, S.K. (1985) Dietary Influences on
    the Toxicity, Mutagenicity and Carcinogenicity of Hydrazines
    and Related Compounds. This Volume.
22. Hayes, J.R. (1985) Effect of Nutrition on the Metabolism and
    Toxicity of Mycotoxins. This Volume.
23. Shinozuka, H., Demetris, A.J., Katyal, S.L. and Perera,
    M.I.R. (1985) Interactions of Barbiturates and a Choline
    Deficient Diet in Promotion of Liver Carcinogenesis. This
    Volume.
24. Herbert, V. (1985) The Inhibition of Some Cancers and the
    Promotion of Others by Folic Acid, Vitamin B[12], and Their
    Antogonists. This Volume.
25. Chow, C.K. (1985) Dietary Vitamin E and Cigarette Smoking,
    This Volume.
26. Milner, J.A. (1985) The Effect of Selenium on Carcinogenesis.
    This Volume.
27. Okano, P., J.P. Whitlock, Jr. (1980) Aryl Hydrocarbon
    Hydroxylase and Benzo-a-pyrene Metabolism in Rodent Liver and
    Human Cells. In: Differentiation and Carcinogenesis in
    Liver Cell Cultures. C. Borek and G.M. Williams, eds.
    Annals of the New York Academy of Sciences Vol. 349. 232-246.

RECEIVED March 15, 1985

Interim Dietary Guidelines to Lower the Risk of Cancer

SUSHMA PALMER

Food and Nutrition Board, Commission on Life Sciences, National Academy of Sciences, Washington, DC 20418

In recent decades, the study of nutritional factors and health has been directed towards investigating the role of dietary constituents in the development and prevention of chronic diseases such as coronary artery disease, hypertension, and cancer. Consequently, in recent years, several public and private organizations concerned with health and nutrition have proposed recommendations to promote health in general or to reduce the risk of particular chronic diseases including cancer. The intent of this paper is to compare those recommendations with interim guidelines to lower the risk of cancer that were proposed in June 1982 by the Committee on Diet, Nutrition, and Cancer of the National Research Council (NRC). A comparison will be made of the areas of consensus and disagreement. Particular emphasis will be placed on the criteria for interpreting scientific evidence relating diet to chronic diseases, on the public policy implications of current knowledge, and the elements of such policy.

At least three major factors need to be examined in contemplating the elements of dietary policy to lower the risk of cancer: the evidence relating diet and carcinogenesis, the criteria for interpreting and translating scientific evidence into dietary recommendations to the public, and the implications of current

0097–6156/85/0277–0011$06.00/0

knowledge about the association of diet and carcinogenesis for the
formulation of dietary guidelines. This paper contains a discussion of each of these factors and outlines the components of such
dietary policy.

Evidence Relating Diet and Carcinogenesis

In the past half a century, scientists and public health officials
have gradually come to realize that the two leading causes of mortality in Western nations, heart disease and cancer, are associated to a certain though unknown extent with life style, including
dietary factors. This association is somewhat better established
for coronary artery disease than it is for cancer. Based on current knowledge, many organizations have offered dietary advice to
the public (1-9). However, the scientific community has reached
no clear consensus about the nature of the association between
diet and chronic diseases and the extent to which dietary modification can decrease the risk, especially cancer risk
(5;6;10;11).
       Part of the uncertainty about cancer stems from long-stand-
ing controversy over the major causes of carcinogenesis (12).
In recent years, however, there appears to be a more consistent
trend. Emphasis seems to have gradually shifted from the assumption that cancer is an inevitable consequence of aging to a
recognition that the environment may play an important role (10;
13-15). A few epidemiologists have suggested that as much as 90%
of all cancer may be related to the environment, and that 40% to
60% of this may be diet-related (14;15). The possibility that
the environment rather than genetic background plays a major role
in susceptibility to certain types of cancer bears the implication that some types of cancer are potentially preventable, possibly through modification of factors such as lifestyle and diet.
       Interest in investigating the relationship between dietary
factors and carcinogenesis dates back to the early part of the
century. Over the past four or five decades, epidemiological
investigations and laboratory experiments in animals have generated abundant data about cancer and its relationship to dietary
patterns, to individual foodstuffs, nutrients, food additives,
and dietary contaminants (16). This vast body of literature was
recently analyzed by the Committee on Diet, Nutrition, and Cancer
of the National Research Council (6), and the committee reached
the major conclusions outlined in Tables I to III.
       These conclusions were reached with the recognition that as
with the general state of knowledge on diet and chronic diseases,
the data base on diet and carcinogenesis is far from complete.
There is a lack of complete understanding of cause and effect and
of the mechanisms involved. This is partly because of attempts
to precisely relate two complex factors, diet and carcinogenesis,

whose nature is itself imprecisely understood. It is difficult
to determine precisely what people eat, how best to measure
dietary intake in relation to the latency period of cancer, and
how to isolate the effects of dietary patterns from those of

Table I. Diet, Nutrition, and Cancer:
General Conclusions (6)

---

1. The differences in the rates at which various cancers occur
    in different human populations are often correlated with
    differences in diet. The likelihood that some of these cor-
    relations reflect causality is strengthened by laboratory
    evidence that similar dietary patterns and components of food
    also affect the incidence of certain cancers in animals.
2. In general, the evidence suggests that some types of diets
    and some dietary components (e.g., high fat diets or the fre-
    quent consumption of salt-cured, salt-pickled, and smoked
    foods) tend to be associated with an increased risk of
    cancer, whereas others (e.g., low fat diets or the frequent
    consumption of certain fruits and vegetables) are associated
    with a decreased risk. The mechanisms responsible for these
    effects are not fully understood.
3. The evidence suggests that cancers of most major sites are
    influenced by dietary patterns. However, the data are not
    sufficient to quantitate the contribution of diet to the
    overall cancer risk or to determine the percent reduction
    that might be achieved by dietary modifications.

---

other environmental factors and genetic influences. Neither the
process of carcinogenesis nor the mechanisms whereby environmental
factors including diet, might promote, initiate or inhibit carcinogenesis are well defined (6;17). However, having considered
all the discrepancies in the data base, the Committee on Diet,
Nutrition, and Cancer found the overall evidence to be sufficiently convincing to propose certain interim dietary guidelines that
have the potential to lower cancer risk. These are shown in Table
IV.

In addition, the committee proposed two guidelines directed at
regulatory agencies such as the Food and Drug Administration that
control the use of food additives and contaminants in the U.S.
diet (Table V).

Criteria for Interpretation of Scientific Data and Formulation of Dietary Policy

As explained in the detailed report (6), the above conclusions and
recommendations were based on evidence from a data base consisting of descriptive as well as analytical epidemiological studies,
and a vast number and variety of animal experiments and in-vitro
tests.

Table II. Diet, Nutrition, and Cancer:
Conclusions on Dietary Macroconstituents (6)

Total Caloric Intake. Neither the epidemiological studies nor the experiments in animals permit a clear interpretation of the specific effect of total caloric intake on the risk of cancer. Nonetheless, the studies conducted in animals show that a reduction in the total food intake decreases the age-specific incidence of cancer. The evidence is less clear for human beings.

Fats and Lipids. Of all the dietary components studied, the combined epidemiological and experimental evidence is most suggestive for a causal relationship between high fat intake and increased occurrence of cancer. The relationship between dietary cholesterol and carcinogenesis is not clearly understood.

Protein. The evidence from both epidemiological and laboratory studies suggests that high protein intake may be associated with an increased risk of cancers at certain sites. However, because of the relative paucity of data on protein compared to fat, and the strong correlation between the intakes of fat and protein in the U.S. diet, no firm conclusion can be drawn about an independent effect of protein.

Carbohydrates. Information concerning the role of carbohydrates in the development of cancer is extremely limited and inconclusive.

Dietary Fiber. There is no conclusive evidence to indicate that total dietary fiber exerts a protective effect against colorectal cancer in humans. Both epidemiological and laboratory reports suggest that if there is such an effect, specific components of fiber, rather than total fiber, are more likely to be responsible.

Alcoholic Beverages. In some countries, including the United States, excessive beer drinking has been associated with an increased risk of colorectal cancer, especially rectal cancer. There is limited evidence that excessive alcohol consumption which causes hepatic injury and cirrhosis, may in turn lead to the formation of hepatomas. Excessive consumption of alcoholic beverages and cigarette smoking appear to act synergistically to increase the risk for cancers of the mouth, larynx, esophagus, and the respiratory tract.

Table III. Diet, Nutrition, and Cancer:
Conclusions on Microconstituents (6)

Vitamins. The laboratory evidence suggests that <u>vitamin A</u> itself and many of the <u>retinoids</u> are able to suppress chemically induced carcinogenesis. The epidemiological evidence is sufficient to suggest that <u>foods rich in carotenes</u> or <u>vitamin A</u> are associated with a reduced risk of cancer.

Limited evidence suggests that <u>vitamin C</u> can inhibit the formation of some carcinogens and that the consumption of <u>vitamin C-containing foods</u> is associated with a lower risk of cancers of the stomach and esophagus.

The data are not sufficient to permit any firm conclusion to be drawn about the effect of <u>vitamin E</u> or the <u>B vitamins</u> on cancer in humans.

Fruits and Vegetables. There is sufficient epidemiological evidence to suggest that consumption of certain vegetables, especially <u>carotene-rich vegetables</u> (i.e., dark green and deep yellow) and <u>vegetables</u> of the <u>Brassica</u> genus (e.g., cabbage, broccoli, cauliflower, and brussels sprouts), is associated with a lower incidence of cancer at several sites in humans. A number of nonnutritive and nutritive compounds that are present in these vegetables also inhibit carcinogenesis in laboratory animals. Investigators have not yet established which, if any, of these compounds may be responsible for the protective effect observed in epidemiological studies.

Minerals. Both the epidemiological and laboratory studies suggest that <u>selenium</u> may offer some protection against the risk of cancer. However, firm conclusions cannot be drawn from the limited evidence.

The data concerning dietary exposure to <u>iron</u>, <u>zinc</u>, <u>copper</u>, <u>molybdenum,</u> <u>iodine</u>, <u>arsenic</u>, <u>cadmium</u>, and <u>lead</u> are insufficient and provide no basis for conclusions about the association of these elements with carcinogenesis.

Food Additives, Contaminants, and Naturally-Occurring Carcinogens. The increasing use of food additives does not appear to have contributed significantly to the overall risk of cancer for humans. However, this lack of detectable effect may be due to their lack of carcinogenicity, to the relatively recent use of many of these substances, or to the inability of epidemiological techniques to detect the effects of additives against the background of common cancers from other causes.

A number of <u>environmental contaminants</u> (e.g., some organochlorine pesticides, polychlorinated biphenyls, and polycyclic aromatic hydrocarbons) cause cancer in laboratory animals. The committee found no epidemiological evidence to suggest that these compounds individually make a major contribution to the risk of cancer in humans. However, the possibility that they may act synergistically and may thereby create a greater carcinogenic risk cannot be excluded.

Table III continued on next page

TABLE III (continued)

Certain naturally-occurring contaminants in food (e.g., aflatoxin and N-nitroso compounds), and nonnutritive constituents
(e.g., hydrazines in mushrooms) are carcinogenic in animals and
pose a potential risk of cancer to humans. These and other
compounds thus far shown to be carcinogenic in animals have been
reported to occur in the average U.S. diet in small amounts;
however, there is no evidence that any of these substances
individually makes a major contribution to the total risk of
cancer in the United States. This lack of sufficient data
should not be interpreted as an indication that these or other
compounds subsequently found to be carcinogenic do not present a
hazard.

Mutagens in Food. Most mutagens detected in foods have not been
adequately tested for carcinogenic activity. Although substances
that are mutagenic are suspect carcinogens, it is not yet possible to assess whether such mutagens are likely to contribute
significantly to the incidence of cancer in the United States.

Table IV. Diet, Nutrition, and Cancer:
Interim Dietary Guidelines (6;17)

- Reduce intake of both saturated and unsaturated fats, from ∿40% to approximately 30% of total calories.
- Include fruits, vegetables, and whole-grain cereal products in the daily diet, especially citrus fruits and carotene-rich and cabbage family vegetables. Avoid high-dose supplements of individual nutrients.
- Minimize consumption of cured, pickled, and smoked foods.
- Drink alcohol only in moderation.

Printed with permission from Cancer Research.

Table V. Guidelines for Regulatory Action (6)

- Minimize contamination of foods with carcinogens from any source. Evaluate food additives for carcinogenicity prior to use. Monitor levels of unavoidable contaminants in the food supply.
- Identify mutagens in food, test them for carcinogenicity; where feasible, minimize their concentration in food.

Sources of Data. The interpretation of the evidence concerning dietary factors and carcinogenesis, and chronic diseases in general, usually encompasses a review of epidemiological studies, animal experiments, and in-vitro tests, and a determination of the quality, preponderance, concordance and the strength of the evidence. In assessing data from human studies, consistency of findings among various population groups and among individuals within a population are important attributes, as is the presence of a gradient in response, and an association that is independent and temporal. In some cases, the effect of modifying dietary exposure might also be known. In animal studies, use of appropriate models that simulate the human condition deserve particular emphasis, especially with respect to semblance of the pathological findings and biological alterations to human disease. Consistency of evidence from experiments in more than one species, replicability in more than one laboratory, and evidence of a dose-response add to the strength of the findings. Furthermore, plausible mechanisms to explain the findings increase the degree of confidence in the evidence (4;17;18). In general, there is agreement about the types of studies that would constitute the data base for investigating the association between diet and chronic diseases.

Criteria for Interpretation of Data and Formulation of Dietary Recommendations. By contrast, there appears to be no unanimity in the scientific community about the degree of importance to attach to data from various types of studies (e.g., how much weight to assign to epidemiological data versus data from animal bioassays,

and the extrapolation of data from animal studies), and there is
no consensus on precisely the type and amount of evidence that is
sufficient to demonstrate a causal association. Furthermore,
there are no universally accepted criteria for determining what
constitutes sufficiently convincing evidence to permit dietary
recommendations to the public. In principle, however, few scientists would disagree that advice to the public is warranted when
the strength, extent, consistency, coherence, and plausibility of
the evidence from lines of investigation ranging from epidemiology
to molecular biology converge to indicate that certain dietary
practices or other aspects of lifestyle promote health benefits
without incurring undue risks (5).

The NRC Committee on Diet, Nutrition, and Cancer abided by
the above principles in evaluating the evidence and formulating
dietary guidelines. Specifically, the committee considered the
evidence from all types of epidemiological studies, but it placed
most confidence in data derived from case-control studies and from
the few cohort studies that have been reported. Instead of rely-
ing on aggregate correlation data, these studies are based on the
collection and analysis of data on individuals; they attain better
control of confounding variables and provide more definitive data.
Particular emphasis was given to the results of case-control or
cohort studies that were designed to examine a specific hypothesis
and to the overall coherence of findings from different types of
studies. In evaluating laboratory experiments, more confidence
was placed in data derived from studies on more than one animal
species or test, on results that have been reproduced in different
laboratories, and on the few data that showed a dose response (6).

The preponderance of the evidence and the degree of concordance between the epidemiological and laboratory evidence determined the strength of the conclusions. Furthermore, concurrence
between epidemiological and laboratory evidence was a prerequi-
site to formulating dietary guidelines as was consistency of the
recommendations with good nutritional practices (6;17).

Implications of Current Knowledge for Dietary Policy

At least three factors need to be considered in determining the
implications of current knowledge for dietary policy:
  ● the certainty of knowledge,
  ● the consistency of guidelines with other dietary
    recommendations, and
  ● the degree of risk and benefit.

Certainty of Knowledge. Investigators would agree that knowledge
concerning the effect of diet on carcinogenesis is far from complete. The NRC Committee on Diet, Nutrition and Cancer had concluded that although there is a preponderance of evidence relating
dietary factors to carcinogenesis and the evidence is overall convincing, current knowledge is not sufficient to demonstrate that
the association is causal. As shown in Table VI, however, the
committee found that of all the dietary factors, the evidence
concerning dietary fat and cancer came closest to pointing toward

Table VI. Dietary Fat and Carcinogenesis:
Some Proposed Hypotheses (<u>19</u>)

- Fat could enhance carcinogenesis by contributing to the formation of peroxides and other reactive forms of oxygen, which could damage DNA.
- A high fat diet may increase excretion of sterol metabolites in the gut, which in turn may promote tumorigenesis in the colonic epithelium.
- Certain fatty acids in the diet could be incorporated into cell membranes, possibly producing changes in cell behavior that are associated with promotion.
- Certain essential fatty acids participate in the synthesis of prostaglandins, and these may influence tumorigenesis.
- A high fat diet could lead to a change in the level of certain hormones that in turn might affect the incidence of breast cancer and some other cancers.
- Lastly, fat may increase cancer rates for reasons that we cannot at present guess, simply because we do not yet know enough about the pathways that lead to cancer.

---

a causal association. For other dietary components, the evidence
was judged to be less certain (6). It is also apparent that although many hypotheses have been proposed, the mechanisms whereby
diet might influence carcinogenesis are largely unknown. For
example, several hypotheses are listed in Table VI to explain how
a high fat diet might lead to increased cancer incidence, however,
there is no conclusive evidence to support any of these hypotheses (19).

Ames (20) recently proposed that the production of oxygen
radicals by certain dietary mutagens and carcinogens and the
quenching of such free radicals by dietary antioxidants such as
ascorbic acid, vitamin E, and selenium may be a major mechanism
to explain the effect of diet on the process of aging and degen-
erative diseases including carcinogenesis. Although some experimental data support this hypothesis, conclusive evidence that
this is a principal mechanism applicable to humans is yet to be
obtained. Thus, evidence to demonstrate a causal association or
data to provide a complete understanding of mechanisms are absent.
However, overall, the evidence for each of the four dietary guidelines in Table IV was judged by the committee to be consistent,
concordant, and biologically plausible (for details see 6 and 17)
and thus to provide the scientific basis and the rationale for
developing interim public policy guidelines.

Consistency of Interim Guidelines with Other Dietary Recommendations. Dietary recommendations to lower the risk of cancer cannot
be viewed in isolation from other guidelines. To what extent do
they conform to nutritional principles to promote health?

Table VII compares the dietary guidelines proposed by the NRC
committee with other dietary recommendations made recently in the
U.S. and shows that:

With the exception of two groups in the U.S., numerous
scientists and organizations listed in Table VII have advised a
reduction in total fat intake for the general population, some
specifying that it should be reduced to about 30% of total
calories. This recommendation is particularly directed at lowering the risk of heart disease, and cancer. Although most groups
favor a reduction in total fat and saturated fats, there appears
to be no agreement about the intake of polyunsaturated fats and
cholesterol, at least in part because of the potential for competing risks. One key issue is whether increasing polyunsaturated fat intake and consequently decreasing serum cholesterol
lowers the risk of heart disease but increases the risk of colon
cancer in males as the results of some studies suggest, or is the
reduction in serum cholesterol in the cases with cancer the
result of metabolic changes due to preexisting, undetected
cancers as other data have suggested? (see 22). Results of a
recent large scale clinical trial to lower serum cholesterol
should shed further light on this issue (23).

Most scientists and organizations have suggested an increase
in complex carbohydrate intake (some have also emphasized dietary
fiber), with a concommitant decrease in simple sugars. These

guidelines generally are intended towards lowering the risk of
chronic conditions including diabetes, dental caries, and cancer.

With some exceptions, scientists and public health organizations have advised a reduction in sodium intake to reduce the
risk of hypertension for the general population.

Maintenance of appropriate body weight to avoid obesity and
decrease the probability of other chronic disorders has also been
universally advised.

Recommendations of the three groups that have specifically
proposed guidelines to lower cancer risk (the National Research
Council [6], the National Cancer Institute [9], and more recently, the American Cancer Society [1]) are generally consistent.
They have suggested lowering total fat intake; moderation in the
consumption of alcohol and smoked and cured foods; and increasing
the consumption of green and yellow, carotene-rich, and cruciferous vegetables; citrus fruits; and whole grain cereal products
and other fiber-containing foods.

Comparison with International Nutrition Policies. As shown in
Table VIII, dietary recommendations issued in Sweden, Norway,
Canada, and Australia are also in general agreement with the
majority of U.S. recommendations.

Thus, overall, there is a high degree of consensus among
diverse groups of scientists and public health organizations
about the type of dietary recommendations, even though some
recommendations were directed towards lowering the risk of particular diseases whereas other groups were concerned with promotion of overall health. However, a few important areas of
controversy persist, particularly about the intake of components
of fat and whether the recommendations should apply to the general population or only to subgroups at high risk for specific
diseases.

This comparison highlights another necessity: the need to
develop a consistent set of criteria for the interpretation of
data on diet and chronic diseases; because the differences in
conclusions made by different groups are in part due to the lack
of clearly defined and universally accepted criteria, both for
the interpretation of scientific data and for the formulation of
dietary guidelines.

The Degree of Risk and Benefit. Dietary guidelines have often
been criticized by the public, educators, and the food industry
for failure to quantify the risks and benefits associated with
the proposed modifications. In the case of cancer, there have
been preliminary attempts at quantification. For example, Wynder
and Gori (15) estimated that 40% to 60% of all cancers are associated with diet. Doll and Peto (10) projected a 10% to 70%
reduction in mortality from cancer with dietary modification,
stating that initially the reduction may be small but that
dietary modification may eventually enable a 35% decrease in mortality. The NRC committee concluded that cancers of most major
sites appear to be influenced by diet. However, the committee
found that the data were neither sufficient to quantify the

Table VII. Dietary Recommendations to the American Public, 1977-1984

	Limit or Reduce Total Fat (% Calories)	Reduce Saturated Fat (% Calories)	Increase Polyunsaturated Fat (% Calories)	Limit Cholesterol (mg/day)	Limit Simple Sugars	Increase Complex Carbohydrates	Increase Fiber	Restrict Sodium Chloride (g/day)	Moderation in Alcohol	Maintain Ideal Body Weight, Exercise	Other Recommendations
Dietary Goals (7) 1977; General	27-33%	Yes	Yes	250-350	Yes	Yes	Yes	<8	Yes	Yes	Reduce additives and processed foods
Surgeon General (4) 1979; General	Yes	Yes	NS[a]	Yes	Yes	Yes	NS	Yes	Yes	Yes	More fish, poultry, legumes; less red meat
AMA (3) 1979; General	No	No	No	No	Yes	NC[b]	NC	12	Yes	Yes	Consider high-risk groups
NCI (9) 1979; Cancer	Yes	NC	No	NC	NC	NS	Yes	NC	Yes	Yes	Variety in diet
USDA-DHEW (8) 1980; General	Yes	Yes	No	Yes	Yes	Yes	Yes	Yes	Yes	Yes	Variety in diet, consider high-risk groups
NAS/FNB (5) 1980; General	For weight reduction only	No	No	No	For weight reduction only	No	No	3 - 8	Yes	Yes	Variety in diet, consider high-risk groups
AHA (2) 1982; Heart Disease	∿30%	To ∿10%	To ∿10%	∿300	Yes	To ∿50% calories	NS	Yes	NS	Yes	Public education

Table VII (continued)

NAS/ DNC (6) 1982; Cancer	~30%	As total fat only	No	NC	NC	Through whole-grains, fruits, and vegetables	NS	Through salt-cured, pickled, smoked foods	Yes	NC	Emphasize fruits and vegetables; avoid high doses of supplements	NC
ACS, 1984 (1) Cancer	~30%	As total fat only	No	NC	NC	Same as NAS (1982)	Yes	Same as NAS (1982)	Yes	Yes	Same as NAS (1982)	Yes

a Not specifically.
b No comment.

Adapted from Refs. 17 and 21

Table VIII.   International Nutrition Policies: 1971–1983

	Maintain Ideal Body Weight	Reduce Total Fat (% Calories)	Reduce Saturated Fat	Increase Poly-unsaturated Fat	Reduce Cholesterol	Reduce Simple Sugars	Increase Complex Carbo-hydrates	Reduce Sodium	Moderation in Alcohol	Other Recommendations
Sweden (24;25) 1971, 1981	Yes	25–35%	Yes	Yes	Yes	By 25%	to 50–60% of calories	NC[a]	Yes	Varied diet, and exercise
Norway (26) 1975	NC	35%	Yes	Yes	NS[b]	Yes	Yes	NC	NC	Increase fiber
Canada (27;28) 1977	Yes	By 25%	Yes	Yes	No	Yes	Yes	Yes	Yes	Increase fiber, exercise
Australia (29;30) 1979, 1983	Yes	Yes	NC	NC	NC	Yes	Yes	Yes	Yes	Increase fiber
USA (8) 1980	Yes	Yes	Yes	No	Yes	Yes	Yes	Yes	Yes	Increase fiber, exercise

[a]No comment.
[b]Not specifically; through decrease in ratio of saturated to polyunsaturated fats.

Adapted from Refs. 17 and 21

contribution of diet to overall cancer risk nor to determine the
percent reduction in risk that might be achieved by dietary modification (6). Despite lack of certainty about the precise quantity of risk, many investigators tend to classify the magnitude
of risk associated with certain dietary patterns as being the
equivalent of the risk due to cigarette smoking, and believe that
in the long run a significant reduction in risk is feasible with
dietary modification.

Some segments of the food industry and some scientists have
suggested that there is insufficient justification for proposing
dietary modification, the benefits of which are unproven and
which may itself pose unknown risks. Proponents of this philoso-
phy cite the lack of a clear association between trends in food
consumption (e.g., fat intake) and changes in cancer incidence
and mortality, the gradual increase in the life span of the U.S.
population despite putative risks from the average American diet,
the lack of a cancer epidemic, and the declining rates of heart
disease. Other scientists contend that the decrease in the rate
of heart disease is associated with a decrease in the intake of
saturated fats (11;31), and despite the lack of a "cancer epidemic," evidence suggests that the risk of cancer can be further
reduced. They cite correlations between dietary variables and
the incidence and mortality from cancers of various sites, supportive evidence from studies of migrants showing changes in
cancer incidence and mortality with adaptation to local dietary
patterns, more definitive evidence from analytical epidemiological studies, and from animal experiments showing a consistent, reproducible reduction in cancer incidence or mortality
with certain dietary modifications (1;6;16). The possibility of
competing risks is at the core of the disagreement, stimulated in
part by limited and inconclusive data associating lower serum
cholesterol with increased risk from colon cancer in men in some
studies (for a review see 22). The scientific basis for these
concerns needs to be considered in the development of public
policy.

Future of Dietary Policy

At least three elements are central to the formulation of a
coherent dietary policy:
- a public health policy (including food safety regulation)
  that is consistent with current knowledge,
- nutrition education programs that are coupled with
  realistic objectives, and
- further research that is focused on clarifying the major
  scientific uncertainties.

The NRC Committee on Diet, Nutrition, and Cancer recently
issued a report suggesting strategies and directions for
research. These directions were developed after consultation
with a large community of scientists (19).

A Consistent Public Health Policy. The first key question in
formulating dietary policy is whether the guidelines should be

directed to the general population or only to special subgroups
that are at high risk? Given the wide range in the intake of
different foods and food groups, it is necessary to consider
whether it is advisable to shift the total distribution curve
(e.g., decrease fat intake and increase fiber consumption for the
entire population) or to truncate the distribution (i.e., reduce
the wide range of intake by limiting the upper and lower
extremes)? Whereas, shifting the total distribution is likely to
benefit a larger percentage of the population even though their
intake may be only slightly below or above the desired
goal, truncating distribution would tend to curtail the risk of a
smaller number, albeit those at greatest risk. Thus, there are
benefits to both approaches. One factor that might affect such a
decision is the size of the population at stake. For example,
total mortality among those with a moderately high serum
cholesterol level would be substantially greater than total
mortality due to extreme elevations in serum cholesterol because
the latter occurs less frequently in the population (32).
Furthermore, truncating the distribution can be more effective if
subgroups at high risk are clearly identified and knowledge is
precise enough to define the risk factors and the degree of risk
for individuals and subgroups.

Another question is whether guidelines about dietary intake
should be quantitated. Although the public and educators have
frequently criticized dietary recommendations for lack of specificity and thus clarity, public health officials and scientists
have tended to refrain from assigning quantities due to scientific uncertainty about causal associations, the mechanisms of
action, and about the degree of risk and benefit. However, it is
apparent thus far that general guidelines such as those shown in
Tables VII and VIII have not enabled public health authori-
ties to formulate a clear set of goals. By contrast, one of the
most widely used and successful set of guidelines are the Food
and Nutrition Board's Recommended Dietary Allowances--that contain a clear and relatively rigid set of standards for nutrient
intake (33). Although the RDA's have been criticized on a few
counts, few scientists and public health officials would question that they are widely and faithfully implemented by public
and private institutions, government agencies, and the food
industry for a variety of purposes.

Yet another question pertains to the nature of food safety
regulation. To what extent should food safety laws be modified
to conform with current knowledge about dietary components and
carcinogenesis? Is it reasonable to continue to base food safety
laws on feasibility of control rather than solely on perception
of risks, e.g., the regulations for the use of food additives are
substantially more rigid than those for naturally occurring
contaminants and nutritive components, even though some scientists would rank their risks in reverse order (e.g., 20)? Is it
feasible legally to institute distinctions between carcinogenic
initiators and promoters? Based on current knowledge, it would
appear that more emphasis needs to be placed on identifying and
modifying exposure to promoters. This is partly because of the

potential for reversibility of the action of promoters and thus the potential for reduction of risk, and partly because the effects of diet appear to occur more often on the later rather than the early stages of carcinogenesis as demonstrated by most animal carcinogenesis bioassays (6). Other aspects of legislation that bear consideration include alterations in the grading of meats to encourage leaner meat production, and better labeling of food products for components of fat and carbohydrates (34). It is highly desirable to seek the cooperation of the food and agriculture industries. Of particular benefit would be encouraging selective breeding of lean animals, to the extent feasible, reduction in the use of chemicals with known or suspected adverse effects, and the promotion of nutritionally more desirable products.

Nutrition Education. Perhaps the single most important aspect of dietary policy is education to divest the public of misconceptions about the myriad of effects attributed to diet, and to encourage behavior that is consistent with scientifically acceptable conclusions and recommendations. Cooperation among nutritionists, the food industry, and educators is essential if this endeavor is to be successful.

The concept of a balanced diet may need to be reexamined in light of new knowledge about the effects of dietary macroconstituents such as fat and fiber. For example, is the concept of food groups that was designed some decades ago to avoid nutrient deficiencies equally well applicable today to lowering the risk of chronic diseases such as cancer? Does current knowledge suggest a need to focus on modifying the proportion of various macroconstituents and thus, food items in the diet? The mechanisms for such modification should also be considered. For example, is it more feasible initially to add food items to the diet (e.g., those with more fiber) than immediate severe reductions (e.g., immediate drastic reduction in fat intake)?

The public needs to be educated about the concept of frequency of exposure and the degree of risk. In this context, the emphasis on greater variety in the diet needs to be expanded to explain the ability of dietary constituents to enhance each others' beneficial effects thus providing a more nutritionally desirable diet, as well as to neutralize the adverse effects of some constituents. Furthermore, the potentially adverse effects of large doses of dietary supplements needs to be emphasized just as much as the potential benefits of supplementation under certain well defined conditions.

Lastly, nutrition education programs need to be coupled with an understanding that dietary factors are not the sole determinants of the risk of chronic diseases, with realistic expectations about the amount of time and effort required to modify food habits, and the likelihood of benefits. Conveying an understanding of the basic concepts about the process of carcinogenesis, its long latency period, and the importance of prevention would further enhance the success of such programs.

Conclusion

It is apparent that substantially more research is needed
to permit definitive conclusions about the effect of dietary
factors on carcinogenesis; perhaps at best current knowledge can
be compared to that about cigarette smoking and lung cancer two
decades ago. However, in the interim, reputable scientists have
judged the evidence to be sufficiently convincing to conclude
that dietary patterns influence carcinogenesis, and even if
absolute proof of benefit is yet to come, that the risk may be
lowered by modifications that are consistent with desirable
nutritional practices. To allow more definitive conclusions and
recommendations, we need additional evidence and more clearly
defined criteria for interpretation of the evidence. In addition
to research to unravel the labyrinth of the process of carcinogenesis, we need to focus scientific attention on a major gap--
general consensus about the point at which scientists should
offer advice to the public, the type and amount of evidence that
is sufficient to justify such action, and the criteria for evaluating such evidence.

Acknowledgments

This work was partially supported by Contract No. NO1-CP-05603
with the National Cancer Institute and is partly based on the
NRC Diet, Nutrition, and Cancer report (6). The opinions about
implications for public policy do not necessarily reflect those
of the Food and Nutrition Board or the National Research Council.

Literature Cited

1. American Cancer Society. "Nutrition and Cancer: Cause and
   Prevention"; American Cancer Society: New York, 1984; p. 15.
2. American Heart Association, Committee on Nutrition. Circulation 1982, 65(4), 839A-854A.
3. American Medical Association, Council on Scientific Affairs.
   J. Am. Med. Assoc. 1979, 242, 2335-8.
4. "Healthy People: The Surgeon General's Report on Health
   Promotion and Disease Prevention," U.S. Department of
   Health, Education, and Welfare, 1979, p. 177.
5. "Toward Healthful Diets," National Academy of Sciences,
   1980.
6. "Diet, Nutrition, and Cancer," National Academy of Sciences,
   1982, p. 496.
7. "Dietary Goals for the United States, Second Edition," U.S.
   Senate Select Subcommittee on Nutrition and Human Needs,
   1977.
8. "Nutrition and Your Health--Dietary Guidelines for
   Americans," U.S. Department of Agriculture and Department
   of Health, Education, and Welfare, 1980, p. 20.
9. "Statement on Diet, Nutrition, and Cancer," by Upton, A. C.,
   Senate Committee on Agriculture, Nutrition, and Forestry,
   October 2, 1979.

10. Doll, R.; Peto, R. <u>J. Natl. Can. Inst.</u> 1981, 66, 1192–1308.
11. Stamler, J. <u>Biometrics</u> 1982, 37 (Suppl.), 95–114.
12. Hiatt, H. H.; Watson, J. D.; Winsten, J. A., Eds.; ORIGINS OF HUMAN CANCER, 3 volumes, Cold Spring Harbor Laboratory: Cold Spring Harbor, New York, 1977.
13. Doll, R. In "Introduction"; Hiatt, H. H.; Watson, J. D.; Winsten, J. A., Eds.; ORIGINS OF HUMAN CANCER, 3 volumes, Cold Spring Harbor Laboratory: Cold Spring Harbor, New York, 1977.
14. Higginson, J.; Muir, C. S. <u>J. Natl. Can. Inst.</u> 1979, 63, 1291–8.
15. Wynder, E. L.; Gori, G. B. <u>J. Natl. Can. Inst.</u> 1977, 58, 825–32.
16. Reddy, B. S.; Cohen, L. A.; McCoy, G. D.; Hill, P.; Weisburger, J. H.; Wynder, E. L. <u>Adv. Can. Res.</u> 1980, 32, 237–345.
17. Palmer, S. <u>Cancer Res. (Suppl.)</u> 1983, 43, 25095–25145.
18. Ahrens, E. H., Connor, W. E. <u>Am. J. Clin. Nutr.</u> 1979, 36, 2621–2748.
19. "Diet, Nutrition, and Cancer: Directions for Research," National Academy of Sciences, 1983, p. 73.
20. Ames, B. N. <u>Science</u> 1983, 221(4617), 1256–64.
21. McNutt, K. <u>Nutr. Rev.</u> 1980, 38, 353–60.
22. Palmer, S.; Bakshi, K. <u>J. Natl. Can. Inst.</u> 1983, 70, 1153–70.
23. Lipid Research Clinics Program. <u>J. Am. Med. Assoc.</u> 1984, 251(3), 351–64.
24. "Diet and Exercise," Stockholm National Board of Health and Welfare, 1972, p. 36.
25. "Swedish Nutrition Recommendations," Swedish National Food Administration, 1981, p. 11.
26. "On Norwegian Food and Nutrition Policy," Royal Norwegian Ministry of Agriculture, 1975.
27. "Recommendations for Prevention Programs in Relation to Nutrition and Cardiovascular Disease," Bureau of Nutritional Sciences, Health Protection Branch, Canadian Department of National Health and Welfare, 1977.
28. Molitor, G. T. "National Nutrition Goals--How Far Have We Gone?;" Chou, M.; Harmon, D. P., Eds.; CRITICAL FOOD ISSUES OF THE EIGHTEES, Pergamon Press: New York.
29. "Nutrition Policy Statements," Commonwealth Department of Health and National Health and Medical Research Council, 1983, p. 39.
30. Langford, W. A. <u>Food and Nutr. Notes and Rev.</u> 1979, 36, 100–03.
31. Walker, W. J. 1983. <u>N. Engl. J. Med.</u> 1983, 308(11), 649–51.
32. Rose, G. <u>Br. Med. J.</u> 1981, 282, 1847–51.
33. "Recommended Dietary Allowances," National Academy of Sciences, 1980, 9th ed.
34. Anonymous. <u>Lancet</u> 1983, 2(8352), 719–21.

RECEIVED August 17, 1984

The Inhibition and Promotion of Cancers by Folic Acid, Vitamin B₁₂, and Their Antagonists

VICTOR HERBERT

Hahnemann University, Philadelphia, PA 19102

For the past two years, our group has been collaborating with that of Dr. Ludwik Gross in the area of these studies, attempting to "switch off" the oncogene for guinea pig leukemia/lymphoma (1). The concept involved is that DNA methylation, and specifically methylation of cytosine in higher eukaryotes can directly suppress gene expression. This concept has been elaborated in several reviews, of which the most recent is by Eick et al. (2) in Analytical Biochemistry 135:165-171, 1983. The first dramatic presentation of possible clinical value of being able to demethylate a gene was the study by Heller and his associates in Chicago suggesting that they could "switch on" the fetal hemoglobin gene using 5-azacytidine, presumably by hypomethylating the fetal globin gene. They collaborated with Ley et al. in a study strongly suggesting that they could, in fact, switch on fetal hemoglobin synthesis with 5-azacytidine (3). This was confirmed by Charache and Dover and their associates at Johns Hopkins University (4) but Nathan and Lethvin and their associates showed that two other S-phase specific cytotoxic agents, hydroxyurea and cytosine arabinoside, could also increase fetal hemoglobin synthesis, Stanatiannopoulos and Poppianopoulou found that cytosine arabinoside can produce identical response in baboons to 5-azacytidine, and Nathan was quoted as concluding that the three drugs "probably act in the same way. Methylation has nothing to do with it" (5).

However, W. French Anderson and his associates were able to show directly in the cell culture system that 5-azacytidine does in fact selectively hypomethylate fetal globin genes, but that other genes, including an oncogene, are remethylated shortly after losing their methyl groups. These superficially divergent results can be reconciled by the concept that hypomethylation causes the persistent hemoglobin, whereas other mechanisms produce the acute increased production of fetal hemoglobin which occurs after 5-azacytidine (or hydroxyurea or cytosine arabinoside (5).

Similarly, different acute and persistent effects may explain

0097-6156/85/0277-0031$06.00/0

why the same antifolate, methotrexate, which can shut down a
lympho-proliferative malignancy, may result years later in the
development of a second malignancy (1). One can speculate that
an acute toxic effect kills the tumor but that the same
methotrexate which acutely toxically kills the tumor, in a long
period of time will result in demethylation of an oncogene, which
can then be expressed as second malignancy.

Other evidence that demethylation can cause the expression of
malignancies comes from studies by Feinberg and Vogelstein at
Johns Hopkins (6) at the Institute Pasteur by Bourgeois and her
associates, who found that glucocorticoids can cause expression
of murine mammary tumor virus (MMTV) by glucocorticoid-induced
methylation of long-terminal repeat sequences (7). Similarly,
Proirier and his associates published a number of studies
delineating the ability of methyl-deficient, amino acid-defined
diets to produce liver tumors in rats treated both with and
without initiating doses of diethylnitrosamine (8, 9). Their
studies indicate that diethylmethyl deficiency markedly promotes
liver carcinogenesis and exhibits complete carcinogenetic
activity in this organ in the rat. Rogers and Newberne had shown
that dietary methyl deficiency enhances the activities of a
number of hepatocarcinogens, and Shinizuka and Lombardi have
found that choline deficiency enhanced the hepatocarcinogenic
activities of several agents.

The concept that deficiency of folate or vitamin B-12, or any
other cause of failure to methylate DNA and/or RNA can activate
malignancy by hypomethylation or oncogenes, and that methylating
oncogenes can inhibit malignancy by making them dormant, is
similar to the concept of "relaxed control" of RNA synthesis. In
the '50s, Mendel and Borek (10) had noted that when an organism
autotrophic from methionine is deprived of methionine, it loses
its ability to suppress synthesis of RNA, which is then
synthesized more rapidly. It was speculated that deficiency of
B-12 or folate could produce similar "relaxed control". It is
possible that some forms of vitamin B-12 and of folic acid may
act as inhibitors of methylation and other forms as promoters of
methylation of RNA and DNA (1). Reduced forms of folic acid are
metabolically active; oxidized forms may be antimetabolites (1).
Hydroxocobalamin is metabolically
active; cyanocobalamin can be a B-12 antimetabolite (1).

Leuchtenberger et al. had reported that inositol inhibited
animal tumor growth but various B vitamins did not (11, 12).
This requires reinvestigation to determine whether inositol can
methylate
oncogenes. Oxidized folate monoglutamate, which is not a
metabolically active form of the vitamin, not only did not
inhibit spontaneous breast cancer in mice but actually produced a
more rapid growth of the primary tumors and a significant
increase in lung metastases. This work requires repeating today,
particularly from the point of view of whether metabolically

inactive folate, that is, oxidized folate, can promote tumor development but metabolically active folate, particularly the very active triglutamates, can promote methylation of oncogenes and thereby inhibit their expression.

For many years, a number of workers have been exploring the question of whether one form of a vitamin can be a growth promoter by acting as a coenzyme (i.e., a promoter of normal and tumor cell

growth) while another form of the same vitamin can attach to the same apoenzyme or other ligand (such as a vitamin transporting protein) and then jam the machinery, just as a key with a tooth missing can fit into a lock and then not turn. The answer to that question is clearly yes. Slight to major differences in the same vitamin structure (i.e., analogues and congeners) both exist in nature and are synthesizable; some of them are antagonists or anti-vitamins which can be created from vitamins by only slightly warping their structure (1).

Farber et al. (13) reported from Harvard giving pteroyltriglutamic acid (teropterin) and pteroyldiglutamic acid (diopterin), both synthesized by U. SubbaRow and his associates at Lederle Laboratories, to 90 patients with various malignancies, noting that "in general, adult patients experienced improvement in energy, appetite, sense of well being...might be ascribed to improved morale resulting from frequent visits, more medical attention..." They also reported inconstant temporary decreases in size of metastases in some tumors and degeneration and necrosis in others.

The apocryphal story is that Dr. Farber was also giving folic acid (the oxidized, stable pharmaceutical form of the vitamin) to children with lymphoproliferative malignancies (lymphocytic leukemia and lymphoma) until one of his residents collected sufficient data to suggest that the children receiving this new vitamin were dying faster than those children not receiving it. This observation allegedly led Dr. Farber to ask the Lederle people to create a warped folic acid molecule which would interfere with folate metabolism in the malignant cells, and this was done by adding an NH_2 group, thereby creating aminopterin. A second alteration, metyhylation in the 10-position, created methotrexate, still one of our most potent anti-cancer agents, particularly effective against childhood lymphoproliferative disorders and trophoblastic malignancies.

There is considerable evidence that rapidly growing neoplastic tissue consumes folate at so rapid a rate that folate deficiency megaloblastosis can occur in the host cells (14, 15). There is also evidence that vitamin B-12 deficiency may slow tumor growth, whether that deficiency results from inadequate absorption or elevated levels in serum of a vitamin B-12 binder which does not deliver the vitamin to tumor tissue (16), but will deliver it to the liver in a calcium-dependent fashion (14, 17-20). Interestingly, granulocytes and liver are a major source

of serum binding proteins for both bitamin B-12 and folic acid
(21), and malignancies of granulocytes and liver may partly
control themselves by releasing into the serum large amounts of
binders for vitamin B-12 and folic acid which bind those vitamins
and thereby prevent delivery to, and nourishment of, the tumor.

Oxidized folate is not only metabolically dead buyt may even
be neurotoxic. For example, a patient with epilepsy who has not
had a convulsion in years because dilantin has produced complete
control, can be thrown into an immediate convulsion with a
megadose of folic acid, because folic acid and dilantin compete
for absorption at the brain cell surface, and too much oxidized
folic acid will block the ability of the brain cell to take up
dilantin, similar to the competition between dilantin and folic
acid for uptake by the gutcell (22).

There appear to be one-way transport systems to remove
oxidized folates from the nervous system (22, 23) and to remove
vitamin B-12 analogues from the body via the bile (24). Some of
the B-12 analogues present in multivitamin/mineral preparations
may block mammalian cell metabolism (25) and since they block
normal cell metabolism, possibly may block malignant cell
metabolism. For a number of years, Russian workers have been
feeding analogues of vitamin B-12 to normal and malignant cells
and showing that these analogues will knock out B-12 metabolism
(25a).

Do the B-12 analogues (which have now been found in human
serum, liver, bile red cells, and brain) (26) play any role in
the promotion or inhibition of carcinogenesis in humans? Levels
of analogue in serum are elevated in some malignancies (1).
Levels of methylated bases in urine are elevated in some
hematologic melignancies (1). In the same hematological
malignancies in which methylated bases are elevated in the urine,
B-12 analogue is elevated in the blood serum (1). We have
recently found enormous quantities of analogues in human stool,
and have been studying whether the analogue in human colon
bacteria is the source of the analogue in human tissues (27). In
preliminary studies, we found two large analogue peaks in human
bile and two similar large analogue peaks in human stool. We are
now attempting to find out whether these peaks are the same
analogue (27). If they are, then the analogue in bile would have
come from the analogue in stool, because the quantity of analogue
present in food is tiny compared to the quantity present in human
stool.

Working with Dr. Ludwik Gross in our first attempts to
methylate oncogenes, we gave 5-methylcytidine (5mC) to guinea
pigs in whom was transplanted guinea pig leukemia/lymphoma (1).
The experiments over a six-month period were unsuccessful in
showing any dramatic inhibition, although there was a
non-statistically significant inhibition. We subsequently began
giving 5-iodocytidine (5IC) to these guinea pigs, having switched
from 5MC because of the evidence that the methyl group is taken

off on passage through the liver, resulting in cytidine alone being incorporated into the DNA and RNA of the oncogene. We though that perhaps iodine would not be removed from the cytidine as easily, and iodocytidine would be incorporated intact into RNA, with the iodine perceived by the cell as if it were a methyl group, as is true for iododeoxyuridine being perceived by cells as if it were methyldeoxyuridine (i.e., thymidine) (1). These studies are not yet completed; preliminary results have been equivocal but teasing.

Evidence that methylation can suppress normal and malignant gene expression, and demethylation can bring about expression, continues to build (28-30), although expression is not always related to state of methylation (31, 32).

Literature Cited

1. Herbert, V. In "Nutritional Factors in the Induction and Maintenance of Malignancy"; Butterworth, C.E., and Hutchinson, M.L., Eds.; Academic Press: New York, 1983, pp. 273-287.
2. Eick, D., Fritz, H.-J., Doerfler, W.: Analyt. Biochem. 1983, 135, 165-171.
3. Ley, T.J., DeSimone, J., Noguchi, C.T., Turner, P. H., Schechter, A.N., Heller, P., Nienhuis, A.W., Blood 1983, 62, 370-380.
4. Charache, S., Dover, G., Smith, K., Talbot, C., Conover, C., Jr., Moyer, M., Boyer, S. Proc. Natl. Acad. Sci. 1983, 80, 4842-6.
5. Kolata, G. Science 1984, 223, 470-1.
6. Feinberg, A.P., Vogelstein, B. Nature 1983, 301, 89.
7. Mermod, J.-J., Bourgeois, S., Defer, N., Crepin, M. Proc. Natl. Acad. Sci. 1983, 80, 110-114.
8. Brown, J.D., Wilson, M.J., Poirier, L.A. Carcinogenesis 1983, 4, 173-177.
9. Mikol, Y.B., Hoover, K.L., Creasia, D., Poirier, L.A. Carcinogenesis 1983, 4.
10. Mandel, L.R., Borek, E. Biochem. Biophys. Res. Comm. 1961, 6, 138.
11. Leuchtenberger, C., Leuchtenberger, R., Laszlo, D., Lewisohn, R. Science 1945, 101, 46.
12. Leuchtenberger, C., Leuchtenberger, R. In: "Nutritional Factors in the Induction and Maintenance of Malignancy"; Butterworth, C.E., and Hutchinson, M.L., Eds.; Academic Press: New York, 1983, pp. 131-148.
13. Farber, S., Cutler, E.C., Hawkins, J.W., Harrison, J.H., Peirce, E.C., Lenz, G.G. Science 1947, 106, 619-621.
14. Herbert, V. "The Megaloblastic Anemias." Grune and Stratton, New York, 1959.

15. Chanaran, I. "The Megalblastic Anemias." Blackwell
    Scientific, St. Louis, 1979.
16. Corcino, J., Zalusky, R., Greenberg, M., Herbert, V. Brit.
    J. Haemat. 1971, 20, 511-520.
17. Herbert, V. J. Clin. Invest. 1958, 37, 646-650.
18. Herbert, V., Spaet, T.H. Amer. J. Physiol. 1958, 195,
    194-196.
19. Allen, R.H. Prog. Hemat. 1975, 9, 57.
20. Beck, W.S. In: "B-12"; Dolphin, D., Ed. John Wiley and Sons:
    New York, 1982, pp
21. Herbert, V., Colman, N. In "Lithium Effects on
    Granulopoiesis and Immune Function"; Rossof, A.H., Robinson,
    W.A., Eds. Plenum Publishing: New York, 1980, pp. 61-78.
22. Colman, N., Herbert, V. In: "Biochemistry of Brain"; Kumar,
    S., Ed. Pergamon Press: New York, 1980, pp. 103, 125.
23. Poncz, M., Colman, N., Herbert, V., Schwartz, E., Cohen,
    A.R. J. Ped. 1981, 98, 76-79.
24. Kanazawa, S., Herbert, V. Trans. Assoc. Amer. Phys. 1984,
    96, 336-344.
25. Kondo, H., Binder, M.J., Kolhouse, J.F., Smythe, W.R.,
    Podell, E.R., Allen, R.H. J. Clin. Invest. 1982,k 70,
    889-898.
25a. Myashcheva, N.W., Quadros, E.V., Matthews, D.M., Linnell,
    J.C. Biochim. Biophys. Acta 1979, 588, 81-88.
26. Kanazawa, S., Herbert, V. Clin. Res. 1982, 30, 540A.
27. Herbert, V., Drivas, G., Manusselis, C., Mackler, B., Eng,
    J., Schwarts, E. Trans. Assoc. Amer. Phys. 1984, 97.
28. Wilson, V.L., Jones, P.A. Cell 1983, 32, 239-246.
29. Christman, J.K., Mendolsohn, N., Herzog, D., Schneiderman,
    N. Cander Res. 1983, 43, 763-769.
30. Harrison, J.J., Anisowicz, A., Gadi, I.K., Raffeld, M.,
    Sager, R. Proc. Natl. Acad. Sci. 1983, 80, 6606-66.0.
31. Gautsch, J.W., Wilson, M.C. Nature 1983, 301, 32-37.
32. Graessman, M., Graessmann, A., Wagner, H., Werner, E.,
    Simon, D.
    Proc. Natl. Acad. Sci. 1983, 80, 6470-6474.

RECEIVED January 23, 1985

The Influence of Fermentable Dietary Fiber on the Disposition and Toxicity of Xenobiotics

J. DONALD DEBETHIZY[1] and ROBIN S. GOLDSTEIN[2]

[1]Rohm and Haas Company, Toxicology Department, Spring House, PA 19477
[2]Smith, Kline, and French Laboratories, L-66, Philadelphia, PA 19101

Fermentable dietary fiber may modulate chemical toxicity by altering the microfloral metabolism of xenobiotics. A series of studies were conducted to assess the influence of fermentable fiber on the toxicity of xenobiotics that require microfloral metabolism to express their toxicity. The hepatic macromolecular covalent binding of 2,6-dinitrotoluene-derived radioactivity and nitrobenzene-induced methemoglobinemia were enhanced in rats fed pectin supplemented purified diets to levels comparable to rats fed cereal-based diets. The increased toxicity of these xenobiotics was associated with a 2- to 3-fold increase in the number of cecal anaerobic bacteria in rats fed the pectin diets. The number of cecal anaerobic bacteria in cereal-based diet-fed rats was similar to rats fed the purified diet supplemented with pectin. Following a single oral dose of Amaranth, the peak plasma concentration of naphthionic acid, a microfloral metabolite of Amaranth, was 5-fold higher in rats fed a pectin-supplemented, purified diet. These studies indicated that feeding diets containing fermentable fibers such as pectin can enhance the toxicity of nitroaromatics by increasing the number of cecal anaerobic bacteria that are required for the microfloral metabolism of these xenobiotics to proximate toxicants.

Dietary fiber has been suggested to play a protective role against chemically-induced toxicity (1) and against colon cancer (2). However, the mechanism(s) by which dietary fiber modulates chemical toxicity or colon cancer has not been well studied. The fiber fraction of the diet is resistant to mammalian digestive enzymes and consequently dietary fiber is not absorbed from the small intestine (3). However, certain types of dietary fiber; specifically fermentable fibers, including the pectic substances and hemicelluloses, are readily digested by the intestinal microflora (4,5). Pectic

0097–6156/85/0277–0037$06.00/0

substances are a family of galacturonic acid polymers which are methoxylated to varying degrees depending on the plant source (6). Hemicelluloses are primarily polymers of the pentose, xylose, with varying amounts of arabinose branching (7). Although hemicellulose constitutes the majority of the fermentable dietary fiber derived from most plant sources, it has not been well studied because it is difficult to extract and isolate from plant cell walls (7). On the other hand, pectin, which is the major component of pectic substances, is easily isolated from apple and citrus fruits as a by-product of the fruit juice industry (8). Therefore, most studies on fermentable fiber have employed pectin as a model fermentable fiber.

Animal feeds as well as human diets vary considerably in the type and quantity of dietary fiber. Wise and Gilbert (9) using modified detergent methods analyzed fourteen commercial rodent diets and found that the total dietary fiber content varied from 8.3 to 22.4%. In fact, it is not unusual for commercially available cereal-based rodent diets to contain 20% dietary fiber on a dry weight basis (10). In general, the fermentable fibers constitute more than half of the total dietary fiber; the remainder composed of the fibers more resistant to fermentation, such as cellulose and lignin (9). Thus, a significant portion of rodent diets has the potential to be fermented in the intestinal tract.

One way in which fermentable fiber could influence chemical toxicity is by altering the microfloral metabolism of xenobiotics. It has been suggested that the fermentable components of dietary fiber significantly influence the intestinal microfloral metabolism of xenobiotics by providing a potential source of energy for microbial growth and activity (11). Using pectin as a model fermentable fiber, Bauer et al. (12) demonstrated that there was a higher incidence of dimethylhydrazine(DMH)-induced tumors of the colon in Sprague-Dawley rats fed pectin-containing purified diets than in rats fed a purified diet alone. These investigators speculated that pectin enhanced the metabolic activation of DMH as suggested by the concomitant elevation of microfloral β-glucuronidase activity in the pectin-fed animals. However, the relationship between microfloral β-glucuronidase activity and DMH-tumorigenicity has been questioned since there is conflicting evidence that hydrolysis of a glucuronide conjugate of DMH is essential for the activation of DMH to a proximate carcinogen (13).

Amaranth Metabolism

Our first indication that fermentable fiber could alter microfloral metabolism was based on studies assessing the influence of dietary fiber types on the disposition of model xenobiotics using pharmacokinetic analysis (14). Amaranth was selected as a model xenobiotic for these studies because it was absorbed only after reduction by gut microflora (15).

In these studies adult, male Wistar rats were fed purified hydrated gelatin diets containing either no fiber or 15% cellulose, lignin, metamucil, or pectin (16). After 28 days on the diet the animals received a single oral dose of Amaranth (1 mmole/kg). Blood samples were collected at various times and the plasma concentration of naphthionic acid (NA), the major microfloral metabolite of

Amaranth, was determined by high pressure liquid chromatography (HPLC) (14).

The fermentable fiber, pectin, elevated the peak plasma concentration of NA 5-fold over the other dietary groups (Figure 1) (17). To determine if the higher plasma concentration of NA was due to enhanced absorption of NA or increased microfloral metabolism of Amaranth, the in vitro metabolism of Amaranth by cecal contents from rats fed the various diets was examined in a preliminary experiment. Cecal contents from animals fed the fiber-containing diets were incubated anaerobically with Amaranth and the amount of NA produced per gram of cecal contents determined by HPLC. Although the specific activity (on a per gram of cecal contents basis) of microfloral Amaranth-azoreductase was lower in pectin-fed animals, the total amount of NA produced per cecum was elevated 2-fold over rats fed the other diets (data not shown). These results suggested that feeding citrus pectin to rats elevated the microfloral metabolism of Amaranth resulting in greater amounts of NA in the plasma. These findings led us to believe that the capacity for microfloral metabolism of xenobiotics is enhanced by feeding pectin.

Dinitrotoluene Hepatotoxicity

Based on the Amaranth studies, it was hypothesized that those chemicals requiring microfloral metabolism to express their toxicity may be more toxic to animals consuming fermentable fiber. 2,6-Dinitrotoluene (DNT) is a hepatocarcinogen in Fischer-344 rats (18) and is genotoxic in the in vivo/in vitro hepatocyte DNA repair assay (19). The hepatic genotoxicity of DNT was found to be dependent upon the presence of gut microflora (20). Long and Rickert (21) demonstrated that DNT is excreted in the bile of male rats as the 2,6-dinitrobenzylalcohol glucuronide. This glucuronide conjugate is hydrolyzed by microfloral β-glucuronidase, permitting DNT to undergo enterohepatic circulation. Evidence also indicated that similar to the hepatic genotoxicity of DNT, hepatic macromolecular covalent binding (CVB) was also dependent upon the presence of gut microflora (22). CVB therefore was used as an endpoint to test the hypothesis that pectin-containing diets could enhance the toxicity of xenobiotics by elevating microfloral metabolism.

In these experiments adult, male Fischer-344 rats were fed a purified diet, AIN-76A, containing 5 or 10% citrus pectin replacing cornstarch or one of two cereal based diets, Purina Rodent Chow 5002 and NIH-07. After 28 days of dietary treatment rats were given a single oral dose of tritiated DNT (10 or 75 mg/kg). Twelve hours after dosing, animals were killed and CVB was determined by exhaustive extraction. The cecum was also excised from these animals and microflora characterized by anaerobic culture techniques (10).

The CVB of DNT-derived radioactivity to hepatic macromolecules was independent of the diet at a dose of 10 mg DNT/kg (Table I). However, at a dose of 75 mg/kg, CVB was increased 40% and 90% by supplementing 5% and 10% pectin to the purified diets, respectively. Livers of animals fed Purina 5002 and NIH-07 exhibited significantly greater CVB than animals fed the purified diet with or without pectin supplementation. CVB was increased approximately sixfold when the dose of DNT was increased from 10 to 75 mg/kg in animals

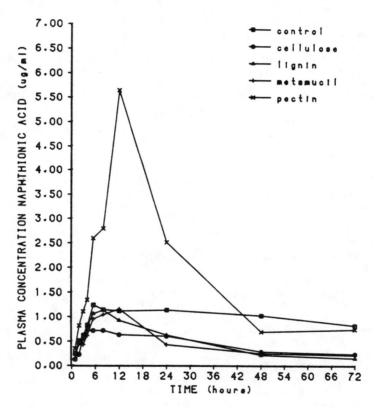

Figure 1.   Concentration of naphthionic acid in plasma from
Wistar rats given a single oral dose of Amaranth (1 mmole/kg)
following feeding purified diets containing no fiber (control)
or 15% (w/w) cellulose, lignin, metamucil, or pectin for 30
days.   Each point represents the mean of six rats.

fed NIH-07, Purina 5002, and purified diet plus 10% pectin, but increased only fourfold in animals fed the purified diet or purified diet supplemented with 5% pectin.

Table I. Effect of Diet on the Hepatic Macromolecular Covalent Binding of DNT

	Hepatic Covalent Binding[1] (nmol equivalents/g liver) After a DNT Dose of	
	10 mg/kg	75 mg/kg
AIN-76A	1.03 + 0.19	3.75 + 0.22[a]
AIN-76A plus 5% pectin	1.21 + 0.23	5.21 + 0.43[b]
AIN-76A plus 10% pectin	1.11 + 0.17	7.06 + 0.71[c]
NIH-07	1.40 + 0.13	9.29 + 0.49[d]
Purina 5002	1.47 + 0.16	8.82 + 0.51[d]

[1] Values are mean ± SE (n=6); means with different superscript are significantly different by Duncan's multiple range test at $p < 0.05$.

The increased CVB in pectin-fed and cereal-based diet-fed animals (compared to purified diet) was correlated with an increase in microfloral enzyme activity. Animals fed the pectin-containing purified diets, NIH-07, or Purina 5002 had significantly higher (two- to threefold) cecal β-glucuronidase and nitroreductase activities than animals fed the purified diet (Table II). The mean specific activities of both enzymes were similar in the pectin-fed groups and cereal-based diet fed groups.

There were no qualitative differences in the species of anaerobic or aerobic bacteria identified among the dietary groups (data not shown). However, both viable colony counts and microscopic counts indicated that there were 2.5- to 3.8-fold more bacteria per gram of cecal contents in animals fed the pectin-containing or cereal-based diets than in cecal contents of animals fed the purified diet (Table III). No consistent diet-related changes were observed in numbers of aerobic organisms, and the increase in cecal bacteria density was limited to anaerobic organisms. All species of anaerobes identified and counted were elevated in pectin-fed and cereal-based diet-fed animals.

These results suggested that dietary pectin induced changes in microflora that affected the activation of DNT at high doses as measured by CVB. The higher CVB observed in these studies suggested that elevation of microfloral β-glucuronidase and nitroreductase activities after feeding diets containing pectin resulted in increased microfloral metabolism of DNT glucuronide conjugate. Because both CVB (22) and genotoxicity (20) of DNT have been shown to be dependent on intestinal microflora, it is possible that

enhancement of the enterohepatic circulation of DNT by the fermentable fiber component of diet could alter the tumorigenicity of DNT
during long-term exposures.

Table II. Effect of Diet on the Weight of Cecal Contents and
Microfloral β-Glucuronidase and Nitroreductase Activities

| Diet | Cecal Contents | Microfloral Enzyme Activity[1,2] | |
		β-Glucuronidase	Nitroreductase
AIN-76A	$3.03 + 0.06^a$	$9.25 + 1.26^a$	$0.06 + 0.01^a$
AIN-76A plus 5% pectin	$2.97 + 0.62^a$	$27.52 + 3.62^b$	$0.21 + 0.05^b$
AIN-76A plus 10% pectin	$4.19 + 1.28^{a,b}$	$26.92 + 5.22^b$	$0.15 + 0.04^b$
NIH-07	$4.41 + 0.33^b$	$20.38 + 2.40^b$	$0.11 + 0.02^b$
Purina 5002	$4.16 + 1.16^{a,b}$	$22.88 + 2.38^b$	$0.13 + 0.07^b$

[1] Enzyme activity expressed as μmol product/g cecal contents/hr.

[2] Values are mean ± SE (n = 3, cecal contents; n = 11,
β-glucuronidase; n = 6, nitroreductase); means with a different
superscript are significantly different by Duncan's new multiple
range test, $p < 0.05$.

Nitrobenzene Toxicity

Although studies suggest that dietary incorporation of fermentable
carbohydrates increases microfloral metabolism of xenobiotics,
Rowland et al. (23) reported that dietary pectin did not uniformly
increase the activity of intestinal microfloral nitroreductases;
that is, dietary pectin increased the cecal nitroreduction of p-
nitrobenzoic acid and metronidazole, but not p-nitrophenol, 2-amino-
4-nitrotoluene, or 4-amino-2-nitrotoluene. The presence of intestinal microflora is known to be essential to the development of
nitrobenzene-induced methemoglobinemia (24). Therefore, the
selective increase in nitroreductase activities by pectin brings
into question whether dietary pectin will influence microfloral
metabolism and red blood cell toxicity of nitrobenzene. These
studies were therefore designed to determine whether alterations in
dietary pectin consumption would affect the microfloral metabolism
and red blood cell toxicity of nitrobenzene. Since the toxicity of
several xenobiotics differs between animals fed cereal-based and
purified diets (25,26), it was also of interest to compare the
metabolism and toxicity of nitrobenzene in these dietary groups.

Table III. Number of Bacteria Present in Ceca of Animals Fed
The Purified Diet, Pectin-Supplemented Diets, and
Two Cereal-Based Diets

	Number of Bacteria ($\log_{10}$ bacteria/g cecal contents)		
	Total Viable[1] Anaerobes	Total Viable Aerobes	Total Bacteria[2] (microscopic counts)
AIN-76A	2.6 + 0.6	0.011 + 0.002	5.3 + 0.8
AIN-76A plus 5% pectin	8.7 + 0.6[3]	0.014 + 0.002	32.8 + 9.8[3]
AIN-76A plus 10% pectin	8.5 + 0.9[3]	0.008 + 0.003	17.0 + 4.0[3]
NIH-07	10.0 + 2.6[3]	0.007 + 0.001	11.5 + 3.4[3]
Purina 5002	7.4 + 0.4[3]	0.009 + 0.002	18.3 + 2.6[3]

[1] Viable counts were obtained by counting and identifying colonies under conditions previously described (10). Values are the mean ± SE for three animals/group.

[2] Microscopic counts include viable and nonviable aerobic and anaerobic bacteria. Values are the mean ± SE for six animals/group.

[3] Significantly different from the AIN-76A-fed group by Duncan's new multiple range test, $p < 0.05$.

Male Fischer-344 rats were fed either AIN-76A (purified diet containing 5% cellulose), AIN-76A with 5% pectin replacing the cellulose, or NIH-07 (cereal-based diet containing 8.4% pectin) for 28 days. Following this period, nitrobenzene (200 mg/kg) was administered by gastric intubation, and methemoglobin concentrations were determined after 1, 2, 4, 8, and 24 hr. Nitrobenzene-induced methemoblobinemia was evident as early as 1 hr, peaked at 4 hr, and diminished thereafter in rats fed the cereal-based diet, NIH-07 (Figure 2). In contrast, nitrobenzene-induced methemoglobimemia was not detectable in rats fed AIN-76A; however, inclusion of 5% pectin in this diet resulted in methemoglobinemia comparable to that of the NIH-07-fed animals at 4, 8, and 24 hr. A dose response relationship for nitrobenzene induced methhemoglobinemia was established with each dietary treatment with doses ranging from 50 to 600 mg/kg. Administration of 400 or 600 mg/kg nitrobenzene resulted in significant diet-related differences in methemoglobinemia (Figure 3). Administration of 600 mg/kg nitrobenzene to animals fed NIH-07 resulted in the highest methemoglobin concentrations; those fed AIN-76A had the lowest, and those fed AIN-76A containing pectin had intermediate methemoglobin concentrations.

The number of anaerobic bacteria in the ceca paralleled the diet-induced changes in methemoglobin response induced by nitro-

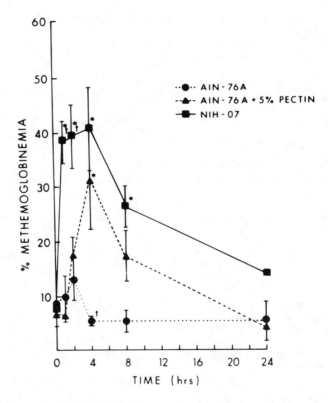

Figure 2.   Influence of diet on the time course of nitro-benzene-induced methemoglobinemia.   Each point represents $\bar{X}$ ± SE of at least three determinations.   Astericks and daggers represent a significant difference from AIN-76A and AIN-76A containing 5% pectin groups, respectively (p < 0.05). "Reproduced with permission from Ref. 27.   Copyright 1984, Academic Press, Inc."

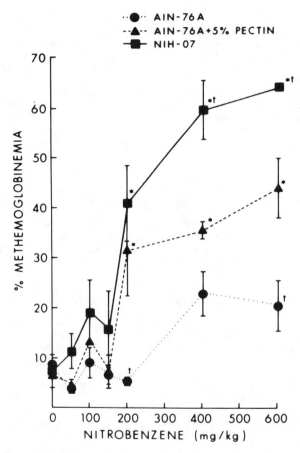

Figure 3.   Influence of diet on the dose-resonse relationship of nitrobenzene-induced methemoglobinemia.   Each point represents $\overline{X}$ ± SE of at least three determinations.   Astericks and daggers represent a significant difference from AIN-76A and AIN-76A containing 5% pectin groups, respectively (p < 0.05). "Reproduced with permission from Ref. 27.   Copyright 1984, Academic Press, Inc."

benzene with the greatest, least, and intermediate in animals fed NIH-07, AIN-76A, and AIN-76A containing 5% pectin, respectively (Table IV). There were no significant diet-related differences in total viable anaerobic or aerobic bacteria in the lumenal contents of the stomach or small intestine (Table IV). As with the DNT studies, there were no diet-related effects on the relative proportion of each of the species present (data not shown).

In vitro reductive metabolism of 14C-nitrobenzene was significantly greater in the cecal contents of rats fed NIH-07 than that in the cecal contents of either of the groups fed the AIN-76A-based diets (Table V). Furthermore, nitrobenzene metabolism by cecal contents tended to be greatest in animals fed NIH-07, least in animals fed AIN-76A, and intermediate in those fed AIN-76A containing pectin. Metabolites of nitrobenzene produced by cecal contents of animals fed NIH-07 and AIN-76A containing pectin included aniline, nitrosobenzene, and azoxybenzene, whereas aniline was the only detectable metabolite observed in animals fed the AIN-76A diet (Table V).

Although these results suggest a similar capacity for microfloral metabolism and methemoglobin formation by nitrobenzene between the NIH-07 and pectin dietary groups, higher doses of nitrobenzene (400 to 600 mg/kg) resulted in a greater degree of methemoglobinemia in the NIH-07 group, suggesting that large doses of nitrobenzene saturate microfloral nitroreductase activity in animals fed purified diets, resulting in decreased methemoglobin production. However, the anaerobic population of the cecum of pectin-fed animals was approximately 92% of the NIH-07-fed animals, while in vitro cecal metabolism of radiolabeled nitrobenzene of pectin-fed animals averaged only 33% of the NIH-07 group, suggesting (a) that the specific activity of microfloral nitroreductases is affected by diet, and/or (b) that dietary constituents other than pectin influence the microfloral metabolism of nitrobenzene.

These studies indicate that intestinal microfloral metabolism and red blood cell toxicity of nitrobenzene is markedly different in animals fed cereal-based versus purified diets. Furthermore, since inclusion of pectin into the purified diet diminishes the magnitude of these effects, differences in dietary composition of fermentable carbohydrates in cereal-based and purified diets may mediate differences in metabolism and toxicity of nitrobenzene (27).

Table IV. Effect of Diet on Microbial Population of Gastrointestinal Tract

| | Number of Bacteria of Cecal Contents (10^8 bacteria/g cecal contents) | | | | | |
| | Total Viable Anaerobes | | | Total Viable Aerobes | | |
Diet	Stomach	Small Intestine	Cecum	Stomach	Small Intestine	Cecum
AIN-76A	0.52 ± 0.04[1]	3.12 ± 0.55	473 ± 54[3]	0.003 ± 0.002	0.005 ± 0.003	0.898 ± 0.048
AIN-76A + 5% Pectin	0.62 ± 0.08	3.08 ± 2.55	963 ± 38[2]	0.014 ± 0.014	0.033 ± 0.018	0.860 ± 0.029
NIH-07	1.17 ± 0.44	6.41 ± 1.45	1050 ± 38[2,3]	0.034 ± 0.019	0.059 ± 0.011	0.845 ± 0.049

[1] All values are expressed as means ± SEM (3).

[2] Significantly different from AIN-76A (p < 0.05).

[3] Significantly different from AIN-76A + pectin (p < 0.05).

Table V.   Influence of Diet on In Vitro Cecal Metabolism
of ^{14}C-Nitrobenzene

Diet	Aniline[1]	Nitrosobenzene	Azoxybenzene	Nitrobenzene
AIN-76A	3 ± 1	0 ± 0	0 ± 0	95 ± 2
AIN-76A + 5% Pectin	11 ± 4	3 ± 2	3 ± 2	78 ± 11
NIH-07	36 ± 10[2,3]	7 ± 0[2,3]	7 ± 1[2]	34 ± 11[2,3]

[1] Data are expressed as % total radioactivity. Values represent
$\overline{X}$ ± SEM of 4 determinations.

[2] Significantly different than AIN-76A ($p < 0.05$).

[3] Significantly different from AIN-76A + 5% pectin ($p < 0.05$).

"Reproduced with permission from Ref. 27. Copyright 1984, Academic
Press, Inc."

Conclusions

These studies indicate: 1) fermentable fiber increases the total
number of viable anaerobic bacteria in the cecum, but not the
stomach or small intestine of rats; 2) the microfloral capacity for
hydrolysis of glucuronide conjugates, for nitroreduction, and for
azoreduction is elevated in fermentable fiber-fed rats; 3) this
increased capacity for microfloral metabolism of nitrobenzene and
dinitrotoluene is correlated with an elevation in the toxicity of
these nitroaromatics; 4) the role fiber plays in the modulation of
chemical toxicity is a function of the fiber-type and the structure
of the toxicant.

Significance

Variation in the fermentable fiber content of diets used in toxicity
studies and in human diets may influence the toxicity of xenobiotics
metabolized by the intestinal microflora. These results emphasize
the importance of characterizing the fiber in diets when investigating the influence of dietary fiber on disease processes and
chemical toxicity.

Acknowledgments

The authors would like to thank the following people who partici-
pated in various aspects of this research: J. P. Chism, T. E. Hamm,
Jr., M. Glover, A. W. Mahoney, D. E. Rickert, J. M. Sherrill, and
J. C. Street. We would also like to thank C. L. Krick for typing
the manuscript. The Amaranth studies were conducted at Utah State
University, Logan, UT and supported in part by grant CA25580 from

the National Cancer Institute, National Institute of Health, Bethesda, MD and grant ES07097 from the National Institute of Environmental Health Science, Research Triangle Park, NC. The DNT and nitrobenzene work was conducted at the Chemical Industry Institute of Toxicology where the authors were postdoctoral Fellows.

Literature Cited

1. Erschoff, B.H. Am. J. Clin Nutr. 1974, 27, 1395.

2. Burkitt, D.P.; Trowell, H.C. "Refined Carbohydrate Foods and Disease"; Academic Press, Inc: New York, 1975.

3. Southgate, D.A.T. Nutr. Rev. 1977, 35, 32-37.

4. Hove, E.L.; King, S. J. Nutr. 1979, 109, 1274-1278.

5. Key, J.E.; Van Soest, P.J.; Young, E.P. J. Anim. Sci. 1970, 31, 1172.

6. McCready, R.M. In "Methods in Food Analysis"; Josslyn, M.A., Ed.; Academic Press: New York, 1970; pp. 565-599.

7. Bauer, W. D.; Talmadage, K. W.; Kaegstra,K.; Albersheim, P. Plant Physiol. 1973, 51, 174-187.

8. Lei, K.Y.; Davis, M.W.; Fang, M.M.; Young, L.C. Nutr. Rept. Intern. 1980, 22, 459-466.

9. Wise, A.; Gilbert, D.J. Drug Nutrient Interactions 1982, 1, 229-236.

10. deBethizy, J.D.;Sherrill, J.M.; Rickert, D.E.; Hamm, T.E. Toxicol. Appl. Pharmacol. 1983, 69, 369-376.

11. Wise, A.; Mallet, A.K.; Rowland, I.R. Xenobiotica 1982, 12, 111-118.

12. Bauer, H.G.; Asp, N.G.; Oste, R.; Dahlqvist, A.; Fredlund, P. E. Cancer Res. 1979, 39, 3752-3756.

13. London, J. F.; Clapp, N. K.; Henke, M.A. Fd. Cosmet. Toxicol. 1981, 19, 707-711.

14. deBethizy, J.D. Ph.D. Thesis, Utah State University, Utah, 1982.

15. Pritchard, A.B.; Holmes, P. A.; Kirschman, J. C. Toxicol. Appl. Pharmacol. 1976, 35, 1-10.

16. deBethizy, J. D.; Street, J. C. Laboratory Animal Science. 1984, 34, 44-48.

17. deBethizy, J. D.; Street, J. C. The Pharmacologist, 1981, 23, 169.

18. Leonard, T. B.; Popp, J. A.   Proc. Amer. Assoc. Cancer Res.
     1981, 22, 82.

19. Mirsalis, J. C.; Butterworth, B. E.   Carcinogenesis 1982, 3,
     241-245.

20. Mirsalis, J. C.; Hamm, T. E.; Sherrill, J. M.; Butterworth,
     B. E. Nature (London) 1982, 295, 322-323.

21. Long, R. M.; Rickert, D. E. Drug Metab. Dispos. 1982, 10,
     455-458.

22. Rickert, D. E.; Long, R. M.; Krakowa, S.; Dent, J. G. Toxicol.
     Appl. Pharmacol. 1981, 59, 574-579.

23. Rowland, I. R.; Mallett, A. K., Wise, A.; Baily, E.
     Xenobiotica 1983, 13, 251-256.

24. Reddy, B. G.; Pohl, I. R.; Krishna, G.   Biochem. Pharmacol.
     1976, 25, 1119-1122.

25. Evers, W. D.; Hook, J. B; Bond, J. T.   Drug Nutrient
     Interactions 1982, 1, 237-248.

26. Mylorie, A. A.; Moore, L.; Olya, B.; Anderson, M. Environ.
     Res. 1978, 15, 57-64.

27. Goldstein, R. S.; Chism, J. P.; Sherrill, J. M.; Hamm, T. E.,
     Jr. Toxicol. Appl. Pharmacol. 1984, 75, 547-553.

RECEIVED January 22, 1985

Influence of Dietary Fiber on Xenobiotics

DAVID KRITCHEVSKY

The Wistar Institute of Anatomy and Biology, Philadelphia, PA 19104

Dietary fiber is a generic term used to describe substances (usually carbohydrate in nature) which are generally impervious to the action of human digestive secretions. Fibers are of specific chemical structure and have unique physiological properties. Dietary fiber, because of its relatively inert nature and bulk can affect absorption of any number of substances by either delaying absorbability or enhancing excretion (because of reduced gastrointestinal transit time). Dietary fiber has been shown to inhibit absorption and diminish deleterious effects of glucascorbic acid, cadmium, strontium-89, nonionic surface active agents, food colorings, such as Amaranth and Tartrazine, and sodium cyclamate.

The effects of dietary fiber on chemically-induced colon cancer in rats are variable being dependent on the carcinogen used and its mode of administration as well as the sex and strain of the rat. In most cases, however, dietary fiber has been found to inhibit carcinogenesis.

Dietary fiber is a generic term used to describe substances which are not susceptible to our own metabolic proceses. The term was coined by Hipsley (1) and refined to its present meaning by Trowell (2). However, as Southgate (3) has pointed out, there is no completely satisfactory definition. Today the designation dietary fiber includes cellulose, hemicellulose, pectic substances, gums, algal products and lignin. All but the last are carbohydrate in nature and all but the last are degradable to some degree by our intestinal flora. These substances have unique chemical structures, different physical properties and specific physiologic effects. It should also be noted that the fiber hypothesis relates to dietary life style rather than specific additions to the diet.

0097–6156/85/0277–0051$06.00/0
© 1985 American Chemical Society

What may have been the first study of fiber effects on xenobiotics was carried out by Woolley and Krampitz (4) in 1943. They
reported that when 10% glucoascorbic acid (an antagonist of ascorbic
acid) was fed to mice maintained on a purified diet, they observed
severe weight loss and severe deficiency symptoms. Addition of 10%
cerophyl (a dehydrated grass preparation) to the diet obliterated
signs of deficiency. Glucoascorbic acid had no effect when added to
a basal ration (containing corn meal, linseed oil meal and alfalfa
leaf meal). Ershoff (5,6) later confirmed these findings and
reported that succulent plants other than alfalfa - orchard grass,
fescue, wheat grass and oat grass - also protected mice from the
effects of glucoascorbic acid.

Dietary fiber has been shown to inhibit the toxic effects of
heavy metals. Wilson and DeEds (7) fed rats diets containing 125
ppm of cadmium chloride and either 3 or 6% fiber. Rats fed 3% fiber
and $CdCl_2$ exhibited poor weight gain, bleaching of teeth and anemia,
whereas rats fed 6% fiber appeared normal.   Paul et al. (8) tested
the effects of calcium alginate on uptake of ^{89}Sr in blood and bone.
Six hours after administration of ^{89}Sr, calcium alginate had inhibited its appearance in the blood by 51% and its uptake in bone by
78%. Uptake of ^{45}Ca by blood and bone was inhibited by 38 and 35%,
respectively. Momcilovic and Gruden (9) have reported that cellulose prevents deposition of ^{85}Sr and ^{47}Ca in the bones of infant
rats.

Chow et al. (10) found that addition of various nonionic surface
active agents to semipurified diets retarded growth of rats fed
those diets. Addition of 5% Tween 60 to a diet containing 22%
casein and 69.5% sucrose retarded growth by 39%, but when the diet
contained 62% soybean meal and 29.5% sucrose, growth was retarded by
only 5%. Soybean meal contains some complex carbohydrate, whereas
casein contains no fiber. Ershoff (11) studied the effects of
cellulose and alfalfa on weight gain and survival in rats fed Tween
20. Rats fed a basal semipurified diet (66% sucrose, 24% casein, 5%
cottonseed oil and 5% mineral mix) gained 85 grams in three weeks.
When 15% Tween 20 was added to the diet, only two rats survived for
3 weeks and their average weight gain was only 30 gm. Addition of
10% cellulose to the Tween 20-containing diet led to 100% survival
but weight gain in the three week period was only 48 g. Replacement
of cellulose with alfalfa meal resulted in 100% survival and optimum
weight gain (98g). In a later study (12), the influence of a
variety of substances was tested in rats fed Tween 60 for 14 days
(Table I). In the absence of fiber, Tween 60-fed rats showed only
33% survival and greatly reduced (by 79%) weight gain. Addition of
2.5% cellulose to the diet increased survival to 50%, but weight
gain was still very low; 5% cellulose gave 67% survival and only
slighly better weight gain; at 10% of the diet, cellulose led to
100% survival but weight gain was still 63% below the control level.
Blond psyllium seed negated the effects of Tween 60 when added to
the diet at a level of 2.5% of the diet. At 10% of the diet, all of
the following substances gave 100% survival (% weight gain of
controls): wheat bran (72); sugar can bagasse (62); cabbage powder
(95); alfalfa meal (96); and carrot root powder (101).

Table I

Influence Of Dietary Additions On Tween 60 Toxicity In Rats
(Six rats per group)

Diet	Weight After 14 Days
Basal	84.2 ± 2.1
Basal + Tween (BT)	18.0 ± 1.6 [a]
BT plus:	
5% Blond Psyllium Seed	80.2 ± 4.3
10% Cellulose	30.8 ± 2.1
10% Wheat Bran	60.8 ± 6.0
10% Bagasse	52.2 ± 4.5
10% Rice Sraw	80.2 ± 3.5
10% Blond Psyllium Seed	80.4 ± 3.1
10% Alfalfa Meal	80.7 ± 2.5

After Ershoff and Thurston (14).

[a] Two survivors

The anti-oxidant 2,5-di-t-butylhydroquinone (DBH) retards weight gain when fed as 0.1-0.2% of a semipurified diet, but addition of similar levels of DBH to a stock diet is without effect. This effect was observed in both Holtzman and Long-Evans rats (13) (Table II). Amaranth (FD and C Red No. 2) is toxic to rats when fed as 5% of a semipurified diet. No rats fed this diet lived as long as 21 days. When the diet also contained 10% pectin, cellulose or alfalfa, however, the dye was not toxic and weight gain was optimum (14). Similar effects of semipurified and commercial diets were observed in Sprague-Dawley rats fed 5% Tartrazine (FD and C Yellow No. 5) or Sunset Yellow FCF (FD and C Yellow No. 6) (15).

Table II

Influence Of Dietary Addition On DBH Toxicity In Rats

Regimen	Holtzman	Long-Evans
Basal (B)	77.3	64.2
B + 0.1% DBH	58.9	42.8 b
B + 0.2% DBH	16.8 a	18.4 b
Stock (S)	86.4	83.3
S + 0.1% DBH	79.6	71.2
S + 0.2% DBH	73.4	63.6

After Ershoff (13)

a: 4/6 survivors
b: 5/8 survivors

Ershoff (16) fed graded levels of sodium cyclamate (2.5, 5 or 10%) to Sprague-Dawley rats of both sexes maintained on either semi-purified or stock diets for three weeks. At 2.5% of the diet, sodium cyclamate retarded weight gain by 31 and 23% in males and females, respectively. At 5% of the diet weight gain was retarded by 71 and 55% and at 10% of the diet no rats survived beyond the first week. It is evident that the female rats fed sodium cyclamate fared better than the males. When added to a stock ration, 2.5 or 5% sodium cyclamate retarded weight gain by 10% in both male and female rats; at 10% of the diet, weight gain was inhibited by 28 and 19% in males and females, respectively. Sodium cyclamate affected weight gain in male Long Evans rats to a lesser extent than in male Sprague-Dawley rats. Apparently biochemical or physiological differences between rat strains affect toxicity of xenobiotics (Table III).

Table III

Influence Of Diet And Sex On Weight Gain In Rats
Fed Sodium Cyclamate (NaC) For 21 Days

Regimen	SD – Male	SD – Female	LE – Male*
Basal (B)	120 ± 8	103 ± 5	120 ± 4
B + 2.5% NaC	82 ± 3	79 ± 4	118 ± 6
B + 5% NaC	35 ± 5 a	46 ± 3	75 ± 6
B + 10% NaC	b	b	c
Stock (S)	119 ± 8	102 ± 5	130 ± 2
S + 2.5% NaC	118 ± 5	96 ± 4	126 ± 3
S + 5% NaC	114 ± 6	91 ± 2	116 ± 5
S + 10% NaC	86 ± 3	82 ± 4	c

After Ershoff (16)
* SD: Sprague-Dawley rats; LE: Long Evans rats

a: 5/6 survivors; b: no survivors; c: not done

Ershoff (14, 16) tested the effects of a vast array of fibers on toxicity of 5% sodium cyclamate. In male rats the most complete protection was afforded by 10% gum Karaya, 10% blond psyllium seed or husk, 20% alfalfa meal and 20% carrot root powder. The most effective substance in female rats was alfalfa meal fed as 15 or 20% of the diet (Table IV).

Fiber was shown to inhibit carcinogenicity of 2-acetylaminofluorene more than thirty years ago (7,17). A recent review (18) has pointed out the lack of consistency in studies of fiber effects on experimental colon carcinogenesis. Investigators use different strains of rat, stock or semipurified diets, and different carcinogens administered orally, subcutaneously or intrarectally (Table V). Ward et al. (19) found cellulose to have no effect on the carcinogenicity of azoxymethane (AOM) in male Fisher rats fed a semipurified diet. Freeman et al. (20), on the other hand, found cellulose to protect male Wistar rats from colon cancer induced by subcutaneous injection of 1,2-dimethylhydrazine (DMH).

Hemicellulose (fed as a high hemicellulose corn bran) also protects rats against DMH-induced colon tumors, but the effect seems to disappear with time (21). Thus, there was a significant protective effect in rats killed one month after the final DMH injection (33% vs. 73% incidence) but not in rats killed 9 months after the final DMH injection (62% vs. 76% incidence). Fisher rats fed semipurified diets containing cellulose, hemicellulose or lignin showed 100, 50, and 70% incidence, respectively, of DMH-induced colon tumors (22).

Wheat bran fed as 20% of the diet has been reported to inhibit DMH-induced colon cancer in male Sprague-Dawley rats fed either a semipurified (23) or stock (24) diets. In both cases, the carcinogen was administered orally. Bran (28%) has also been found to inhibit DMH-induced colon carcinogenesis in male rats for the Chester Beatty strain fed a stock diet and given the carcinogen by subcutaneous injection (25). Cruse et al. (26) found 20% bran to have no effect in chow-fed female Wistar rats given subcutaneous injections of DMH. Bauer et al. (27) reported that bran (20%) fed to male Sprague-Dawley rats as part of a semipurified diet enhanced colon carcinogenesis caused by DMH injection. They found that carrot powder also enhanced tumorigenesis. Degraded carageenen has also been reported to enhance DMH-induced colon carcinogenesis (28). Wheat bran fed at the 40% level protects mice from DMH-induced colon cancer (29) but addition of 7-9% agar to the diet enhances carcinogenesis (30).

Watanabe et al. (31) tested the effects of alfalfa, pectin and bran on colon tumors induced in female Fisher rats by subcutaneous injection of AOM or intrarectal instillation of methylnitrosourea (MNU). The fibers were fed as 15% of the diet. When AOM was used, alfalfa had no effect but both pectin and bran inhibited tumor formation. When the carcinogen was MNU, alfalfa had an enhancing effect and pectin and bran had none (Table VI). These data suggest interaction between type of fiber and route of carcinogen administration. An explanation for these observations may lie in the findings that different fibers show varying capacities to bind bile

Table IV

Influence Of Dietary Addition On Weight Gain In Rats
Fed 5% Sodium Cyclamate

Regimen	Weight Gain, g, After 14 Days
Basal (B)	77.5 ± 5.4
B + 5% Na Cylcamate (BC)	19.2 ± 3.6 a
BC plus 10%	
Wheat Bran	36.2 ± 4.3
Locust Bean Gum	38.2 ± 4.6
Agar	53.4 ± 5.1
Gum Karaya	71.4 ± 3.4
Alfalfa Seed	45.8 ± 2.8
Blond Psyllium Seed	83.2 ± 3.9
Bagasse	48.0 ± 3.1
Cabbage Powder	58.4 ± 2.9
Carrot Root Powder	58.2 ± 2.8

After Ershoff and Marshall (12)

a: 5/24 survivors

Table V

Influence Of Bran On Dimethylhydrazine-Induced Colon Cancer In Rats

Strain	Sex	Diet	% Bran	Effect	Ref.
S-D	M	SP	20	P	23
S-D	M	C	20	P	24
C-B	M	C	28	P	25
W	F	C	20	N	26
S-D	M	SP	20	E	27

S-D: Sprague-Dawley; C-B: Chester Beatty; W - Wistar; M: male; F: female; SP: semipurified; C: commercial; P: protects; N: no effect; E: enhances

Table VI

Influence Of Fiber (15%) On Colon Cancer Induced By AOM Or MNU

Fiber	AOM	MNU
Alfalfa	53	83
Bran	33	60
Pectin	10	59
Control	57	69

After Watanabe et al. (31).

AOM: azoxymethane administered subcutaneously
MNU: methylnitrosourea instilled intrarectally

Female Fisher rats were used.

acids and salts (32,33) and that fibers show a tendency to disrupt
the colonic and jejunal epithelium which parallels their bile acid
binding capacity (34,35). Partially denuded colonic tissue could be
very susceptible to a locally instilled carcinogen. Fibers also
show varying capacities to bind mutagens (36,37).

Just as there is a male-female difference in susceptibility to
the effects of sodium cyclamate (16), there is a difference between
male and female Sprague-Dawley rats in their susceptibility to
DMH-induced colon cancer and to the effects of bran on tumor incidence (38). Male rats given 15 mg/kg of DMH exhibited an 80% incidence of tumors and a 75% incidence of multiple tumors, whereas
females given the same dose of carcinogen exhibited a 20% incidence
of tumors with no multiple tumors. Addition of 20% bran to the diet
reduced tumor incidence by 50% in both groups. When the dose of
carcinogen was 30 mg/kg, tumor incidence was 100% in male rats and
30% in females. Addition of 20% bran to the diet led to a 29%
increase of multiple tumors in male rats and a 17% reduction in
females. Overall tumor incidence was not affected.

The foregoing indicates that much remains to be learned concerning the effects of fiber on the metabolic influences of xenobiotics. Very little has been done to elucidate influences of types
of fiber and to relate them to fiber structure. The sex differences
observed have not been exploited to learn what there is about the
male-female difference (hormones, blood chemistries) which could be
used to make dietary fiber a more effective protective agent in
males.

Literature Cited

1. Hipsley, E.H. Br. Med. J. 2: 240 (1953).
2. Trowell, H. Am J. Clin. Nutr. 29: 417 (1976).
3. Southgate, D.A. In: "Dietary Fiber in Health and Disease", ed.
    G.V. Vahouny and D. Kritchevsky, Plenum Press, NY, 1982, pp.
    1-7.
4. Woolley, D.W. and L.D. Krampitz. J. Exp. Med. 78: 333 (1943).
5. Ershoff, B.H. Proc. Soc. Exp. Biol. Med. 87: 134 (1954).
6. Ershoff, B.H. Proc. Soc. Exp. Biol. Med. 95: 656 (1957).
7. Wilson, R.H. and F. DeEds. Arch. Ind. Hyg. Occup. Med. 1: 73
    (1950).
8. Paul, T.M., S.C. Skoryna and D. Waldron-Edward. Can Med. Ass.
    J. 95: 957 (1966).
9. Momcilovic, B. and N. Gruden. Experientia 37: 498 (1981).
10. Chow, B.F., J.M. Burnett, C.T. Ling and L. Barrows. J. Nutr.
    49: 563 (1953).
11. Ershoff, B.H. J. Nutr. 70: 484 (1960).
12. Ershoff, B.H. and W.E. Marshall. J. Food Sci. 40: 357 (1975).
13. Ershoff, B.H. Proc. Soc. Exp. Biol. Med. 112: 362 (1963).
14. Ershoff, B.H. and E.W. Thurston. J. Nutr. 104: 937 (1974).
15. Ershoff, B.H. J. Nutr. 107: 822 (1977).
16. Ershoff, B.H. Proc. Soc. Exp. Biol. Med. 141: 857 (1972).
17. Engel, R.W. and D.H. Copeland. Cancer Res. 12: 211 (1952).

18. Kritchevsky, D.   Cancer Res. 43: 2491S (1983).
19. Ward, H.M., R.S. Yamamoto and J.H. Weisburger. J. Natl. Cancer Inst. 51: 713 (1973).
20. Freeman, H.J., G.A. Spiller and Y.S. Kim. Cancer Res. 38: 2912 (1978).
21. Freeman, H.J., G.A. Spiller and Y.S. Kim. Carcinogenesis 5: 261 (1984).
22. Klurfeld, D.M., M.M. Weber and Kritchevsky. Unpublished observation.
23. Wilson, R.B., D.P. Hutcheson and L. Wideman. Am. J. Clin. Nutr. 30: 176 (1977).
24. Barbolt, T.A. and R. Abraham. Proc. Soc. Exp. Biol. Med. 157: 656 (1978).
25. Fleiszer, D., J. MacFarlane, D. Murray and R.A. Brown. Lancet 2: 552 (1978).
26. Cruse, J.P., M.R. Lewin and C.G. Clark. Lancet 2: 1278 (1978).
27. Bauer, H.G., N.G. Asp, R. Oste, A. Dahlqvist and P.E. Fredlund. Cancer Res. 39: 3752 (1979).
28. Iatropoulos, M.J., L. Goldberg and F. Coulston. Exp. Mol. Pathol. 23: 386 (1975).
29. Chen, W.F., A.S. Patchefsky and H.S. Goldsmith. Surg. Gynecol. Obstet. 147: 503 (1978).
30. Glauert, H.P., M.R. Bennink and C.H. Sander. Food Cosmet. Toxicol. 19: 281 (1981).
31. Watanabe, K., B.S. Reddy, J.H. Weisburger and D. Kritchevsky. J. Natl. Cancer Inst. 63: 141 (1979).
32. Kritchevsky, D. and J.A. Story. J. Nutr. 104: 458 (1974).
33. Story, J.A. and D. Kritchevsky. J. Nutr. 106: 1292 (1976).
34. Cassidy, M.M., F.G. Lightfoot, L.E. Grau, T. Roy, D. Kritchevsky and G.V. Vahouny. Dig. Dis. Sci. 25: 509 (1980).
35. Cassidy, M.M., F.G. Lightfoot, L.E. Grau, J.A. Story, D. Kritchevsky and G.V. Vahouny. Am. J. Clin. Nutr. 34: 218 (1981).
36. Barnes, W.S., J. Maiello and J.H. Weisburger. J. Natl. Cancer Inst. 70: 757 (1983).
37. Moorman, W.F.B., J.J. Moon and R.E. Worthington. J. Food Sci. 48: 1010 (1983).
38. Barbolt, T.A. and R. Abraham. Tox. App. Pharmacol. 55: 417 (1980).

RECEIVED August 30, 1984

Effect of Dietary Factors on Drug Disposition in Normal Human Subjects

ELLIOT S. VESELL

Department of Pharmacology, The Pennsylvania State University, College of Medicine, Hershey, PA 17033

In normal human subjects, several dietary manipulations have been identified that can alter the disposition of such model drugs as antipyrine, phenacetin, and theophylline. Other environmental factors were kept as constant as possible, and each subject served as his own control. Nutritional factors thus far investigated in this way include: 1) varying the proportions of protein, carbohydrate and fat in a daily diet of 2500 calories; 2) charcoal broiling of beef; 3) high intake of cruciferous vegetables; 4) daily doses of theobromine acetate; 5) obese subjects on a diet of 15 gms carbohydrate/day for 10 days. These and related studies showed clearly that physicians should take dietary factors that influence drug disposition into consideration before arriving at the appropriate dose of some drugs. In different countries and regions of the U.S.A. particular dietary practices such as vegetarianism may make certain subjects and groups especially susceptible or resistant to the therapeutic as well as the toxic effects of drugs. Future studies should address this different question: to what extent do these isolated single factors interact with each other in the normal diet and thereby contribute to the well recognized large interindividual variations that occur in drug metabolism and disposition? Experimental designs are described that could help to define what role dietary factors play in accounting for these large interindividual variations.

Beginning in 1976, the laboratories of Kappas at Rockefeller University and Conney at Roche published in collaboration several pioneering experiments that demonstrated an effect of different dietary factors on drug disposition. Antipyrine, theophylline, phenacetin, and acetaminophen served as model drugs and were given to carefully selected normal volunteers before, during, and after a single dietary manipulation lasting from 3 to 14 days (see 1-5 for

0097–6156/85/0277–0061$06.00/0
© 1985 American Chemical Society

reviews of these studies). All other environmental factors during the studies were controlled as rigidly as possible. Because the results of these now classical dietary studies are clear and have been reviewed frequently (1-5), they will be summarized only briefly here. Instead other aspects of the relationship between dietary factors and variations in drug metabolism will be described, and the design of experiments to solve these problems will be discussed.

To summarize briefly, in studies performed as described above on 5 of the dietary factors shown in the outer circle of Fig. 1, it was possible to show that a) on a diet of 2500 calories per day a high ratio of protein (44%) to carbohydrate (35%) enhanced antipyrine and theophylline metabolism, whereas a high ratio of carbohydrate (70%) to protein (10%) retarded biotransformation of these drugs (6). Substitution of fat for carbohydrate did not significantly change these results (7). b) Ingestion of charcoal broiled beef increased the rate of antipyrine and theophylline metabolism (8), but not that of acetaminophen (9). The rate of biotransformation of phenacetin was unchanged, although charcoal broiled beef produced a large first pass effect, thereby appreciably reducing plasma phenacetin concentrations (10). c) Cruciferous vegetables in large amounts induced the metabolism of antipyrine and theophylline (11) and the glucuronidation of acetaminophen (12). d) Theobromine acetate given in high concentrations as the salt retarded the rate of its own biotransformation (13). Theobromine is a major constituent of chocolate. However, this dose of theobromine given as chocolate rather than the salt failed to alter its own metabolism, presumably because of its reduced bioavailability in chocolate. e) Starvation of obese subjects for 10 days failed to alter antipyrine or tolbutamide disposition (14), but in Indian (15) and Sudanese (16) children with protein calorie malnutrition antipyrine metabolism was impaired. Nutritional rehabilitation of these children restored antipyrine kinetics to normal values.

A few of the factors shown in the outer circle of Fig. 1 have not been studied in human subjects. Those have been demonstrated in laboratory animals to affect drug metabolism and disposition.

To What Extent Do Dietary Factors Contribute to Interindividual Variations in Drug Metabolism?

The preceding studies, each performed on a different dietary factor, were carefully controlled. Thus, only a single variable was altered independently of all others. Furthermore, subjects were painstakingly selected so that their hepatic cytochrome P-450 dependent monooxygenases would be under stable, near basal conditions (neither markedly induced nor inhibited through the potential influence of numerous environmental perturbations) (1-5). For example, none of the subjects took any drug regularly. None smoked cigarettes or consumed ethanol chronically. A single dietary manipulation could be introduced under these well defined, uniform environmental conditions. Then any alteration in rate of metabolism of a model drug, such as antipyrine or theophylline, could serve as a reliable, sensitive index of the effect of that specific nutritional change on the hepatic drug-metabolizing capacity of the subject.

Use of each carefully selected subject as his own control eliminated not only all genetic but most extraneous environmental

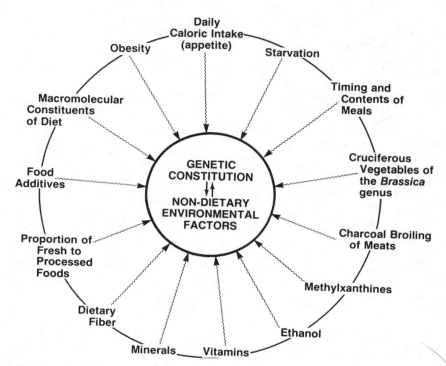

Figure 1. This circular design suggests the possibility of dynamic interactions among the several well-established or suspected dietary factors that may influence drug response in humans. Arrows from each factor in the outer circle are wavy to indicate that effects of each dietary factor on drug response may occur at multiple sites and through different processes. The inner circle suggests that effects of dietary factors may be modified by many other environmental, as well as by genetic, factors.

sources of variation in drug metabolism. Therefore, the alteration observed in the disposition of a model drug after imposition of a single dietary manipulation could reasonably be ascribed to that nutritional change alone.   Furthermore, this experimental design permitted results to be verified in several ways. Firstly the effect could be reproduced either in the same or in other subjects. Secondly, dose-response relationships could be generated between the particular dietary factor investigated and the subsequent change in metabolism of the model drug. Results of the experiments described above on dietary factors have been reproduced.

Questions arise, nevertheless, about how far these results on dietary factors in normal subjects under near basal conditions extend to other, more complicated, dynamic circumstances such as those that prevail among patients whose environments may be rapidly changing in complex ways.   What portion of the interindividual variation that exists among such patients and also among normal subjects with unrestricted life styles can be attributed to dietary factors? Most likely this question cannot be answered simply. Probably among all subjects complex interactions of numerous factors explain the totality of interindividual variation that occurs in rates of drug metabolism. In some subjects, dietary considerations may play a major role; in others, smoking; in others, age; in others, genetic factors; in still others, interactions among these and other factors.

This discussion emphasizes the complexity of such interactions that may occur when all subjects are included. Interactions can take place not only among different factors, but also among the dietary factors themselves (Fig. 1). The magnitude of the alteration in drug metabolism produced by single dietary factors in subjects under carefully controlled environmental conditions needs to be compared to the magnitude of the total interindividual variation in rates of metabolism of these same model drugs before imposition of any dietary change.   Since several dietary manipulations can change a subject's rate of drug metabolism, it might be expected that these dietary factors should account for a large proportion of the extensive variations observed among normal subjects. However, the latter does not necessarily follow from the former well established observations, and it remains to be determined whether such extrapolations are valid.

With respect to the changes in antipyrine and theophylline metabolism after imposition of diets high in cruciferous vegetables and charcoal broiled beef, relatively small alterations, in the range of 10% to 20% of basal values, are caused by these dietary manipulations. Such changes are an order of magnitude less than those observed among normal, carefully selected subjects of the same age and sex, who are unmedicated, nonsmokers and not chronic consumers of ethanol (17,18). Figs. 3 and 4 in Alvan (19) illustrate the 6-fold interindividual variations that occur in antipyrine clearance when a representative number of subjects are investigated.   Thus, these particular dietary factors appear to play only a very small role in accounting for the 6-fold interindividual variations in antipyrine metabolism among normal subjects under basal environmental conditions. Although each factor by itself may play a small role, in combination with other factors a very much larger synergistic effect could emerge. Figure 1 was designed to suggest this possibility. Here each dietary factor is displayed as if in dynamic interaction with other factors.

While the magnitude of change contributed by large shifts in the proportion of protein to carbohydrate on an isocaloric diet is larger than that from diets high in cruciferous vegetables, it is still considerably less than the 6-fold interindividual variations commonly encountered when antipyrine kinetics are compared in at least 12 normal subjects (17,18). Here again it might appear initially that even a very marked manipulation in the ratio of protein to carbohydrate might be insufficient to contribute substantially to the much larger interindividual variations that occur among normal subjects in rates of drug metabolism. Superficially, such a conclusion might seem to be supported by the observation of no change in antipyrine clearance after starvation of obese subjects.

Studies on starvation, however, are compatible with a major effect of changing the proportion of the macromolecular constituents of isocaloric diets. This reconciliation of seemingly contradictory results offers an opportunity to stress the complex effects of several dietary factors and the possibility for interactions among them.

Why does starvation fail to change antipyrine metabolism, whereas switching the proportion of carbohydrate to protein results in profound alterations of antipyrine metabolism? Possibly the body can detect the former dietary manipulation better than the latter. Through detection of the gross diet change of starvation for a limited time, the body can compensate by providing from another source the amino acids required for protein synthesis. In contrast, the body may be unable to detect, and hence compensate for, a much more subtle switch in the proportion of calories supplied as either carbohydrate or protein. If this change is uncompensated, depletion of protein could reduce rates of synthesis of hepatic drug-metabolizing enzymes, which in turn could cause retention of antipyrine and theophylline.

Although fasting in rodents greatly reduces rates of hepatic metabolism of some drugs (20-22), no change in drug metabolism occurred in obese, otherwise healthy, human subjects after 7 to 10 days on a diet in which the total daily carbohydrate intake was under 15 gm (14). This diet induced ketoacidosis, as well as weight loss that ranged from 4 to 15 kg. When uncorrected for body weight, the apparent volume of distribution (aVd) of both antipyrine and tolbutamide was significantly lower after fasting than before, presumably because during fasting the early loss of body weight is mainly from body water, rather than from fat stores or muscle mass (14). The extent of decrease in the aVd was proportional in each subject to the loss of body weight. Therefore, when correction was made for body weight, fasting had no effect on the aVd of either antipyrine or tolbutamide. These results, extended to other hepatic microsomal oxidations, including those for sulfisoxazole, isoniazid, and procaine (23), disclosed that when allowance was made for body weight, neither half-life values nor rates of hepatic metabolism of these drugs changed in otherwise normal obese subjects fasted for 7 to 10 days.

General conclusions on failure of absolute fasting to alter hepatic drug metabolism in normal subjects or in subjects without liver dysfunction were extended by a study of 7 female patients with confirmed classic anorexia nervosa (24). In these patients prolonged refusal to eat produced differing degrees of dehydration, hyponatremia, hypochloremia, hypokalemia, and anemia. Compared with age and sex matched normal nurses who served as controls, when these values were corrected for body weight, the anorexic patients had normal antipyrine kinetics.

A study on Asian Indian subjects (25) revealed that in 15 men suffering from nutritional edema - a severe manifestation of protein deficiency and resultant hypoalbuminemia - the mean plasma antipyrine half-life of 12.8 hours did not differ significantly from that of age and sex matched nonsmoking controls (11.2 hours), but was higher than that of age and sex matched smoking controls (8.9 hours). The same study examined another group of 13 undernourished, underweight men without edema. Their short mean antipyrine half-life of 8.6 hours, similar to that of smoking controls (8.9 hours), could be due to the fact that some smoked cigarettes, some drank ethanol, and some were agricultural laborers exposed to pesticides known to induce hepatic drug-metabolizing enzymes. Thus, in this study, severe malnutrition did not alter antipyrine disposition, supporting the observations already described for patients with anorexia nervosa or for obese but otherwise normal subjects after a 7 to 10 day fast. However, several problems, including chronic exposure of some subjects to inducing chemicals, render the results inconclusive.

In a significant contribution to this topic, phenylbutazone pharmacokinetics were measured in 4 normal male Asian Indian controls (mean age, 30) and in 5 undernourished hypoalbuminemic male Asian Indian subjects (mean age, 36), none of whom smoked cigarettes or consumed ethanol for prolonged periods (26). Compared to controls, the malnourished group exhibited shorter mean plasma phenylbutazone half-lives, but a larger mean phenylbutazone aVd and metabolic clearance. These changes in phenylbutazone disposition in undernutrition presumably arose as a result of reduced binding of phenylbutazone to albumin, with a corresponding increase in availability of drug for metabolism and elimination. The results need to be confirmed in studies on larger groups of undernourished subjects since the conclusions could be important therapeutically. Nutritionally deprived hypoalbuminemic patients who receive drugs highly bound to albumin may require dosage adjustment due to enhanced rates of elimination.

Renal elimination of certain drugs can be decreased by fasting or starvation (23). Also, since concentrations of free fatty acids in plasma rise dramatically after 12 hours of fasting and since these free fatty acids bind albumin with an avidity capable of displacing many highly bound drugs, fasting for 24 to 72 hours would be expected to accelerate the rate of elimination of such highly bound drugs as bishydroxycoumarin, diazepam, phenylbutazone, phenytoin, and warfarin. Drug removal from the body would be hastened because displacement of drug from albumin by free fatty acids makes the previously bound, and hence sequestered, drug immediately available for both metabolism and renal elimination, as in the case of undernutrition accompanied by hypoalbuminemia.

This discussion of starvation illustrates the complex problems of interpreting the results of even well controlled experiments on single dietary manipulations. It also shows the difficulties of extrapolating results from one set of environmental conditions to another. Clearly, such extrapolation is hazardous in assessing the contribution of any single dietary factor to large interindividual variations in metabolism of model drugs. Other approaches must be developed to avoid the problems inherent in these extrapolations. The final two sections of this review describe other attempts to answer this important question.

A Statistical Approach to Determine Causation of Large Interindividual Variations in Rates of Drug Metabolism

The approach of studying each environmental factor independently of all others under rigidly controlled conditions has advantages enumerated in the preceding section. The principal advantage consists of the use of each subject as his own control before and after imposition of single dietary factors, whose effects can then be estimated sensitively and verified by repetition of the entire experiment in the same subject at a later time as well as by construction of a dose-response curve. However, as we have also seen, this method does not permit easy extrapolation to a different circumstance and a different question: how much of the total extensive interindividual variation observed in drug metabolism in a large nonbasal population can be accounted for by each dietary factor alone?

An entirely statistical approach to this question has been attempted. In gathering 128 factory workers in London, the investigators deliberately chose subjects with differing environments; in their words, "the aim in this study was to use individuals drawn from the Community and to include a range of race and environment" (27). Antipyrine was then given once to each of 128 London factory and office workers. A critical, but as yet unproven, assumption of this approach is that in subjects who are environmentally perturbed, antipyrine kinetics obtained only once are representative and reproducible. A computerized program based on multiple regression analysis was employed to relate the antipyrine clearance of each subject to numerous anthropometric and biochemical indices of nutritional status (27). Five variables correlated independently with antipyrine clearance: race, contraceptive pill usage, smoking status, ponderal index (body weight/height^2) and serum albumin concentration (27). Because the coefficients for race and diet were virtually identical, the authors concluded that it was impossible to analyze the role of one factor independently of the other. The majority of their Asian Indian subjects were vegetarians, whereas their population of White Londoners almost all ate meat and, furthermore, were confounded by additional environmental perturbations such as cigarette smoking and ingestion of oral antifertility agents.

Recognizing that firm conclusions regarding the role of dietary factors in causing large interindividual variations in antipyrine kinetics were impossible in this mixed, and hence hopelessly confounded, experimental situation, the investigators decided to use this same statistical method but with another group of subjects. This second group was considered more amenable to investigation by multiple regression analysis because it was racially homogeneous, thereby permitting the role of diet to be assessed without interference from the unresolvable differences they encountered in their first population of 128 racially mixed subjects. The subjects of this second study were 36 healthy adult Indo-Pakistani immigrants to Britain. Among these 36 subjects, antipyrine clearance was much slower in the 16 lactovegetarians (0.54 ± 0.06 ml min^{-1} kg^{-1}) than in the 20 regular meat eaters (0.91 ± 0.07 ml min^{-1} kg^{-1}) (28). Since absence of meat

from the diet was associated with a significantly smaller daily intake
of dietary protein, which in the 16 lactovegetarians was abnormally
low by Western standards, the investigators concluded that this
difference in daily protein intake was the principal cause of the
differences observed in antipyrine clearance (28).

As the authors recognized, however, their methods are open to
numerous criticisms. For example, as they state: "Retrospective
dietary assessments made at a single interview, even when this is
conducted by an experienced dietician, are open to criticism since
they rely heavily upon the memory of the subject interviewed, the
estimates of quantity made by the dietician, and the subsequent
expression of those quantities in mass units. The opportunity for
error is clearly increased when the interview is conducted through an
interpreter" (28).

Very high standard deviations were calculated for the 16
lactovegetarians. Since extensive interindividual variations in
antipyrine kinetics persist within a population uniform with respect
to this particular dietary factor, factors other than protein intake
must cause them. The authors attempt to provide some possible sources
for these interindividual variations: "significant correlations
occurred between antipyrine clearance and age, sex, religion, smoking,
haemoglobin, kilocalories, carbohydrate, and fat. No significant
correlation was observed between antipyrine clearance and weight,
coffee/tea index, alcohol intake or plasma albumin" (28). But the
authors did not attempt to relate the socioeconomic or educational
level of subjects to their dietary habits, particularly their protein
intake. This and additional confounding factors might influence their
results.

Even for this limited group of 36 Indo-Pakistani, the methodology
employed left the major conclusion open to question because, as the
authors state, "when non-vegetarians alone were considered, there was
no significant correlation between antipyrine clearance and daily meat
intake, raising the possibility that one or more other dietary factors
might be of greater importance. Moreover, many of the variables
correlated significantly with each other as well as with clearance.
Stepwise multiple regression analysis was therefore performed and
identified smoking, age and fat intake as independent correlates with
clearance" (28).

Other discrepancies merit attention. Again, according to the
authors, since "daily protein intake was significantly lower amongst
vegetarians, while daily fat intake was similar in the two subgroups,
it was surprising that regression analysis identified fat intake as
the only independent dietary correlate with antipyrine clearance"
(28). This anomaly should be considered not only in light of the
carefully controlled dietary studies (7) that assigned a small role to
fat in affecting antipyrine kinetics but also in connection with the
inconsistency of the present results on albumin with these of the
authors' previous study (27). Collectively, these difficulties render
questionable the statistical approach used here and elsewhere (29).

In an earlier study using multiple regression analysis to
determine the basis of interindividual variations in antipyrine
clearance among 49 Gambians (29), the principal causative factor
identified was the number of cola nuts chewed per day (r = 0.4).
However, in a prospective study on an entirely different population of
carefully controlled, environmentally stable normal male subjects

living in south central Pennsylvania, chewing cola nuts failed to alter antipyrine clearance (30). These apparently conflicting results are not necessarily contradictory because of the multiple genetic and environmental differences between the groups investigated. However, their divergence emphasizes the crucial role played by the criteria used to select methods to analyze data, as well as subjects to receive drugs.

Because the British group applied extensively their statistical method to determine causation of large interindividual pharmacokinetic variations without describing its strengths and weaknesses, others have attempted to assess critically the application of multiple regression analysis for this particular purpose (31,32). While this statistical method has great potential, it requires considerable modification beyond its initial applications in this area (27-29), if that potential is to be realized (31,32). Thus far, its applications in pharmacokinetics (27-29) have been disappointing because those who have employed it neither formulated nor addressed, much less demonstrated fulfillment of, several fundamental assumptions inherent in its use (31, 32).

Several fundamental assumptions of the particular model used are dubious when applied to investigations of sources of interindividual differences in antipyrine kinetics. Four major concerns arise.

Firstly, the numbers studied in most investigations have been small and do not represent formal probability samples from a known population. Thus, the true representative character of the results is questionable, and the robustness of this model remains to be established through a demonstration that the results obtained with it can be replicated in another sample group drawn from the same larger population. The seriousness of this reservation arises from the multiple environmental factors that could exert some effect and the difficulty in obtaining a sufficiently large group of subjects to represent adequately most pertinent environmental factors. In fact, as indicated below, replicability of results has not been obtained with this model.

Secondly, this method fails to account for the majority of the intersubject variability in antipyrine disposition that exists among even those few subjects in whom the method has been applied. For example, when smoking and oral contraceptive use were considered alone (33), only 9% of the total variance in antipyrine kinetics among 207 normal volunteers was accounted for; none of the other factors examined by multiple regression analysis could provide a clue as to what was responsible for the other 91% of the variance.

The third and possibly most serious flaw in the particular multiple regression model lies in the assumption that it accurately accounts for the large intersubject variability in antipyrine kinetics that arises in response not only to any single environmental factor acting alone but also to several such factors acting concomitantly. The multiple regression analysis model used to assess sources of phenotypic variation in antipyrine kinetics is sensitive only to variations that exhibit a linear relationship (27,29,33). Distribution curves of antipyrine clearances themselves, as well as of environmental effects on antipyrine clearance, are not entirely linear. Nonlinear portions of this variability are insensitive to resolution by the model that was selected. Other more sensitive models based on multiple regression analysis might have been, and still can be, employed to resolve non-linear systems or non-linear portions of linear systems, providing that these independent variables are properly represented, e.g. by forming products or powers. However, with respect to phenotypic variations in antipyrine kinetics, our present knowledge of the current distribution properties produced by each environmental factor is too incomplete to permit its appropriate representation as a linear or non-linear function. The following considerations suggest that this fundamental assumption of linearity of the model based on multiple regression analysis is incorrect.

Individual responses to many environmental factors are unpredictable and highly variable. For example, induction of hepatic drug-metabolizing enzymes has been shown to be highly variable even though apparently normal subjects are exposed to similar doses of an inducing agent given by the same route.

Hence, large interindividual variations exist in the extent to which the activities of the hepatic mixed-function oxidases are enhanced by the same dose of certain inducing agents administered by the same route. Similarly, large interindividual variations occur in the magnitude of enzyme inhibition produced by a drug administered in the same dose by the same route to normal subjects under near basal conditions. The computer model cannot decipher from a single antipyrine kinetic measurement the sources for these large interindividual differences beyond the few specific environmental factors that the investigators have considered. Accordingly, it appears that such a model, by applying an average value for any given factor to all subjects, corrects inaccurately for variable responses to induction or inhibition and is therefore biased when applied to the investigation of a genetic hypothesis. This model overcorrects certain subjects for the influence exerted by an environmental factor on antipyrine clearance, while undercorrecting other subjects, thereby yielding contradictory conclusions.

When several concomitantly acting factors influence antipyrine metabolism in environmentally perturbed subjects, the extent of the variability produced probably exceeds that expected from the results of carefully controlled experiments in subjects under near basal conditions where only one factor is changed at a time. Although the antipyrine test can identify such departures from expectation due to interactions among factors, the model based on multiple regression analysis, by contrast, assumes that the net effect of all factors can be accounted for simply by adding the effects of each individual factor taken alone. Thus, the particular model based on multiple regression analysis that was selected for use cannot detect synergism from interacting factors.

It must be emphasized that the potential of multiple regression analysis to resolve sources of pharmacokinetic variations is much greater than has been realized by the particular 'canned' model used previously. The technique itself is both sensitive and powerful. However, for multiple regression analysis to be used appropriately, a model must be developed that encompasses non-linear as well as linear relationships (34). Error terms especially need to be appropriately modelled, rather than treated in a simply additive manner as in previous applications of this method.

Fourthly, in view of the preceding 3 major weaknesses in the model, it is not surprising that the results obtained with it differ markedly from much previous work on age, sex and genetic constitution.

For example, on the 3 occasions where regression analysis was applied, 3 divergent conclusions were reached on the effect of sex on antipyrine metabolism. Despite different populations in each study, ethnic differences alone probably do not explain the discrepancies. Possibly too much reliance has been placed on the statistical significance of 'p values' derived from the model based on multiple regression analyses, particularly when the correlations themselves are low and the subjects are under highly perturbed environmental conditions (35,36). Whereas the results of such studies on causes of variability in antipyrine kinetics may provide valuable clues, the conclusions and clues drawn from the model that uses multiple regression analyses should be validated by a carefully controlled, prospective experiment before safe acceptance.

In an application of this model for assessing factors that cause large interindividual variations in the clearance of theophylline (37), the authors clearly recognized its limitations and this requirement that the conclusions be tested by a prospective controlled experiment: "The factors identified as important in theophylline body clearances are associations found by retrospective statistical analysis which need not imply a cause-and-effect relationship, especially where a pathophysiological or drug interaction rationale does not exist. Often these factors need further confirmation by prospective examination of cohorts of subjects with the disease or history in question."

The relationship between intraindividual and interindividual variation merits discussion because recent approaches either ignored the former or assumed that it was negligible compared with the latter (27,29,33). The magnitude of intraindividual variation is not always small. The more environmentally perturbed the subjects investigated, the larger the intraindividual variability relative to interindividual variability, although the former can never exceed the latter. The magnitude of intraindividual variation also depends on the drug under study, being low for drugs with low hepatic extraction ratios (such as phenylbutazone and antipyrine) and high for drugs with high hepatic extraction ratios (e.g. phenacetin) (38). A similar conclusion was reached earlier (39) in a study that stressed large intraindividual variations in subjects of pharmacokinetic studies on clindamycin, ephedrine, ethosuximide, lincomycin, and warfarin. Interpretation of the values for intraindividual variation in the subjects of that study is difficult because no information concerning specific environmental conditions of the subjects was provided.

A Third Approach to Assessment of Dietary Contributions to Interindividual Variations in Drug Disposition

The magnitude of interindividual variation reported can depend on the drug selected for study, the number of subjects studied, the particular population from which the subjects are drawn, and the 'condition' of the subjects, including their present and past health, genetic constitution, age, sex, diet, and exposure to environmental chemicals and drugs that induce or inhibit hepatic mixed-function oxidases. As suggested in the preceding section, results of such published studies also reflect the specific method used and the degree to which the assumptions underlying each method are fulfilled.

Accordingly, this review stresses the characteristics of each method and the assumptions upon which it is based.

It should be emphasized that when subjects are under basal environmental conditions with respect to the many factors that can affect hepatic drug oxidation and when accordingly their hepatic drug-metabolizing enzymes are relatively uninduced and uninhibited, large interindividual variations still remain. Although well established, this important fact is often ignored. Thus, under near basal conditions interindividual pharmacokinetic variations cannot be attributed safely to any obvious environmental influence. Furthermore, numerous twin and family studies have indicated that these large interindividual pharmacokinetic variations in subjects under near basal environmental conditions arise from genetic factors (17,18,31,32,36). Nevertheless, under other conditions, where environmental factors are permitted to exert a differential (unequal) influence on the subjects of a study, this pattern of genetic transmission can be concealed. The major portion of the interindividual variation observed can then be mistakenly attributed solely to environmental sources, because underlying genetic factors that are also operative become unrecognizable. Accordingly, the answer to the difficult question of what role nutritional factors play in maintaining large interindividual pharmacokinetic variations in normal subjects living unrestricted life styles depends on the characteristics of the subjects selected, the extent of their environmental perturbation, and the particular combination of environmental factors exerting their effects on these subjects at any given time.

To elucidate these precise relationships a different approach from those undertaken thus far is recommended. This approach incorporates parts of several methodologies described in the preceding sections. The part adopted from studies that employed multiple regression analysis is selection of normal subjects under unrestricted life styles. The part adopted from carefully controlled studies on subjects under uniform near basal environmental conditions is manipulation of single nutritional factors independently of all others with repeated administrations of the model drug to obtain kinetic measurements before, during and after this single dietary change.

Such an experimental design should permit assessment of the influence of the single dietary change, generally withdrawal of a particular element, on the kinetics of the model drug. For example, in normal subjects living an unrestricted life style, substitution for several weeks of a vegetarian diet for one in which meat plays a principal part could be assessed with respect to antipyrine kinetics. All other dietary and environmental factors of the subjects in such a study would have to remain as constant as possible. In separate experiments effects of cruciferous vegetables and charcoal broiled beef could be estimated by prohibiting each from the diet for several weeks and comparing the kinetics of a model drug before, during and after such a period of withdrawal.

The influence of such variables as age, sex, smoking, ethanol, oral antifertility agents, total calories, the relative proportion of the macromolecular constitutents of the diet, exercise, and environmental exposure to certain prevalent chemicals would eventually need to be recognized and to some extent tested before the generality of any conclusions drawn in one group of subjects could be extended to other groups. Also, as previously emphasized, normal subjects under perturbed environmental conditions are more variable on repetition of their kinetic values than subjects under near basal environmental conditions. Therefore, the suggested experimental design needs to establish in each subject the extent of intraindividual variation. That is, kinetic values should be measured in each subject several times prior to the dietary manipulation. Possibly in some subjects the magnitude of intraindividual variation may reach, or perhaps exceed, that obtained after imposition of a specific dietary change. Such studies are laborious, time-consuming and technically difficult to undertake, but they may represent the next step in the extension of the conclusions on dietary factors from normal subjects under near basal environmental conditions to subjects under environmentally perturbed conditions.

In this connection a study revealed markedly altered therapeutic responses secondary to a change in drug kinetics produced by switching the proportion of macromolecular constituents in the diet. In 14 children with asthma, theophylline kinetics were accelerated by a diet high in protein, and retarded by a diet high in carbohydrate (40). Of particular interest with respect to this discussion was the observation that within each of the 3 dietary groups the extent of interindividual variation was similar (3-fold) (40). Therefore, under none of these 3 different dietary conditions did the proportion of the macromolecular constitutents of the diet alone account for the 3-fold interindividual variations observed in theophylline clearance. More studies of this kind need to be performed to determine what proportion of the total interindividual pharmacokinetic variation arises from dietary factors. A major recent advance is the demonstration that parenteral nutrition is associated with altered antipyrine metabolism and that the extent of this change exhibits large interindividual variations (41).

Literature Cited

1. Anderson, K.D.; Conney, A.H.; Kappas, A. <u>Nutr. Rev.</u> 1982, 40, 161-171.
2. Conney, A.H.; Buening, M.K.; Pantuck, E.J.; Pantuck, C.B.; Fortner, J.G.; Anderson, K.E.; Kappas, A. In "Environmental Chemicals, Enzyme Function and Human Disease"; Evered, D.; Lawrenson, G., Eds.; PRECEDINGS OF THE CIBA FOUNDATION SYMPOSIUM No. 76, Excerpta Medica, Amsterdam, 1980; p. 147.
3. Conney, A.H.; Pantuck, E.J.; Kuntzman, R.; Kappas, A.; Anderson, K.E.; Alvares, A.P. <u>Clin. Pharmacol. Ther.</u> 1977, 22, 707.
4. Kappas, A.; Alvares, A.P.; Anderson, K.E.; Garland, W.A.; Pantuck, E.J.; Conney, A.H. In "Microsomes and Drug Oxidation"; Ulrich, V.; Roots, I.; Hildebrand, A.; Estabrook, R.W.; Conney, A.H., Eds.; Pergamon Press, New York, 1977, p. 703.
5. Vesell, E.S. <u>Rational Drug Ther.</u> 1980, 14, No. 5, 1.
6. Kappas, A.; Anderson, K.E.; Conney, A.H.; Alvares, A.P. <u>Clin. Pharmacol.</u> <u>Ther.</u> 1976, 20, 643.
7. Anderson, K.E.; Conney, A.H.; Kappas, A. <u>Clin. Pharmacol. Ther.</u> 1979, 26, 493.
8. Kappas, A.; Alvares, A.P.; Anderson, K.E.; Pantuck, E.J.; Pantuck, C.B.; Chang, R.; Conney, A.H. <u>Clin. Pharmacol. Ther.</u> 1978, 23, 445.

9. Anderson, K.E.; Schneider, J.; Pantuck, E.J.; Pantuck, C.B.; Mudge, G.H.; Welch, R.M.; Conney, A.H.; Kappas, A. Clin. Pharmacol. Ther. 1983, 34, 369.
10. Conney, A.H.; Pantuck, E.J.; Hsiao, K.-C.; GArland, W.A.; Anderson, K.E.; Alvares, A.P.; Kappas, A. Clin. Pharmacol. Ther. 1976, 20, 633.
11. Pantuck, E.J.; Pantuck, C.B.; Garland, W.A.; Min, B.H., Wattenberg, L.W.; Anderson, K.E.; Kappas, A.; Conney, A.H. Clin. Pharmacol. Ther. 1979, 25, 88.
12. Pantuck, E.J.; Pantuck, C.B.; Anderson, K.E.; Wattenberg, L.W.; Conney, A.H.; Kappas, A. Clin. Pharmacol. Ther. 1984, 35, 161.
13. Drouillard, D.D.; Vesell, E.S.; Dvorchik, B.H. Clin. Pharmacol. Ther. 1978, 23, 296.
14. Reidenberg, M.M.; Vesell, E.S. Clin. Pharmacol. Ther. 1975, 17,650.
15. Narang, R.K.; Mehta, S.; Mathur, V.S. Amer. J. Clin. Nutr. 1977, 30, 1979.
16. Homeida, M.; Karrar, Z.A.; Roberts, C.J.C. Arch. Dis. in Childhood 1979, 54, 299.
17. Penno, M.B.; Dvorchik, B.H.; Vesell, E.S. Proc. Natl. Acad. Sci. USA 1981, 78, 5193.
18. Penno, M.B.; Vesell, E.S. J. Clin. Invest. 1983, 71, 1698.
19. Alvan, G. Clin Pharmacokin. 1978, 3, 155.
20. Dixon, R.L.; Shultice, R.W.; Fouts, J.R. Proc. Soc. Exp. Biol. Med. 1960, 103, 333.
21. Kato, R.; Gillette, J.R. J. Pharmacol. Exp. Ther. 1965, 150, 279.
22. Furner, R.L.; Feller, D.D. Proc. Soc. Exp. Biol. Med. 1971, 137, 81b.
23. Reidenberg, M.M. Clin. Pharmacol. Ther. 1977, 22, 729.
24. Bakke, O.M.; Aanderud, Syversen, G.; Bassøe, H.H.; Myking, O. Brit. J. Clin. Pharmacol. 1978, 5, 341.
25. Krishnaswamy, K.; Naidu, A.N. Brit. Med. J. 1977, 1, 538.
26. Adithan, C.; Gandhi, I.S.; Chandrasekar, S. Ind. J. Pharmacol. 1978, 10, 301.
27. Fraser, H.S.; Mucklow, J.C.; Bulpitt, C.J.; Kahn, C.; Mould, G.; Dollery, C.T. Brit J. Clin. Pharmacol. 1979, 7, 237.
28. Mucklow, J.C.; CAraher, M.T.; Henderson, D.B.; Chapman, P.H.; Roberts, D.F.; Rawlins, M.D. Brit. J. Clin. Pharmacol. 1982, 13, 481.
29. Fraser, H.S.; Bulpitt, C.J.; Kahn, C.; Mould, G.; Mucklow, J.C.; Dollery, C.T. Clin. Pharmacol. Ther. 1976, 20, 369.
30. Vesell, E.S.; Shively, C.A.; Passananti, G.T. Clin. Pharmacol. Ther. 1979, 26, 287.
31. Vesell, E.S.; Penno, M.B. Clin. Pharmacokin. 1983, 8, 378.
32. Vesell, E.S. Clin. Pharmacol. Ther. 1984, 35, 1.
33. Blain, P.G.; Mucklow, J.C., Wood, P.; Roberts, D.F.; Rawlins, M.D. Brit. Med. J. 1982, 284, 150.
34. Cohen, J.; Cohen, P. "Applied Multiple Regression/Correlation Analysis for Behavioral Sciences"; Erlbaum Assoc., Hillsdale, N.J., 1975, p.
35. Modell, W. Clin. Pharmacol. Ther. 1981, 30, 1.
36. Vesell, E.S. Clin. Pharmacol. Ther. 1982, 31, 1.
37. Jusko, W.J.; Gardner, M.J.; Mangione, A.; Schentag, J.J.; Koup, J.R.; Vance, J.W. J. Pharmacol. Sci. 1979, 68, 1358.

38. Alvares, A.P.; Kappas, A.; Eiseman, J.L.; Anderson, K.E.; Pantuck, C.B.; Pantuck, E.J.; Hsiao, K.-C.,; Garland, W.A.; Conney, A.H. Clin. Pharmacol. Ther. 1979, 26, 407.

39. Wagner, J.G. J. Pharmacokinet. Biopharm. 1976, 1, 165.

40. Feldman, G.H.; Hutchinson, V.E.; Pippenger, C.E.; Blumenfeld, T.A.; Feldman, B.R.; Davis, W.J. Pediatrics 1980, 66, 956.

41. Pantuck, E.J.; Pantuck, C.B.; Weissman, C.; Askanazi, J.; Conney, A.H. Anesthesiology 1984, 60, 534.

RECEIVED November 30, 1984

Free Radical Involvement in Chronic Diseases and Aging

The Toxicity of Lipid Hydroperoxides and Their Decomposition Products

WILLIAM A. PRYOR

Departments of Chemistry and Biochemistry, Louisiana State University, Baton Rouge, LA 70803

Six chronic diseases are most important in limiting the lifespan of humans, and there now is strong evidence for the involvement of free radicals in several of these. For example, emphysema, which is largely a disease of smokers, results from the oxidation of an antiprotease; this oxidation is caused by radicals and by powerful oxidants that result from the interaction of compounds with radicals that are present in gas phase cigarette smoke. Radicals also are implicated in cancer: Some chemical procarcinogens are activated to carcinogenic forms via radical-mediated reactions; promotion involves radicals; and many antioxidants are anticarcinogenic. Radicals also appear to be involved in atherosclerosis and arthritis. Lipid hydroperoxides, either in foodstuffs or produced endogenously, can be a source of radicals in vivo. Surprisingly, there are relatively few reports on the toxicity and biological effects of lipid hydroperoxides and other peroxidic materials in food, and this literature is reviewed. This article also presents the details of a system, consisting of linoleic acid in SDS micelles, that can be used to test the effectiveness of antioxidants.

At this symposium on the effects of toxins in food, I would like to review three related areas that bear on this theme. Firstly, I will discuss recent evidence supporting the hypothesis that free radicals contribute to important chronic diseases in man and exert an important life-shortening effect. Secondly, I will review data on the toxicity of lipid hydroperoxides and their decomposition products, since lipid hydroperoxides can be a source of free radicals in vivo. And lastly, I will review a system under study in our laboratory in which quantitative data on lipid peroxidation and antioxidants is being obtained using linoleic acid in SDS micelles.

Free Radical Involvement in Chronic Diseases and Aging

In a recent review of the chronic diseases that contribute most
importantly to limiting human lifespan, Fries and Crapo (1) list the
six diseases shown in Table I. It is interesting that there is
beginning to be evidence for an important contribution of free
radical processes in many of these six diseases, and much of this
evidence is quite new. I will briefly review the evidence for free
radical involvement in each of these processes.

Table I. Chronic diseases of humans (p. 83 of Reference 1)

Disease	Are Radicals Involved?
Emphysema	Definitely: The oxidation of an anti-protease by radicals and other species induced by smoke contributes to smoker's emphysema.
Atherosclerosis	Very probably: There is good evidence for some involvement of radicals in controlling PG/TX ratios.
Cancer	Probably: There is good evidence for substantial involvement of radicals in the activation of certain procarcinogens and in promotion.
Osteoarthritis Cirrhosis Diabetes	Evidence beginning to emerge for some involvement of radicals in these diseases.

Emphysema

An overwhelming percentage of the persons who suffer from emphysema
are smokers, and there now is very strong evidence that emphysema is
caused by the inactivation of alpha-1-protease inhibitor (alPI) in
the lung by oxidants in smoke (2). Smoke causes pulmonary alveolar
macrophages (PAM) to be activated, so smokers lungs contain higher
concentrations of superoxide and hydrogen peroxide than do those of
non-smokers and these oxidants are known to inactivate alPI (2). In
addition, free radicals in smoke (such as nitrogen dioxide) react
with hydrogen peroxide to form strongly oxidizing materials that
inactivate alPI (3-6). Recently, we have found that other species
that are formed in gas-phase smoke inactivate a1PI; one such species
may be the peroxynitrates that are produced from the reaction of
peroxyl radicals with nitrogen dioxide, as shown in Equation 1 (6).

$$NO_2 + ROO^\cdot \longrightarrow ROO-NO_2 \qquad\qquad (1)$$

Thus, emphysema represents a major chronic disease in which there is
strong evidence for free radical involvement. The hope remains that

this insight ultimately will lead to strategies for protection of the lung against this type of oxidative damage.

Atherosclerosis

The arachidonic acid cascade produces hydroperoxide-containing products such as PGG and 15-HPETE. These hydroperoxides are reduced to alcohols by a peroxidase that is associated with prostaglandin cyclooxygenase activity (7,8). In this process, an oxidant is formed that causes suicide inactivation of some enzyme systems; prostacyclin (PGI) synthetase but not thromboxane (TXA) synthetase is inhibited (9,10). Thus, high hydroperoxide levels may lead to a high TXA/PGI ratio, leading to diseases associated with hypertension and atherosclerosis. This peroxide-mediated mechanism for vessel-wall injury also can be initiated by endotoxin (11). Interestingly, cigarette smoke alters the metabolism of arachidonic acid in rat aortas, platelets and lungs in a manner that results in increased TXA and decreased PGI, also creating a condition that favors the development of cardiovascular disorders (12). Cigarette smoke contains a variety of oxidizing species that could be involved in these effects (3,5,13).

There is increasing evidence for the involvement of superoxide radicals and other oxy-radicals in ischemic injury of tissue (14-16) including myocardial injury (17). It appears that antioxidants and radical scavengers may play a role in reducing tissue damage during the reprofusion phase of surgical procedures or in shock (18).

Cancer

The evidence for radical involvement in some types of chemically-induced carcinogenesis is now quite strong (8,19-25). Many chemicals are metabolized to carcinogens by processes that do not seem to involve free radicals; a well-understood example is the oxidation of benzo(a)pyrene [B(a)P] to the diol epoxide by the cytochrome P450 system. However, the oxidation of B(a)P and other polynuclear aromatic hydrocarbons (PAH) to carcinogenic compounds can involve radicals. This statement, while once controversial, now has ample evidence (19,22,25). Although it is clear that some products arise from radical-mediated metabolism of PAH, the involvement of these products in tumorigenesis is less clear; nevertheless, I believe that such evidence does now exist (18,19). In addition, the phenomenon of tumor promotion appears to involve radicals and radical precursors, although the mechanisms are not at all clear as yet (26,27,28).

Originally it was hoped that electron-spin resonance (ESR) could be used as a technique for detecting early stages of tumor development. However, this hope, to date at least, has not been realized (29). There is some very recent evidence, however, that some tumors do possess a highly anomolous ESR signal (30).

Another line of evidence that free radicals may be involved in chemical carcinogenesis is that antioxidants often act as anti-cancer compounds. Many types of chemical carcinogens, in a variety of organs and in many animal species, are protected against

by an extensive series of antioxidants (25,31,32). While it is not
yet clear that all of these compounds act as anti-cancer compounds
because of their antioxidant properties, it seems reasonable that
some of them do. In the mouse-skin test, where peroxides act as
promoters, antioxidants again show protective effects (33).

Systems that produce superoxide, such as human neutrophils,
give a positive Ames test (34), suggesting a connection between
radical-forming activity and mutagenesis.

Another area in which free radical reactions may contribute to
carcinogenicity is the reactions of nitrogen dioxide (a reactive
free radical) with PAH. The striking observation has been made that
even PAH that are not themselves carcinogenic may form strongly
mutagenic compounds when they react with nitrogen dioxide (35-38).
In fact, pyrene is nitrated by NO_2 to form 1-nitropyrene and
1,8-dinitropyrene, both of which are mutagenic; in fact, the dinitro
compound is among the most mutagenic substances yet discovered (39).
This area is of considerable current interest since diesel engines
produce more particulate matter than do gasoline engines, and the
PAH absorbed in these particles undergo nitration to form nitro-PAH
compounds. We have begun a study of the animal toxicity of these
types of compounds (40).

Osteoarthritis, Cirrhosis and Diabetes

Although evidence for free radical involvement in these diseases is
less strong, there are some indications that radicals might be
implicated (41-43).

The Wear and Tear Theory

The wear and tear theory of aging postulates that random processes
produce deleterious changes in biomolecules with time, and that
these changes contribute to cellular aging. Most forms of this
theory propose that changes gradually occur in enzymes, that these
"bad" enzymes then lead to "bad" DNA, which leads to "bad" RNA, and
finally inaccurate enzymes. This spiral eventually produces an
error catastrophy and death (44,45). Since plastics, paper, and
rubber gradually decay in air due to autoxidation, it seems
reasonable to postulate that tissue would as well. Of course a
living system, unlike inert materials, possesses impressive repair
mechanisms to overcome this damage. Nevertheless, it is reasonable
to presume that random oxidative damage would accumulate over the
life of an organism, and in some cases, overwhelm the repair
mechanisms. The evidence for the accumulation of inaccurate enzymes
with time is still rather controversial (44). However, there does
appear to be no doubt that random errors do accumulate in
biomolecules with time (46), and it seems reasonable that free
radical reactions would contribute to this. For example, I have
already reviewed the evidence for the inactivation of a1PI by
radicals. This occurs by the oxidation of the methionine residues
to methionine sulfoxide. This oxidation also has been postulated to
occur in any protein or enzyme containing methionine residues (47),
again suggesting a connection between free radicals and the random
processes associated with aging.

The finding, originally discovered by Harman (48), that antioxidants extend the mean life span of small mammals is impressive evidence for radical involvement in some of the processes that contribute to aging. The correlations of enzyme levels that protect against radical damage (such as superoxide dismutase) and the lifespan of species also is evidence for the involvement of radicals in the aging process (49).

Detection of Free Radicals Directly in Toxicology Research Using ESR

Certainly the most powerful evidence for the presence of free radicals is to directly detect the radicals by ESR, and the use of ESR in toxicology is beginning to prove to be extremely useful. Reviews of this powerful new technique can be found by Mason (24), by Kalyanaraman and Sivarajah (23), Docampo and Moreno (50), O'Brien (51), and Cavalieri and Rogan (19). From our present viewpoint, a most interesting report was published in 1983 by Trapp et al. (52). These workers have shown that both the diet and the age of Drosophila effects the intensity of the ESR signal obtained from wild-type flies. Twenty live flies are placed in an ESR tube, and a single near-Lorentzian line is observed at a g-value of 2.0040 with an intensity of approximately 10^{16} spins per fly. The ESR signal intensity decreases for all of the flies with age, no matter what the diet. However, if certain types of carcinogens are incorporated in the diet (at a 1% level), then the ESR intensity is reduced even more. Carcinogens that are known to involve free radicals in their metabolic conversions (such as benzo(a)pyrene and acetylaminofluorine) show this behavior, but so do carcinogens that may not involve free radical activity. The possibility of using ESR as a monitor of the toxicity of food in simple organisms such as fruit flies, although perhaps promising, is in its infancy.

Sugars and proteins give a "browning" reaction when heated together and it appears that the products produced in this reaction may be toxic (53,54,55). These so-called Maillard reaction products (56) have an ESR signal (57-59). Cigarette tar also has a strong ESR signal (61) that is similar in g-value to the signal of Maillard reaction products although the chemical nature of the two radicals appears to be different (56,61).

How are Free Radicals Produced In Vivo?

Free radicals can be produced in living organisms by two distinctly different processes. Firstly, all aerobic organisms continually produce a high flux of superoxide radicals, and these radicals can be converted to more damaging free radicals, such as the hydroxyl radical, by processes that are not yet entirely understood (62). The second mechanism for free radical production involves the metabolism of xenobiotics (63,64). Since I have reviewed these topics rather extensively recently, I will not discuss them again here. However, I would like to briefly review a topic that is relevant to this symposium; namely, the toxicity of lipid peroxides.

The Toxicity of Lipid Hydroperoxides

In 1982, the American Chemical Society sponsored a symposium at its annual meeting in Kansas City entitled "Xenobiotics in Foods and Feeds," and 23 major contributions were presented (65). The fact that the ACS is again presenting a major symposium on this subject in 1984 clearly indicates that the role of toxic substances in the food we eat is of major concern to both the lay public and the scientific community.

Since the heating of fats and fat-containing foods is an extremely common occurrence in food preparation, and since heating fats in air produces lipid hydroperoxides, it is surprising that there has been so little study of the toxicity of these types of materials. In fact, Addis et al. (66) remark in their contribution to the 1982 ACS Symposium that: "It is obvious that studies on toxicity and carcinogenicity of lipid oxidation products, as they occur in food, are in their infancy." These authors go on to discuss a number of areas of current interest including the toxicity of aldehydic products, including malonaldehyde, from the autoxidation of lipids; the toxicity of lipid hydroperoxides; and the toxicity and atherogenicity of cholesterol oxidation products. The toxicity of cholesterol oxidation products also has been reviewed recently in detail by Leland Smith (67), and I will not discuss this subject further.

The Armed Forces have a considerable interest in the oxidative degradation of foods since they need to be able to store foods for long periods of time. For this reason, the US Army Research Office aided in the organization of a symposium entitled "Autoxidation in Food and Biological Systems" that was held in Natick, Massachusetts in October 1979. The proceedings of this symposium were published, with 33 contributions from leading research groups (68).

When fats are heated, autoxidation occurs and lipid hydroperoxides are produced (64,68,69).

$$LH + O_2 \xrightarrow{\text{Heat}} LOOH$$
(lipid)

Since fats are commonly heated in many types of food preparation, the ingestion of lipid hydroperoxides must be a relatively common phenomenon, despite the fact that these materials are known to be toxic. Methyl linoleate hydroperoxide when injected i.v. in the rat at a level of 30mg/100g body weight kills the animals within 24 hours (70). Ten times the dose that is toxic when injected i.v. does not cause death when taken orally, suggesting that a reductase is present that catalyzes the reduction of lipid hydroperoxides as the materials are transported through the gut wall. Interestingly, when lipid hydroperoxides are given to rats by i.v. injection, the lung is the principal organ affected. The toxicity of methyl linoleate ozonide is found to be similar, and both the hydroperoxide and the ozonide produce effects that resemble those observed when animals breathe ozone-containing air, a remarkable observation (70).

The toxicity of a number of hydroperoxides and peroxides were investigated some years ago by a group that believed that the lethality of radiation could be largely explained as being due to the lipid peroxidation that it induces (71). These data are shown in Table II. It has been suggested (72) that these data were not corrected for deaths due to peritonitis, and further study in this area might be worthwhile, particularly since this early report (71) appears to be the only structure-activity study of peroxide toxicity.

Table II. The toxicity of a number of peroxides in mice (injected ip).

Compound	LD_{50} (umole)[a]
Autoxidized Linoleic Acid	7
Disuccinoyl Peroxide	10
3-Cyclohexene Hydroperoxide	15-20
Benzoyl Peroxide	20
Autoxidized Squalene	20-50
Autoxidized Ethyl Linoleate	45-60
Tetralin Hydroperoxide	40
tert-Butyl Hydroperoxide	60-70
tert-Butyl Peroxide	1080

[a] Various strains. Horgan, Philpot et al. *Biochem. J.* **67**:551 (1957).

As might be expected, lipid hydroperoxides are more toxic in vitamin E-deficient animals (73). In the rabbit, the LD_{50} for methyl linoleate hydroperoxide is approximately 2 mg (74). Using methyl linoleate hydroperoxide-1-^{14}C, it is found that 78% of the radioactivity is excreted in the breath as CO_2 and 4% in the urine after 22 hours. The lungs (3%), the liver (7%), and the blood (3% at two hours) concentrate most of the activity that is retained (74). Interestingly, triglycerides in these tissues and in kidney contain both trienoic and dienoic polyunsaturated fatty acids (PUFA) and hydroxy-PUFA, again suggesting the presence of a reductase (74). Ethylbenzene hydroperoxide also is metabolized by reduction to the alcohol (60).

In conclusion, the toxicity of lipid hydroperoxides suggests that these materials are extremely toxic. These peroxidic materials could be a potent source of free radicals *in vivo*.

The Toxicity of Decomposition Products of Lipid Hydroperoxides

Not only are lipid hydroperoxides themselves toxic, but their
decomposition products also can be extremely toxic. This is an area
of intense research, and considerable progress has been made in
separating and analyzing the very complex mixtures that result from
the autoxidation of even very simple lipids using new and powerful
analytical methods. Frankel and his coworkers have been among the
groups reporting detailed analyses of the products of autoxidation
of lipids and PUFA and comparing these products with those produced
by the reaction of singlet oxygen (75).
The aldehydic products from the autoxidation of PUFA have
always been of interest, since the thiobarbituric acid (TBA) test
detects malonaldehyde (or malonaldehyde precursors) with
considerable sensitivity (76-78) and since malonaldehyde itself is
mutagenic (77). More recently, Esterbauer and his coworkers have
shown that 4-hydroxy-2-alkenals, and particularly
4-hydroxy-2-nonenal, are extremely cytotoxic (76,77,79).
In the coming years, it is clear that the toxicity of the
products of lipid autoxidation will come under intense scrutiny;
that is, not only are the free radicals that are produced during the
autoxidation toxic, but some of the stable molecules also are, and
these products can explain the occurrence of damage at some distance
from the site of autoxidation (63).

Cooxidation of Lipids with Other Materials

Lipid hydroperoxides would be expected to induce the oxidation of
other, less oxidative-prone materials (80,81).

$$\text{Biological} \xrightarrow[\text{air}]{\text{LOOH}} \text{Cooxidation} \qquad (2)$$
$$\text{compound}$$

The influence of lipid peroxides on the cooxidation of other
biological materials has been studied to some extent (56,59,82), but
the toxicity of cooxidation products has received only limited study
so far (83,54). This clearly is an area where much more work is
necessary.

A Technique for the Quantitative Study of Antioxidants

It is interesting to consider the concentrations of free radicals
that result from lipid hydroperoxides in an in vitro model system.
For example, my group has been studying the autoxidation of linoleic
acid in SDS micelles at $37^\circ C$. We initiate the autoxidation by the
decomposition of an initiator, as shown in Equation 3.

$$R-N=N-R \longrightarrow 2R^\cdot + N_2 \qquad (3)$$

These $R^\cdot$ radicals rapidly react with oxygen in an aerated system,
and a peroxyl radical is formed, Equation 4.

$$R^{\cdot} + O_2 \longrightarrow ROO^{\cdot} \tag{4}$$

This peroxyl radical can then abstract reactive hydrogen atoms from the substance undergoing autoxidation.

In order to make my discussion specific, and so I can give actual rate constants and concentrations of free radicals, I will illustrate using data from the linoleic acid-SDS micelle system. We are using this system to assess the relative antioxidant potentials of vitamin E, BHT, and new synthetic antioxidants and anti-inflammatory agents (84). To perform these calculations, I have leaned on texts (85,86) and excellent reviews of autoxidation by Mill and Hendry (87) and Howard (88), publications by Ingold and coworkers (89,90) and our own data (84). When linoleic acid undergoes autoxidation, the ROO˙ radicals are formed in eq 4 attack linoleic acid as shown in Equation 5. In this equation linoleic acid is abbreviated as LH, where the H is one of the reactive, doubly allylic hydrogens, and the linoleyl radical, L˙, is the conjugated dienyl radical. Equations 3-5 constitute the <u>initiation sequence</u>.

$$ROO^{\cdot} + LH \longrightarrow ROOH + L^{\cdot} \tag{5}$$

The carbon-centered radical, L˙, reacts with oxygen to give the peroxyl radical, Equation 6.

$$L^{\cdot} + O_2 \xrightarrow{k_o} LOO^{\cdot} \tag{6}$$

These peroxyl radicals then attack another molecule of linoleic acid to abstract an allylic hydrogen and produce the conjugated diene hydroperoxide, LOOH, Equation 7.

$$LOO^{\cdot} + LH \xrightarrow{k_p} LOOH + L^{\cdot} \tag{7}$$

Equations 6 and 7 are the <u>propagation sequence</u>; note that they constitute a chain. Each primoridal radical R˙ initiates a chain of reactions 6-7, and the ratio of the number of product molecules produced (LOOH) to primordial radicals that initiate the chain is called the kinetic chain length, KCL.

Equations like 6 and 7 are called <u>propagation reactions</u> since they propagate the chain; as long as equations like these occur, the number of radicals is conserved and the reaction will keep going until the substrate is used up. However, radical chains are stopped by reactions called terminations. In the absence of an antioxidant, termination occurs by collision of any two of the radicals involved.

$$2LOO^{\cdot} \xrightarrow{k_t} \text{non-radical products (NRP)} \tag{8a}$$

$$LOO^{\cdot} + L^{\cdot} \longrightarrow NRP \tag{8b}$$

$$2L^{\cdot} \longrightarrow NRP \tag{8c}$$

For autoxidations conducted under 1 atmosphere of air, the ratio of peroxyl to alkyl radicals is very high, so Equation 8a is the only important termination (p. 291 in Reference 85).

The Rate Constants and Concentrations of Free Radicals in The Autoxidation of Linoleic Acid in Micelles

A steady-state analysis can now be performed for the autoxidation of linoleic acid. The rate of initiation is given by eqs 3-5 and can be simply written as R_i. At the steady-state, the rate of initiation must equal the rate at which termination occurs; otherwise the process either would stop or would continue to increase in rate and eventually explode! Thus, we can write Equation 9.

$$R_i = 2k_t [LOO^\bullet]^2 \tag{9}$$

Most of the linoleic acid is used in the propagation step, Equation 7. (This is the so-called long-chain approximation.) Thus, the rate of autoxidation, R_{oxi}, is given by Equation 10 (85,86).

$$R_{oxi} = k_p [LOO^\bullet][LH] \tag{10}$$

Equations 9 and 10 can be combined to give Equation 11.

$$R_{oxi} = \frac{k_p}{(2k_t)^{0.5}} [LH][R_i]^{1/2} \tag{11}$$

(The factor of two occurs since each termination destroys two free radicals, and rate constants are written on a per radical basis by convention.) Using Equation 9 and the values of the rate constants given in Table II, we can solve for the concentration (91) of the main chain-carrying species, the peroxyl radical. In our studies, $R_i = 3 \times 10^{-7}$ M s^{-1}, a typical value for an in vitro autoxidation. Therefore, we obtain 2×10^{-7} M as the steady-state concentration of the peroxyl radical, Equation 12.

$$[LOO^\bullet] = (R_i/2k_t)^{0.5} = 2 \times 10^{-7} \text{ M} \tag{12}$$

This value for the concentration of LOO$^\bullet$ is just at the borderline of detectability of most ESR spectrometers; thus, only in special cases can a standing concentration of peroxyl radicals be observed in autoxidations (93). (Oxygen, if present, also broadens the signal and makes it more difficult to observe radicals by ESR.)

We also can now calculate the concentration of L$^\bullet$, the carbon-centered radicals. Another steady-state relationship is that the two chain reactions must occur at the same rate; that is, the chain consists of Equation 6 and Equation 7 occurring alternatively, so each time one occurs the other then follows. That means that the material passed through these steps must be equal and their rates must be equal.

Table III.   Rate constants adopted for kinetic calculations on the autoxidation of linoleic acid at 37°C in SDS micelles.

eq	Symbol	Value	Notes
6	k_o	2×10^9 M^{-1} sec^{-1}	Taken from Reference 94. I have neglected the reverse of reaction 6.
7	k_p	62 M^{-1}sec^{-1}	These are the values for homogeneous solution at 30° C (p. 92 of Reference 88). The values at 37°C are expected to be similar within the accuracy of these illustrative calculations. However, k_t in a micelle may be smaller than the homogeneous value since diffusion from the micelle may be rate limiting (95).
8	$2k_t$	9×10^6 M^{-1}sec^{-1}	
3-5	R_i	3×10^{-7} M sec^{-1}	The initiation rate in the micelle, for the system described here (and in 84).
7	[LH]	0.63 M	Linoleic acid molarity in the micelle, assuming the reagent associates entirely with the lipid phase (84).
17	[InH]	5×10^{-4} M	Ditto for α-tocopherol (84).
17	k_{inh}	2×10^5 M^{-1} sec^{-1}	For α-tocopherol as the inhibitor; data obtained in Reference 84.

$$k_p[LOO^{\bullet}][LH] = k_o[L^{\bullet}][O_2] \tag{13}$$

The value of k_o is 2×10^9 (94), so the L$^{\bullet}$ concentration is given by eq 14, where 0.63 M is the concentration of linoleic acid in our micelles and 1×10^{-3} M is taken as the initial oxygen concentration in the oil phase of the micelle.

$$[L^{\bullet}] = \frac{(62)\ (2 \times 10^{-7})\ (0.63)}{(2 \times 10^9)\ (10^{-3})} = 4 \times 10^{-12}\ M \tag{14}$$

We see that the LOO$^{\bullet}$ is much greater than the L$^{\bullet}$ concentration because of the high rate of reaction 6.

We also can calculate the kinetic chain length; this is equal to the rate of the autoxidation process (and thus to the rate of either propagation step) divided by the rate of primary radical production, Equation 15.

$$\text{KCL} = \frac{k_p[\text{LOO}^{\cdot}][\text{LH}]}{R_i} = \frac{(62)\,(2 \times 10^{-7})\,(0.63)}{3 \times 10^{-7}} = 26 \qquad (15)$$

Thus, 26 molecules of linoleic acid undergo autoxidation when a single free radical is introduced into this model membrane system (96). That much damage might well be enough to destroy the membrane and produce cell lysis and death; however, we must remember that in the real system, the polyunsaturated fatty acids (PUFA) would be protected by antioxidants such as vitamin E.

Inhibited Autoxidation

Inhibitors such as   -tocopherol are effective antioxidants because they rapidly trap peroxyl radicals to give a stabilized radical that does not continue the chain, Equation 16.

$$\text{LOO}^{\cdot} + \text{InH} \xrightarrow{k_{inh}} \text{LOOH} + \text{In}^{\cdot} \qquad (16)$$

In fact, in the case of vitamin E, the inhibitor radical that is produced (In$^{\cdot}$) reacts with a second peroxyl radical to form non-radical products (NRP), Equation 17:

$$\text{LOO}^{\cdot} + \text{In}^{\cdot} \longrightarrow \text{NRP} \qquad (17)$$

(Inhibitors like this are said to have a stoichiometric factor of 2; that is, 2 radicals are stopped per molecule of inhibitor.) We can calculate the fraction of the peroxyl radicals that undergo reaction 7 and continue the chain versus those that react with tocopherol, Equation 16, ultimately to terminate the autoxidation. In this calculation (Equation 18), the concentration of peroxyl radicals cancels out (97). We will use the concentration of tocopherol that we use in our micelle studies and the value of k_{inh} that we measure for tocopherol (84).

$$\frac{2R_{16}}{R_7} = \frac{2k_{inh}\,[\text{LOO}^{\cdot}][\text{InH}]}{k_p\,[\text{LOO}^{\cdot}][\text{LH}]} = \frac{(2)\,(2 \times 10^5)\,(5 \times 10^{-4})}{(62)\,(0.63)} = 5 \qquad (18)$$

Thus, even though there is much more linoleic acid than tocopherol, 5/6 = 83% of the peroxyl radicals react with inhibitor and the chain reaction is greatly slowed, as shown in Figure 1.

   We can now calculate the concentration of the peroxyl radicals in this inhibited autoxidation. The principal termination reaction is now reaction with vitamin E, rather than reaction 8a as had been previously true. Therefore, we can write Equations 19 and 20, giving the new concentration of peroxyl radicals as 2×10^{-9}. Thus, the inhibitor acts to keep the peroxyl radical concentration about 100-fold lower than it was in the uninhibited autoxidations. (Compare Equations 12 and 20.)

$$R_i = R_{inh} = nk_{inh}[\text{LOO}^{\cdot}][\text{Inh}] \qquad (19)$$

$$[LOO^{\cdot}] = \frac{3 \times 10^{-7}}{(2)\,(2 \times 10^{5})\,(5 \times 10^{-4})} = 2 \times 10^{-9}\ M \tag{20}$$

We also can now calculate the new kinetic chain length. The formula is given in eq 15, and we only need to supply the new concentration of the peroxyl radical. This is done in Equation 21.

$$KCL = \frac{(62)\,(2 \times 10^{-9})\,(0.63)}{(3 \times 10^{-7})} = 0.3 \tag{21}$$

Thus, when the inhibitor is present the chain length is very small.

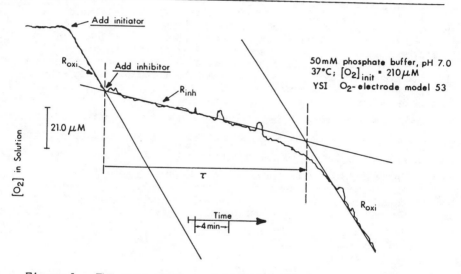

Figure 1. The autoxidation of linoleic acid in SDS micelles. The initiator is first injected into the bulk buffer phase and then the antioxidant is injected. The oxygen-electrode trace shown is for alpha-tocopherol as the antioxidant ([84]).

The Kinetics of the Inhibited Autoxidation

I have used a value of k_{inh}, the rate constant for reaction 16, of 2 x 10^{5} M^{-1} sec^{-1} in the calculations above. How was this value determined? Figure 1 shows a plot of oxygen concentration (determined using an oxygen electrode) versus time when linoleic acid undergoes autoxidation in SDS micelles at 37°C and with α-tocopherol as the inhibitor. First let me describe the advantages of this system for studying autoxidation and then let me describe the data that are acquired in order to calculate k_{inh}.

Ingold and his coworkers have described an autoxidation system in which styrene is oxidized to styrene polyperoxide in chlorobenzene as a solvent (90). This obviously is a far cry from a biological lipid bilayer system, but Ingold has argued convincingly of the merits of this system. (It gives a single product, has a high value of k_p and the reversal of reaction 16 can be neglected, and the rate constants are well characterized.) If a system is studied that is a close model for in vivo autoxidation (such as red blood cells, a classical model system), initiators and inhibitors cannot be injected into the bulk aqueous phase and produce an instantaneous response, since diffusion into the bilayer from the aqueous phase is too slow. [Even an egg lecithin bilayer vesicle system gives this problem (89).] Our system, on the other hand, is an extremely useful halfway house.

In our system, the rate of autoxidation of linoleic acid, is essentially zero in the absence of the initiator. (Notice the flatness of the oxygen trace at the far left in Figure 1 before the initiator is added.) Our system produces classical inhibition kinetics. Initiator can be injected into the bulk aqueous phase and the autoxidation starts instantly. When the vitamin E is injected, it also produces an instantaneous effect. The rate of autoxidation before the vitamin E is added, R_{oxi}, is also observed after all the vitamin E has been used. (See Figure 1.) The two quantitites that we need to measure to obtain a value of k_{inh} are shown on this plot; they are τ, the length of the inhibition period, and R_{inh}, the rate of autoxidation in the presence of the inhibitor (98).

We can derive the necessary equations as follows. We can combine Equation 19 and the definition of the rate during the inhibition period, given in Equation 22, to give Equation 23.

$$R_{inh} = k_p \, [LH][LOO^{\cdot}] \tag{22}$$

$$R_{inh} = k_p \, [LH] \, \frac{R_i}{n \, k_{inh} \, [InH]} \tag{23}$$

Notice that the rate of autoxidation during the inhibition period, R_{inh}, shows a first power dependence on R_i, and not the square root dependence that was observed in Equation 11; this is because the $LOO^{\cdot}$ radicals are scavenged by the inhibitor, InH, rather than undergoing a bimolecular termination reaction.

We can simplify Equation 23 as follows. The lag time, τ, is defined as shown in Equation 24.

$$\tau \equiv \frac{n[InH]}{R_i} \qquad \text{(in sec)} \tag{24}$$

That is, γ is the ratio of the total number of radicals that is scavenged (n [InH]) divided by the rate at which radicals are being produced, R_i. (This definition perhaps is not obvious at first glance, but notice that it does have the correct units, seconds, since the numerator is in mole/liter and the denominator is a rate in moles/liter-sec.) If Equation 24 is substituted into Equation 23, we obtain the final equation, Equation 25.

$$R_{inh} = \frac{k_p[LH]}{k_{inh} \gamma} \tag{25}$$

Since both the rate during the inhibition period, R_{inh}, and γ can be directly measured from traces like Figure 1, and since the linoleic acid concentration in the micelle can be calculated from the dimensions of the micelle and the total amount of the linoleic acid that is added, a knowledge of k_p allows the calculation of k_{inh}. Alternatively, the ratio of k_{inh}/k_p can be obtained.

Table IV. A comparison of k_{inh} data from our laboratory (84) with literature data.

Compound	$k_{inh} \times 10^{-4}$ ($M^{-1} s^{-1}$)	
	Our value (84)	Literature Values
α-Tocopherol	18	234[a], 51[b], 15[c]
BHT	3.0	3.6[c], 1.2[a]
BHA[e]	2.4	--
DBP[f]	0.94	6.0[c], 2.2[d]

[a] Styrene autoxidation in chlorobenzene, 30°C. Reference 90.
[b] Methyl linoleate autoxidation in t-butanol, 37°C. Reference 99.
[c] Ethylbenzene autoxidation in o-dichlorobenzene. 25°C.
    Reference 100.
[d] Stryene autoxidation in styrene, 65°C. Reference 101.
[e] 2(3)-tert-butyl-4-methoxyphenol.
[f] 2,6-di-tert-butylphenol.

Our group is measuring values of k_{inh} for a series of natural and synthetic antioxidants and for non-steroidal anti-inflammatory drugs using this new test system (84); some selected results are presented in Table IV along with the corresponding values obtained by other investigators. These data were obtained from a wide variety of experimental systems and the difference among the reported values should not be overinterpreted until further data have been obtained. There is, however, a uniform agreement that α-tocopherol is superior to the synthetic antioxidants.

Acknowledgment
The research in my Laboratory described in this review was supported by the National Institutes of Health (HL-16029 and HL-25820), the National Science Foundation, and the National Foundation for Cancer Research. I also wish to acknowledge contributions by Drs. D.F. Church, L. Castle, M.M. Dooley, M.J. Kaufman, K. Uehara and M. Tamura.

Literature Cited

1. Fries, J.F. and Crapo, L.M. In "Vitality and Aging"; W.H. Freeman and Company: San Francisco, Ca., 1981.
2. Janoff, A., Carp, H., Laurent, P., and Raju, L. Am. Rev. Respir. Dis. 1983, 127, S31–S38.
3. Church, D.F., Crank, G., Chopard, C., Govindan, C.K., and Pryor, W.A. Fed. Proc. 1982, 41, 2346.
4. Dooley, M.M. and Pryor, W.A. Biochem. Biophys. Res. Comm. 1982, 106, 981–987.
5. Pryor, W.A., Chopard, C., Tamura, M., and Church, D.F. Fed. Proc. 1982, 41, 2346.
6. Pryor, W.A., Dooley, M.M., and Church, D.F. 1984, (in press).
7. Gale, P.H. and Egan, R.W. In "Free Radicals in Biology"; Pryor, W.A., Ed.; Academic Press: New York, 1984; Vol. VI, Chapter 1.
8. Marnett, L. In "Free Radicals in Biology"; Pryor, W.A., Ed.; Academic Press: New York, 1984; Vol. VI, Chapter 3.
9. Ham, E.A., Egan, R.W., Soderman, D.D., Gale, P.H., and Kuehl, F.A. J. Biol. Chem. 1979, 254, 2191–2194.
10. Moncada, S. and Vane, J.R. Brit. Med. Bull. 1978, 34, 129–134.
11. Yoshikawa, T., Murakami, M., Furukawa, Y., Kato, H., Takemura, S., and Kondo, M. Thromb. Haemostas. 1983, 49, 214–216.
12. Lubawy, W.C., Valentovic, M.A., Atkinson, J.E., and Gairola, G.C. Life Sci. 1983, 33, 577–584.
13. Pryor, W.A., Tamura, M., and Church, D.F. J. Am. Chem. Soc. 1984 (in press).
14. Bulkley, G.B. Surgery 1983, 94, 407–411.
15. McCord, J.M. Surgery 1983, 94, 412–414.
16. Parks, D.A., Buckley, G.B., and Granger, D.N. Surgery 1983, 94, 415–422.
17. Gardner, T.J., Stewart, J.R., Casale, A.S., Downey, J.M., and Chambers, D.E. Surgery 1983, 94, 423–427.
18. Parks, D.A., Bulkley, G.B., and Granger, D.N. Surgery 1983, 94, 428–432.
19. Cavalieri, E.L. and Rogan, E.G. In "Free Radicals in Biology"; Pryor, W.A., Ed.; Academic Press: New York, 1984; Vol. VI, Chapter 10.

20. Cornwell, D.G. and Marisaki, N. In "Free Radicals in Biology"; Pryor, W.A., Ed.; Academic Press: New York, 1984; Vol. VI, Chapter 4.

21. Floyd, R.A. In "Free Radicals in Biology"; Pryor, W.A., Ed.; Academic Press: New York, 1980; Vol. V, pp. 187-206.

22. Floyd, R.A., Editor. In "Free Radicals in Cancer"; Marcel Dekker: New York, 1982.

23. Kalyanaraman, B. and Sivarajah, K. In "Free Radicals in Biology"; Pryor, W.A., Ed.; Academic Press: New York, 1984; Vol. VI, Chapter 5.

24. Mason, R.P. In "Free Radicals in Biology"; Pryor, W.A., Ed.; Academic Press: New York, 1982; Vol. V, pp. 161-196.

25. Ts'o, P.O.P., Caspary, W.J., and Lorentzen, R.J. In "Free Radicals in Biology"; Pryor, W.A., Ed.; Academic Press: New York, 1982; Vol. III, pp. 251-300.

26. Emerit, I. and Cerutti, P.A. Proc. Natl. Acad. Sci. 1982, 79, 7509-7513.

27. Slaga, T.J., Klein-Szanto, A.J.P., Triplett, L.L., Yotti, L.P., and Trosko, J.E. Science 1981, 213, 1023-1025.

28. Birnboim, H.C. Science 1982, 215, 1247-1249.

29. Swartz, H.M. In "Submolecular Biology and Cancer"; CIBA SYMPOSIUM NUMBER 67 (NEW SERIES), Elsevier Publisher: New York, 1979.

30. Benedetto, C. In "Free Radicals, Lipid Peroxidation, and Cancer"; McBrien, D.C.H. and Slater, T.F., Eds.; Academic Press: New York, 1982, pp. 27-54.

31. Shamberger, R.J., Baughman, F.F., Kalchert, S.L., Willis, C.E., and Hoffman, G.C. Proc. Natl. Acad. Sci. 1973, 70, 1461-1463.

32. Wattenberg, L.W. J. Natl. Cancer Insti. 1972, 48, 1425-1430.

33. Heckler, E., Fusenig, N.E., Kunz, W., Marks, F., and Thielmann, H.W., Eds. In "Cocarcinogenesis and Biological Effects of Tumor Promoters"; Raven Press: New York, 1982.

34. Weitzman, S.A. and Stossel, T.P. Science 1981, 212, 546-547.

35. Schmitt, R.J., Buttrill, Jr., S.E., Ross, D.S. J. Amer. Chem. Soc. 1984, 106, 926-930.

36. Kohan, M., Claxton, L. Mut. Res. 1983, 124, 191-200.

37. Pryor, W.A., Gleicher, G.J., Church, D.F. 1984, (submitted for publication).

38. Pitts, J.N., Van Chauwenberghe, K.A., Grosjean, D., Schmid, J.P., Fitz, D.R., Belser, W.L., Knudson, G.B., Hynds, P.M. Science 1978, 202, 515-519.

39. Mermelstein, R., Kiriazides, D.K., Butler, M., McCoy, E.C., Rosenkranz, H.S. Mut. Res. 1981, 89, 187-196.

40. Pryor, W.A., Yoshikawa, T. 1984, (unpublished).

41. Blake, D.R., Hall, N.D., Bacon, P.A., Dieppe, P.A., Halliwell, B., and Gutteridge, J.M.C. Lancet 1981, 1142-1144.

42. Cohen, G. and Greenwald, R.A. In "Oxy-Radicals in Their Scavenger Systems, Molecular Aspects"; Elsevier: New York, 1983; Vol. I.

43. Greenwald, R.A. and Cohen, G. In "Oxy-Radicals in Their Scavenger Systems, Cellular and Molecular Aspects"; Elsevier: New York, 1983; Vol. II.

44. Laughrea, M. Exp. Gerontol. 1982, 17, 305-317.

45. Strehler, B.L. In "Time Cells and Aging"; Academic Press: New York, 1977; 2nd Edition, p. 25.

46. Man, E.H., Sandhouse, M.E., Burg, J., and Fisher, G.H. Science 1983, 220, 1407-1408.
47. Brod, N. and Weissbach, H. Arch. Biochem. Biophys. 1983, 223, 271-281.
48. Harman, D. In "Free Radicals in Biology"; Pryor, W.A., Ed.; Academic Press: New York, 1982; Vol. V, pp. 255-271.
49. Cutler, R.G. In "Free Radicals in Biology"; Pryor, W.A., Ed.; Academic Press: New York, 1984; Vol VI, Chapter 11.
50. Docampo, R. and Moreno, S.N.J. In "Free Radicals in Biology"; Pryor, W.A., Ed.; Academic Press: New York, 1984; Vol VI, Chapter 8.
51. O'Brien, P.J. In "Free Radicals in Biology"; Pryor, W.A., Ed.; Academic Press: New York, 1984; Vol VI, Chapter 9.
52. Trapp, C., Waters, B., Lebendiger, G., and Perkins, M. Biochem. Biophys. Res. Comm. 1983, 112(2), 602-605.
53. Lee, T.C. and Chichester, C.O. In "Xenobiotics in Foods and Feeds"; Finley, J.W. and Schwass, D.E., Editors; American Chemical Society: Washington, DC, 1983; Chapter 23.
54. C. Eriksson, Ed. In "Progress in Food and Nutrition Science: Maillard Reactions in Food"; Pergamon Press: New York, 1981; Vol.5, Numbers 1-6.
55. Waller, G.R., and Feather, M.S., Eds. In "The Maillard Reaction in Foods and Nutrition" American Chemical Society Symposium Series 215; American Chemical Society: Washington, DC, 1983.
56. Mauron, J. Prog. Food Nutr. Sci. 1981, 5, 5-35.
57. Pryor, W.A. and Church, D.F. 1982, (unpublished).
58. Namiki, M. and Hayashi, T. In "The Maillard Reaction in Foods and Nutrition" American Chemical Society Symposium Series 215; Waller, G.R., and Feather, M.S., Eds.; American Chemical Society: Washington, DC, 1983; pp 21-46.
59. Namiki, M. and Hayashi, T. Prog. Food Nutr. Sci. 1981, 5, 81-91.
60. Climie, I.J.G., Hutson, D.H., and Stoydin, G. Xenobiotica 1983, 13, 611-618.
61. Pryor, W.A., Hales, B.J., Premovic, P.I., and Church D.F. Science 1983, 220, 425-427.
62. Gutteridge, J.M.C., Rowley, D.A., and Halliwell, B. Biochem. J. 1982, 206, 605-609.
63. Pryor, W.A. New York Acad. Sci. 1982, 393, 1-30.
64. Pryor, W.A. In "Free Radicals in Biology and Aging"; Armstrong D. and Harman, D., Eds.; Raven Press: New York, 1984; Chapter XX.
65. Finley, J.W. and Schwass, D.E., editors (1983): In Xenobiotics in Foods and Feeds, American Chemical Society Symposium Series #239, American Chemical Society, Washington, DC.
66. Addis, P.B., Csallany, A.S., and Kindom, S.E. In "Xenobiotics in Foods and Feeds"; Finley, J.W. and Schwass, D.E., Editors; American Chemical Society: Washington, DC, 1983; Chapter 5.
67. Smith, L.L. In "Cholesterol Autoxidation"; Plenum Press: New York, 1981.
68. Simic, M.G. and Karel, M., Editors. In "Autoxidation in Food and Biological Systems"; Plenum Press, New York, 1980.
69. Ames, B.N. Science 1983, 221, 1256-1264.
70. Cortesi, R. and Privett, O.S. Lipids 1972, 11, 715-721.

71. Horgan, V.J., Philpot, J. St.L., Porter, B.W., and Roodyn, D.B. Biochem. J. 1957, 67, 551-558.
72. O'Brien, P. 1984, Remark made in discussion period following this contribution at the ACS meeting.
73. Privett, O.S. and Cortesi, R. Lipids 1972, 7, 780-787.
74. Findlay, G.M., Draper, H.H., and Bergan, J.G. Lipids 1970, 5, 970-975.
75. Frankel, E.N. Prog. Lipid Res. 1982, 22, 1-33.
76. Esterbauer, H. and Slater, T.F. IRCS Medical Sci. 1981, 9, 749-750.
77. Schauenstein, E., Esterbauer, H., and Zollner, H. In "Aldehydes in Biological Systems"; Pion Publishers: London, England, 1977.
78. Pryor, W.A., Stanley, J.P., and Blair, E. Lipids 1976, 11, 370-379.
79. Benedetti, A., Comporti, M., and Esterbauer, H. Biochim. Biophys. Acta, 1980, 620, 281-296.
80. Pryor, W.A. In "Free Radicals in Biology"; Pryor, W.A., Ed.; Academic Press: New York, 1976; Vol. I, pp. 1-43.
81. Benedetti, A., Esterbauer, H., Ferrali, M., Furceri, R., and Comporti, M. Biochim. Biophys. Acta 1982, 711, 345-356.
82. Desai, I.D., and Tappel, A.L. J. Lipid. Res. 1963, 4, 204-207.
83. Dworschak, E. CRC Crit. Rev. Food Sci. Nut. 1980, 13, 1-40.
84. Pryor, W.A., Kaufman, M.J., and Church, D.F. 1984, (to be submitted).
85. Pryor, W.A. In "Free Radicals"; McGraw Hill Book Co.: New York, 1966.
86. Walling, C. In "Free Radicals in Solution"; John Wiley and Sons: New York, 1957.
87. Mill, T. and Hendry, D.G. In "Chemical Kinetics"; Bamford, C.H. and Tipper, C.F.H., Eds.; Elsevier Scientific Publishing Co.: New York, 1980; pp. 1-83.
88. Howard, J.A. In "Advances in Free-Radical Chemistry"; Williams, G.H., Ed.; Academic Press: New York, 1972; pp. 49-174.
89. Barclay, L.R.C. and Ingold, K.U. J. Am. Chem. Soc. 1981, 103, 6478-6485.
90. Burton, G.W. and Ingold, K.U. J. Am. Chem. Soc. 1981, 103, 6472-6477.
91. Our system uses 14% linoleic acid in an SDS micelle. This percentage of linoleic acid roughly equals that found in a biological membrane. However, micelles are only about 30A in diameter whereas cells are many orders of magnitude larger. The advantage of micelles is that diffusion into them is so rapid that initiator and inhibitors can be injected into the bulk aqueous phase and they equilibrate into the linoleic micelle layer too fast for any delay to be observed in our kinetic traces. (See Figure 1 and Reference 92.)
    In this article I have calculated concentrations of linoleic acid, vitamin E, the initiator, and O_2 in the micelle, since this is where the autoxidation occurs. Thus, the concentrations quoted in the text are 100 times larger than the values that would be obtained if the solution were assumed to be a single homogeneous phase and average concentrations were used. Similarly, therefore, the value of R_i I have used is 100 times larger than the value calculated from the rate of

disappearance of the initiator averaged over the entire
solution.

92. Turro, N.J., Zimmt, M.B., and Gould, I.R. J. Am. Chem. Soc.
1983, 105, 6347-6349.
93. Pryor, W.A., Ohto, N., and Church, D.F. J. Am. Chem. Soc. 1983,
105, 3614-3622.
94. Maillard, B., Ingold, K.U., and Scaiano, J.C. J. Am. Chem. Soc.
1983, 105, 5095-5099.
95. Henglein, A. and Proske, T. J. Am. Chem. Soc. 1978, 100,
3706-3709.
96. Remember these calculations are only approximate and meant to
be merely illustrative.
97. The factor of 2 occurs in Equation 18 since each inhibitor
stops 2 kinetic chains.
98. Because the chain lengths are not large in inhibited runs and
because one O_2 is used in Equation 4 in the initiation
sequence, the long-chain approximation used in Equations 10 and
11 is no longer correct, and R_{inh} is defined as $(R_{oxi} - R_i)$,
where $R_{oxi} = -dO_2/dt$.

99. Niki, E., Yamamoto, Y., and Kamiya, Y. In "Oxygen Radicals in
Chemistry and Biology"; Bors, W., et al., Ed.; Walter de
Gruyter and Co.: Berlin, Germany, 1984.
100. Niki, E., Tanimura, R., and Kamiya, Y. Bull. Chem. Soc. Jpn.
1982, 55, 1551-1555.
101. Howard, J.A., and Ingold, K.U. Can. J. Chem. 1963, 41,
2800-2806.

RECEIVED August 17, 1984

Xenobiotic Adduct Formation with DNA or Glutathione Following Oxidation by Lipid Peroxidation or Hydrogen Peroxide-Peroxidase

M. RAHIMTULA, W. MARSHALL, B. GREGORY, and P. J. O'BRIEN

Departments of Biochemistry and Chemistry, Memorial University of Newfoundland, St. John's, Newfoundland, Canada

Prostaglandin synthetase, peroxidase or lipid peroxidation have been shown to oxidise arylamine xenobiotics to reactive species that bind extensively to DNA. The binding could be an initial event in the toxic or carcinogenic process. Evidence is presented that cation radicals are involved in the formation of the various oxidation products and DNA adduct formation with the carcinogen aminofluorene. Furthermore methylaminoazobenzene (butter yellow) was found to form the same major GSH adduct as is formed in vivo.

The metabolic activation of carcinogenic arylamines is widely believed to involve N-hydroxylation by the cytochrome P450-dependent mixed function oxidase system of the liver. Subsequent conjugation, transport in the blood or bile and hydrolysis in the non hepatic target organ results in binding of an electrophilic species to DNA of the target organ (1,2). However recently a wide range of xenobiotics have been found to act as hydrogen donors for the peroxidase activity of prostaglandin H synthase during the oxygenation of polyunsaturated fatty acids (3). In the process the xenobiotic undergoes a one electron oxidation to free radicals and reactive species that can also bind extensively to DNA, RNA or protein (4,5). Extrahepatic tissues usually contain high levels of prostaglandin H synthase or peroxidase so that metabolic activation in the target organ itself is an attractive alternative theory for the initiation of carcinogenesis.

Experimental Methods

Materials: N-(ring-^{14}C)-Methylaminobenzene was synthesized as described (6) and had a specific activity of 0.54 mCi/ mol with a purity of 99%. 2-(9-^{14}C-Aminofluorene was prepared from 2-(9-^{14}C)-acetylaminofluorene (specific activity 50 mCi/nmol) that was purchased from New England Nuclear (Boston, Mass.). The latter was incubated with carboxyesterase II, and the 9-^{14}C-2-aminofluorene formed was extracted with ethylacetate and purified by high pressure liquid chromatography (7). (ring-^{14}C)-Benzidine (specific activity of 25.7 mCi/nmol) was purchased from New England Nuclear (Boston, Mass.). The following reagents were purchased from Sigma Chemical Co. (St. Louis, MO): horseradish peroxidase (type VI), protease (type XI), calf

thymus DNA (type I) and butylated hydroxyanisole. Hydrogen peroxide
was obtained from BDH Chemicals (Toronto, Canada). 2,3,6-Trimethyl-
phenol was purchased from Aldrich Chemical Co. All other chemicals
were of the highest grade available.

Peroxide catalyzed aminofluorene oxidation

The incubation mixtures (2 ml) consisted of 0.1M Tris-HCl buffer
pH 6.5, 10 µg of horseradish peroxidase (type VI), 100µM (^{3}H)-2-AF,
100µM H_2O_2 and water. The reaction was started by the addition
of H_2O_2 and terminated after 1 minute by the addition of 100µM
ascorbate and extraction with ethyl acetate. The products were
then separated by thin layer chromatography.

Lipid peroxide catalyzed azo dye oxidation

The incubation mixture consisted of 0.1M Tris-HCl pH 6.5, hematin
(0.02 mM) and 0.1 mM of DAB, MAB and AB. The reaction was started
by the addition of linoleic acid hydroperoxide (0.1 mM) and terminated
after 5 minutes at 20°C by extraction with ethyl acetate. The
azo dyes and their metabolites were separated and quantified
by high performance liquid chromatography.

TLC of Aminofluorene products

The ethyl acetate extracts of the reaction mixture were concentrated
under nitrogen and applied to 250µ Silica Gel G plates (Analtech).
The solvent used for the mobile phase was $CHCl_3$-ethyl acetate
(8:2). The plates were examined under an ultraviolet lamp and
the bands were scraped clear into separate tubes. The products
were then dissolved in ethyl acetate or n-butanol and analyzed
by UV-visible spectrophotometry and the spectra from 254-450
nm were compared with those of authentic standards. Radioactivity
levels were determined and the products were analyzed by mass
spectrometry.

Mass Spectrometry

Products were analyzed using a VG Micromass 7070HS mass
spectrometer equipped with VG 2035 data system. Samples were
introduced using a direct insertion probe whose temperature could
be increased to 400°C; the ion source temperature was maintained
at 220°C. Ions were generated by 70eV electron bombardment.
Scanning was performed over a mass range of 800-35 at scan rates
of 1-7 sec/decade. Low resolution spectra were obtained at resolving
power 1000; mass calibration was achieved using a calibration
file previously made using perfluorokerosene. High resolution
spectra were obtained at resolving power 7-10,000 in the presence
of perfluorokerosene and using a perfluorokersene accurate mass
calibration file containing at least 50 lock mass reference peaks.
Accurate masses were then obtained by averaging data from several
consecutive scans.

HPLC of azo dye metabolites

An HPLC method was developed for the separation of DAB, MAB and
AB. A Waters HPLC system was used with a µ-Bondapack C-18 reverse
phase column (25 cm in length) using a 50% methanol in water

to 100% methanol linear gradient during 20 minutes at a flow rate of 1 ml/min at 20°C. The HPLC system consisted of a model UGK injector, two model 6000A solvent delivery pumps and a model 660 solvent programmer. Absorbance at 405 nm was continuously monitored. Fractions were collected on a LBK fraction collector at a rate of 5 fractions/min. Eluant fractions were mixed with Atomlight scintillation fluid (New England Nuclear, Boston, Mass) and radioactivity was determined on a Beckman model LS-330 liquid scintillation spectrometer with quench correction. The retention times were as follows:-DAB (15.6'), 4'-OH-DAB (12.0'), MAB (13.1'), AB (10.0'), 4'-OH-MAB (9.5') and 4'-OH-AB (5.5').

DNA binding

DNA (3 mg) or polyribonucleotides (3 mg) were included in the above reaction mixtures. The reaction was stopped by extraction with an equal volume of ethyl acetate-acetone (2:1) and the organic solvent was removed. This extraction was repeated three times. The residual organic solvent in the aqueous layer was then removed by bubbling with nitrogen. Sodium dodecyl sulfate solution (10%, 200ul) and protease (0.5 mg) were added and the mixture allowed to incubate at 37°C for 30 min to digest any possible contaminating protein. Water saturated phenol (1 ml) and water saturated $CHCl_3$ (1 ml) were then added and the mixture was shaken vigorously. After centrifuation, the aqueous phase was transferred to a new test tube. The DNA or polyribonucleotides were subsequently precipitated by the addition of NaCl (5M, 100ul) and ethanol (6 ml). After centrifugation, the supernatant was discarded. The DNA or polyribonucleotides were dissolved in water (1 ml), reprecipitated with NaCl (5 M, 100ul) and ethanol (2.5 ml), washed with ethanol (1 ml) and ether (1 ml) and dried under nitrogen. The isolated macromolecule was then dissolved in water (1 ml) and aliquots were used for the determination of the radioactivity of bound ^{14}C-aminofluorene and the UV-visible absorbance spectra of the bound adduct. The concentration of the DNA or polyribonucleotide in an aliquot was also determined (8).

The peroxide oxidation of MAB in the presence of GSH and identification of products

The incubation mixture consisted of 2 ml of 0.1M acetate buffer pH 6.0, 0.2 mM of ^{14}C-MAB, 0.2 mM GSH, 0.2 mM H_2O_2 and peroxidase (10ug). The reaction was started by the addition of H_2O_2 and was stopped after 1 minute at 20°C by shaking with an equal volume of water-saturated ethyl acetate resulting in extraction of MAB and its products into the organic phase with the GSH adduct remaining in the aqueous phase. The aqueous phase was further extracted with water-saturated chloroform and centrifuged. Formaldehyde was determined in the aqueous phase by Nash reagent (9). The GSH adduct was then extracted with water-saturated n-butanol, concentrated under nitrogen and run on a cellulose TLC plate. The solvent used for the mobile phase was n-propanol: H_2O (7:3). The major band had an R_f of 0.8 and its ultraviolet and visible absorption spectra was similar to that of GS-CH_2-AB synthesized from AB as described previously (10). An n-butanol extract of the peroxide formed, GS-CH$_2$-AB, was made 1N with respect to HCl. After standing for 30 mins at 37°C, AB was found to be the principal product as determined by HPLC and UV-visible spectroscopy. Previously, GS-CH$_2$-AB was characterized by its acidic decomposition to stoichiometric amounts of AB (10). Furthermore, if the incubated acidified n-butanol extract was extracted twice with equal volumes of aqueous 0.27 mM semicarbazide, stoichiometric amounts of GSH and HCHO were formed in the aqueous phase as determined by the Ellman reagent (11) and the Nash reagent (9) respectively.

Results

As can be seen from Table I, linoleic acid hydroperoxide in the presence of hematin rapidly catalyzed the N-demethylation of dimethylaminoazobenzene to form methylaminoazobenzene. N-methylamino-azobenzene was also N-demethylated to aminoazobenzene. However aminoazobenzene disappeared rapidly in this system and no other basic dye product was detected in the mixture. Instead a polymeric material appeared at the interface following extraction of the reaction mixture with ethyl acetate. A similar N-demethylation occurred with H$_2$O$_2$ and peroxidase (0.1ug). At higher peroxidase concentrations other products were formed. Formaldehyde was also readily detected in the reaction mixture with Nash reagent following extraction of the interfering highly coloured products with ethyl acetate.

TABLE I.   METABOLISM OF AMINOAZO DYES BY LINOLEIC ACID HYDROPEROXIDE
           AND HEME

Incubation Mixture	Percentage of azo dye and its metabolites			
	DAB	MAB	AB	Recovery
DAB + heme + LAHPO	3.78	42.1	3.0	82.9
MAB + heme + LAHPO	--	70.4	10.6	81.0
AB + heme + LAHPO	--	--	26.1	26.1

The incubation mixture contained in a final volume of 2.0 ml: Tris-HCl buffer 0.1M (pH 6.5), LAHPO (0.1 mM), heme (20 M) and azodye (0.05 mM). The reaction was started by the addition of LAHPO and terminated after 15 minutes at 37°C by extraction with diethyl ether. Azo dyes and their metabolites were separated and quantified by high performance liquid chromatography.
     In the presence of glutathione, HCHO and AB formation were inhibited and water-soluble GSH adducts were formed if the peroxidase

concentration was 1-10ug. TLC chromatography of a butanol extract of the GSH adducts showed that the major band had an R_f identical to that of synthetic GS-CH$_2$-AB. Furthermore the band had an identical UV-visible spectra to that of synthetic GS-CH$_2$-AB and on acid treatment, both formed stoichiometric amounts of GSH, HCHO and AB. Upon addition of HCl to the butanol extract, a transient magenta colour, presumably due to protonated GS-CH$_2$-AB, was observed before fading to the spectrum of pink protonated AB. On neutralization, a spectrum of neutral AB was obtained. Two other adducts were also observed if the incubation time or the peroxidase concentration or H$_2$O$_2$ concentration was increased. Linoleic acid hydroperoxide with hematin at pH 6.5 also oxidized MAB in the presence of GSH to GS-CH$_2$-AB.

At pH < 6 or at higher peroxide concentrations, other GSH adducts were also formed but have not yet been identified. Presumably they are formed by further oxidation of GS-CH$_2$-AB and/or GSH adduct formation with other MAB oxidation products. Under optimal conditions in the H$_2$O$_2$-peroxidase system, 83% of the MAB could be recovered as GS-CH$_2$-AB as calculated from a molar extinction coefficient for GS-CH$_2$-AB of 22,600 M^{-1} at 395 nm in methanol: water 1:1.

DNA binding during aminofluorene catalyzed oxidation by peroxide

As shown in Table II, the oxidation of aminofluorene by peroxide and peroxidase readily results in adduct formation with DNA or polyribonucleotides. Polyriboguanylic acid and polyriboadenylic acid were much more effective than polyribouridylic acid or poly-ribocytidylic acid in forming adducts with aminofluorene oxidation products. One equivalent of H$_2$O$_2$ with respect to aminofluorene was required. The nature of the reactive species involved in DNA binding was next investigated. In Table II, it can be seen that DNA binding was prevented by ascorbate or NADPH. However, examination of the oxidation products separated by TLC showed that aminofluorene oxidation was prevented by ascorbate or NADPH. The peroxide-peroxidase mediated oxidation of ascorbate or NADPH monitored at 270 nm or 340 nm respectively was slow at pH 7 with peroxide peroxidase. However they were rapidly oxidized on the addition of aminofluorene. This suggests that ascorbate and NADPH protect the DNA by reducing the activated oxidation products to aminofluorene.

The phenolic antioxidants 2,3,6-trimethylphenol and butylated hydroxyanisole also markedly prevented DNA binding. The reaction mixture was pink in colour and stable over time. Chromatography of the ethyl acetate extractable oxidation products formed in the presence of 2,3,6-trimethyl- phenol however showed that most of the radioactivity was concentrated in a pink band with an R_f of 0.8. This product was not formed in the absence of either aminofluorene or H$_2$O$_2$. The formation of other aminofluorene products were markedly inhibited. Glutathione and N-acetyl cysteine products also markedly prevented DNA binding. Chromatography of the oxidation products showed a marked inhibition of oxidation product formation. Most of the radioactivity was recovered in

TABLE II. DNA OR POLYRIBONUCLEOTIDE ADDUCT FORMATION WITH
AMINOFLUORENE FOLLOWING OXIDATION BY PEROXIDES

REACTION CONDITIONS	Macromolecule Binding pmoles/mg
DNA	358+31
DNA + Ascorbate (50uM)	0+1
DNA + NADPH (50uM)	4+1
DNA + 2,3,6-trimethylphenol (5uM)	41+4
DNA + Butylated Hydroxyanisole (5uM)	21+7
DNA + Glutathione (50uM)	53+5
DNA + N-Acetylcysteine (50uM)	32+3
Polyriboadenylic Acid	85+9
Polyriboguanylic Acid	389+30
Polyribouridylic Acid	10+2
Polyribocytidylic Acid	23+2

Reaction Conditions: - ^{14}C-Aminofluorene (0.05 mM), H_2O_2 (0.05
mM), peroxidase (10ug), 0.1 M Tris-HCl buffer pH 6.5 with and
without denatured DNA or polyribonucleotides (0.5 mg) were incubated
for 1 minute and extracted with ethyl acetate. DNA and polyribonucleotides were isolated as described in methods. All values
are mean $\pm$ S.D., n=4.the aqueous layer following ethyl acetate
extraction.

Aminofluorene product identification

The addition of H_2O_2 to the mixtures containing 2-AF and peroxidase
at pH 6.5 resulted in the rapid formation of a blue colour with
an absorption maxima at 385 and 615 nm which reached a maximum
in about 30 sec. The intensity of this colour was directly
proportional to the enzyme and aminofluorene concentrations.
One equivalent of H_2O_2 with respect to aminofluorene was required.
The blue colour faded after this and became light brown after
5 mins. The blue colour disappeared upon extraction with ethyl
acetate. The yellow extract was concentrated and applied to
a TLC plate. The R_f of the various products is shown in Table
III. Azofluorene was readily identified by its absorption spectra
and mass spectrometry. The UV-visible absorption spectra had
maxima in ethanol at 278 and 380 nm with shoulders at 362 and
396 nm. The mass spectrum showed a molecular ion at m/e 358.1463

with a base peak at m/e 165 as a result of cleavage of the fluorene-nitrogen bond with charge retention on the aromatic fluorene ring. Ions at m/e 181 may arise from cleavage between the nitrogens of some hydrazofluorene running with the same R_f. A similar mass spectra for azofluorene was recently reported (7). $C_{26}H_{18}N_2$ requires an m/e of 358.1470.

TABLE III. THE EFFECT OF DNA ON THE PRODUCTS FORMED BY THE OXIDATION

OF AMINOFLUORENE BY PEROXIDASE-H_2O_2

PRODUCTS	Absorbance maxima	R_f	% radioactivity		
			without DNA	with DNA	with DNA +2,3,6-(CH$_3$)phenol
"INDOANILINE"	525 nm	0.82	---	---	81
AZOFLUORENE	380 nm	0.75	27	10	4
PRODUCT I	295,330nm	0.48	9	2	2
AMINOFLUORENE	290 nm	0.4	9	12	5
PRODUCT II	290,355nm	0.31	32	19	2
PRODUCT III	355,540nm	0.2	7	10	1
"ORIGIN"	---	0	10	4	2
AQUEOUS	355 nm	---	1	38	1
INTERPHASE	---	---	5	4	2

Reaction conditions: $-^{14}$C-Aminofluorene (0.15 mM), H_2O_2 (0.15 mM), peroxidase (10 μg), 0.1 M Tris-HCl buffer pH 6.5 with and without DNA (3 mg) + 2,3,6-tri-CH$_3$-phenol (0.15 mM) were incubated for 1 minute. Ascorbate (0.2 mM) was added to stop the reaction and the mixture was extracted with ethyl acetate. The extract was concentrated and chromatographed on Silica Gel G plates with CHCl$_3$-ethyl acetate (8:2) as solvent.

Azofluorene formation was decreased if the reacting mixture contained DNA. Two other products decreased by the presence of DNA was a band (R_f 0.31) II which turned brown-green within several hours of running the plate and a band (R_f 0.48) I which turned blue-green after running the plate. Ascorbate was needed to be added to the reaction mixture before extraction to observe band I. This suggests that I unlike II is fully oxidised in the reaction mixture. Oxidation of both products by H_2O_2 and peroxidase resulted in the rapid formation of the same transient blue intermediate as was observed with aminofluorene. Product I however bound much more rapidly to DNA than Product II and unlike Product II could not be removed from the DNA by extraction with 1% sodium dodecyl sulfate. Product II showed a UV absorption spectra in an acetonitrile solution of 355 nm with a shoulder at 290 nm. Mass spectra showed a molecular

ion at m/e 360 and a small peak at m/e 180 presumably from a
fragment resulting from cleavage of a nitrogen to fluorene ring
bond. The product was similar in R_f, UV spectra and mass spectra
with 2'-amino-2,3'-difluorenylamine synthesized from azoxyfluorene
according to the literature (12). Furthermore oxidation of products
I and II by H_2O_2 and peroxidase resulted in the rapid formation
of the same transient blue colour as was observed with aminofluorene.

The pink band (R_f 0.8), formed when 2,3,6-trimethylphenol
is present in the reaction mixture, had an absorption maxima
at 286 and 510 nm. Mass spectra of the isolated product showed
a molecular ion at m/e 313 (with M+2 reduction product peak).
Fragments at m/e 298   presumably arise from the phenolic
portion of the adduct whereas peaks at m/e 180 and 165 results
from cleavage of the nitrogen to fluorene bond with charge retention
on the difluorenylamine or fluorenyl fragment respectively.
If the 2,4,6-trimethylphenol was added at 30 sec the major product
was isolated as a purple band (R_f 0.76). The absorption maxima
was at 286 and 528 nm and the isolated product showed a molecular
ion and base peak at m/e 493 with an M+2 reduction product peak.
The above fragments at m/e 180 and 165 were also observed.
Suggested structures are shown in Figure 2.

Table IV. The effect of pH on the nature of the products formed

by aminofluorene oxidation.

PRODUCTS	% radioactivity		
	pH 5	pH 6.5	pH 7.4
AZOFLUORENE	5	29	51
AMINOFLUORENE	11	9	11
PRODUCT I	11	8	6
PRODUCT II	52	36	18
POLYMER (interphase)	17	14	8
AQUEOUS	3	4	6

Reaction conditions: - as described in Table III.

In Table IV it can be seen there is a marked pH dependence with
regard to the qualitative nature of the products formed. The
reaction was stopped at 30 secs with ascorbate and extracted
with ethyl acetate. At pH 5 a 52% conversion to aminodifluorenylamine
with little azo formation was seen. At pH 7.4 however azofluorene
formed 51% of the products.

Absorption spectrum of the DNA adduct and reaction mixture

The difference in absorption spectra of bound denatured DNA was determined using identical concentrations from unbound denatured DNA as estimated by a sugar analysis. The pale green aminofluorene bound DNA had an absorption maxima at 295 with a shoulder at 350 nm. A similar amount of DNA binding was formed if the DNA was added 30 secs after starting the reaction. However little binding occurred at 5 minutes. A similar DNA adduct was formed when 2′-amino-2,3-difluorenylamine was substituted for aminofluorene in the peroxidase-H_2O_2-DNA reaction mixture. However the absorbance of this DNA adduct at 350 nm was greater than 295 nm. These results suggest that the aminofluorene bound DNA adducts include aminodifluorenylamine complexes as well as monomer aminofluorene adducts.

The effect of DNA on the initial spectral change of the reaction mixture was also investigated. In the absence of DNA a blue color (385 and 610 nm) rapidly formed, reached a maximum at 30 secs and faded. In the presence of DNA a bright blue color (390 and 670-710 nm) formed more slowly but persisted for 5-10 minutes. Similar results were obtained with aminodifluorenylamine which suggests that the blue color is a DNA complex of the imino-difluorenylamine.

Discussion

Carcinogenic aminoazo dyes were previously found to increase the latent period of linoleate peroxidation and that DAB was a more effective antioxidant than MAB (13). Furthermore, as autoxidation of the linoleic acid proceeded, N-demethylation of DAB and MAB occurred. Demethylation of DAB also occurred in vitro when DAB is dissolved in cottonseed oil and mixed with ground brown rice (14). Our results clearly indicate that a linoleic acid hydroperoxide-hematin system readily N-demethylates DAB to MAB and MAB to AB. Previously, it was found that in this system, HCHO formation by N-demethylation of DAB was faster than that obtained with MAB (15). Similar results are now reported during the H_2O_2-peroxidase catalyzed oxidation of DAB and MAB. Peroxidase and H_2O_2 have previously been reported to catalyze the N-dealkylation of other arylamines (16, 17).

When DAB is given to uninduced rats, glutathione in the liver plays a major role in its detoxification as GSH conjugates form the major biliary metabolites. GSH depletion in vivo markedly decreased the biliary excretion. The detoxification of DAB is believed to proceed by N-demethylation to MAB which undergoes N-methyl oxidation to an N-methylol or methimine which is required to be conjugated with GSH to form the adduct GS-CH_2-AB if the MAB N-methyloxidation is to proceed at a rapid rate in vivo. Thus biliary AB levels also fall with GSH depletion indicating that the presence of AB in bile may be artifacts due to the decomposition of GS-CH_2-AB and 4′sulphonyloxy-GS-CH_2-AB (18). The GSH adducts were first discovered on the addition of GSH to a rat liver homogenate system catalyzing the N-demethylation of 3-methyl-DAB which resulted in the formation of a water soluble labile dye (19). This was later characterized as GS-CH$_2$-AB and was formed in vitro by incubating MAB, NADPH, NADH and GSH with rat liver microsomes. Its formation was inhibited by a cytochrome P450 inhibitor which suggests that it was formed during a cytochrome P450 catalyzed N-demethylation (10). Other investigators have confirmed the involvement of cytochrome P450 isoenzymes in DAB metabolism in the rat (Levine and Lu, 1982). Our results show that lipid peroxides or hydrogen peroxide, in the presence of a heme catalyst or peroxidase, respectively readily oxidize MAB to GS-CH$_2$-AB in the presence of GSH in nearly stoichiometric amounts. It is therefore unlikely that the depression of DAB metabolism by the in vivo depletion of hepatic glutathione is due to lipid peroxidation (20). It would however be interesting to ascertain whether Kupffer cells play a role in the detoxification of DAB by the liver as these cells have very high peroxidase activity in their endoplasmic reticulum and line the bile ducts (21). It remains to be seen whether cytochrome P450 is responsible in vivo for the detoxification by the liver.

Another consequence of these findings is that the same adduct can be formed by a free radical mediated pathway from MAB following a one electron oxidation by peroxides as that formed from methylol or methimine by a two electron oxidation catalyzed by cytochrome P450. Clearly identification of the GSH adducts of carcinogens in vivo may not distinguish both metabolic activation systems. It is also still not clear whether cytochrome P450 and peroxidases form common intermediates during N-demethylation reactions (22-24).

Deacetylated aminofluorene: DNA adducts form most of the DNA adducts formed in vivo following ^{14}C-acetylaminofluorene administration (25). Acetylaminofluorene is not readily oxidized by peroxidases or prostaglandin synthetase. However, mixed function oxidase catalyzes the formation of N-hydroxyacetylaminofluorene which is an effective substrate for a one electron catalyzed oxidation activation. Dismutation of the nitroxy radicals to N-acetoxy-AAF would however result in acetylated DNA adducts. The lack of acetylated DNA adduct formation in nonhepatic target tissues appears therefore to argue against a free radical mediated carcinogenesis (27). However, we have recently shown that a one electron oxidation activation mechanism for acetylaminofluorene exists which should result in the formation of deacetylated aminofluorene: DNA adducts (28). The mechanism involves the initial N-deacetylation by a microsomal deacetylase to aminofluorene. All target tissues contain deacetylase but the target organ Zymbal gland contains particularly high levels of deacetylase activity (29).

We previously compared the properties of the reactive species involved in DNA binding by N-OH-aminofluorene, N-acetoxy-acetyl-aminofluorene and the aminofluorene products formed by a peroxidase catalyzed oxidation (28). The marked differences in reactivity suggested that different species were involved and that nitrenium ions were not responsible for the peroxidase catalyzed activation. The identity of the products formed following a peroxidase catalyzed oxidation is still not clear. Other investigators have shown the formation of nitrofluorene and azofluorene but most of the product was polymeric in nature (7). The results presented here however show that the principle product first formed is 2-aminodifluorenylamine.

The following reaction sequence is suggested and outlined in Fig. 1. Aminofluorene is oxidized initially to cation radicals which undergo "head to tail" dimerization and further oxidation to produce 2-iminodifluorenylamine which reacts with itself to form polymers. This dimer is also formed during electrochemical oxidation (30). At a neutral pH, the formation of azofluorene suggests that "head to head" dimerization occurs to form hydrazo-fluorene which is readily oxidized to azofluorene. The lack of azofluorene formation at pH 5 may be due to the acid lability of hydrazofluorene (31) or may reflect the unlikelihood of N-N-coupling if the cation radicals at pH 5 are charged as a result of protonation (32).

The DNA binding was readily prevented by the biological hydrogen donors NADH, GSH and ascorbate and by phenolic antioxidants. The biological hydrogen donors apparently act by reducing the aminofluorene oxidation products responsible. However, in the case of 2,3,6-trimethylphenol, the phenol reacted with the amino-fluorene cation radical to form an adduct radical which would yield the "indoaniline derivative" on further oxidation. The proposed structure of this adduct as supported by mass spectrometry is shown in Figure 2. The other adduct isolated was presumably formed from 2-iminodifluorenylamine. Recently other investigators using NMR spectroscopy have confirmed similar structures for aminofluorene adducts with butylated hydroxyanisole and xylenol formed with a peroxidase- H_2O_2 reaction mixture (7).

The nature of the DNA adduct remains to be determined. However the spectrum of the isolated DNA is similar to that of the DNA adduct formed when 2-aminodifluorenylamine is oxidized by a peroxidase-H_2O_2 reaction mixture. Furthermore a similar DNA adduct is formed when DNA is added at a time when the blue imino derivative is maximal. Furthermore in the presence of DNA much less extractable azofluorene, aminodifluorenylamine or polymer was formed suggesting that DNA reacts with the amino-fluorene cation radical and 2-iminodifluorenylamine.

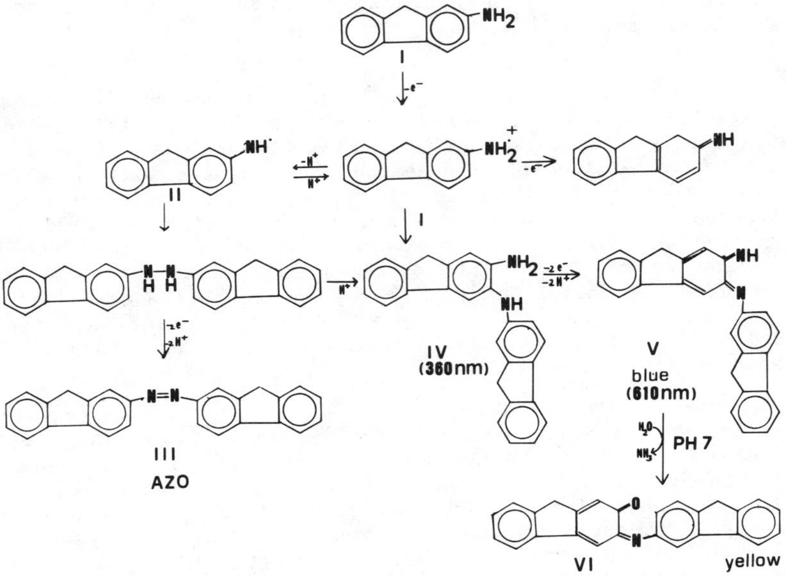

Figure 1.   A reaction scheme for peroxidase catalysed aminofluorene oxidation.

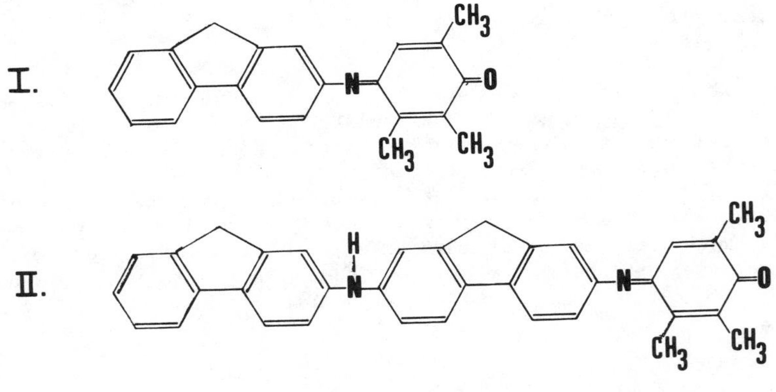

Figure 2.   Proposed structures of aminofluorene / 2,3,6-$(CH_3)_3$-
phenolic adducts   (quinonoid forms).

Literature Cited

1. Miller, E.C. and Miller, J.A. Cancer (1981) 47, 2327-2345.
2. Kadlubar, F.F., Miller, J.A. and Miller, E.C. Cancer Res. (1977), 37, 805-814.
3. Marnett, L.J., and Eling, T.E. In Reviews in Biochemical Toxicology (Hodgson, E., Bend, J.R., and Philpot, R.M., eds.) (1983) Vol. 5. pp. 135-172, Elsevier Biomedical, New York.
4. O'Brien, P.J. in Free Radicals in Biology, W. Pryor, W.E. Academic Press, N.Y. (1984). Vol. VI, 289-322.
5. Eling, T.E., Boyd, J.A., Reed, G.A., Mason, R.P. and Siwarajah, K. Drug Metab. Rev. (1983), 14, 1023-1053.
6. Meunier, M. and Chauveau, J. Int. J. Cancer (1970), 6, 463-469.
7. Boyd, J.A., Harvan, D.J. and Eling, T.E. J. Biol. Chem. (1983) 258, 8246-8254.
8. Ashwell, G. Methods in Enzymology (1957), 3, 73-105.
9. Werringloer, J. Methods in Enzymology, (1978) 52, 297.
10. Ketterer, B., Srai, S.K.S., Waynforth, B., Tullis, D.L., Evans, F.E. and Kadlubar, F.F. Chem. Biol. Interacns. (1982), 38, 287-302.
11. Habeeb, A.F.S.A. Methods in Enzymology (1976), 25, 457.
12. Cislak, F.E., Eastman, I.M. and Senior, J.K. J. Amer. Chem. Soc. (1927), 49, 2318.
13. Rusch, H.P. and Miller, J.A. Proc. Soc. Exp. Biol. and Med. (1948), 68, 140-143.
14. Kensler, C.J., Magill, J.W. and Sugihara, K. Cancer Res (1947), 7, 95-100.
15. O'Brien, P.J. In "Lipid Peroxides in Biology and Medicine", (1982). Kazi, K., Ed., Academic Press, N.Y. pp. 317-338.
16. Gillette, J.R., Dingall, J.V. and Brodie, B.B. Nature (London), (1958), 181, 891-899.
17. Griffin, B.W. and Ting, P.L. Biochem. (1978), 17, 2206-2212.
18. Coles, B., Srai, S.K.S., Waynforth, H.B. and Ketterer, B. Chem.-Biol. Interacns. (1983), 47, 307-323.
19. Mueller, G.C. and Miller, J.A. J. Biol. Chem. (1953), 202, 579-586.
20. Levine, W.G. Life Sciences (1982), 31, 779-784.
21. Levine, W. and Lu, A.Y.H. Drug Metab. Dispos. (1982), 10, 102.
22. Angermuller, S. and Fahimi, H.D. Histochem (1981), 71, 33-44.
23. O'Brien, P.J. Pharmacol. Therap. (1978), 2A, 517-537.
24. Kedderis, G.L. and Hollenberg, P.F. J. Biol. Chem. (1953), 258, 8129-8138.
25. Beland, F.A., Allaben, W.T. and Evans, F.E. Cancer Res. (1980) 40, 834-840.
26. Floyd, R.A. In "Free Radicals in Biology", (W. Pyror, ed.) Academic Press, New York, 1980, Vol. IV, p.187-198..
27. Allaben, W.T., Weiss, C.C., Fullerton, N.F. and Beland, F.A. (1983), Carcinogenesis, 1983, 4, 1067-1074.
28. Marshall, W. and O'Brien, P.J. In "Icosanoids and Cancer" Ed. Thaler, D.H., Raven Press, New York (In press).

29. Irving, C.C. (1979) In "Carcinogenesis: Identification and
    Mechanisms of Action". (A.C. Griffin and C.R. Shaw, eds),
    pp. 211–227, Raven Press, New York.
30. Yasukouchi, K., Taniguchi, I., Yamaguchi, H., Miyaguchi,
    K. and Hone, K. Bull. Chem. Soc. Japan (1979), 52, 3208–3212.
31. Fletcher, T.L. and Nankung, M.J. J. Org. Chem (1970) 35,
    4231.
32. Boyd, J.A. and Eling, T.E. Submitted for publication.

RECEIVED March 15, 1985

Antioxidants and Malonaldehyde in Cancer

RAYMOND J. SHAMBERGER

Department of Biochemistry, Cleveland Clinic Foundation, Cleveland, OH 44106

Selenium, vitamin C, vitamin E, BHT (butylated hydroxytoluene), BHA (butylated hydroxyanisole) and several compounds with antioxidant properties have been shown to inhibit chemically induced carcinogenesis and mutagenesis. Of the natural antioxidants selenium has been shown to be the most effective against chemically induced carcinogenesis in a large number of animal test systems. In two epidemiological studies selenium in blood bank and forage crop selenium has been inversely correlated with human cancer mortality. Large amounts of vitamins E and C also inhibit chemically induced carcinogenesis in some test systems. Antioxidants may interfere with the formation of a product of peroxidative fat metabolism, malonaldehyde which has been shown to be mutagenic and carcinogenic. In addition, antioxidants may also reduce the interaction of DNA with mutagens and carcinogens from pyrolyzed food. The objective of this report is to summarize some of the evidence relating antoxidants, dietary fat, malonaldehyde and pyrolyzed food.

SELENIUM

Even though selenium itself is not an antioxidant, selenium is an important cofactor for the enzyme, glutathione peroxidase, which has been shown to break down hydrogen peroxide (1) as well as organic hydroperoxides (2). The reactions may well be important in removing peroxides which might interact with and damage DNA.

$$2GSH + H_2O_2 \; \rightarrow \; GSSG + 2H_2O \qquad (1)$$

$$2GSH + ROOH \; \rightarrow \; GSSG + ROH \qquad (2)$$

0097–6156/85/0277–0111$06.00/0

Selenium has been shown to be an unusually important dietary chemopreventative.   In general, the dietary chemopreventative effects have been demonstrated between 0.5 and 1.0 ppm. However, most animals have a dietary requirement of 0.1 to 0.2 ppm of selenium.   The dietary requirement seems to be lower than the amount needed for the optimal chemopreventative effect and therefore may not be related to a minimal nutritional requirement. On the other hand, one could also postulate that cancer is a nutritionally related disease and that the real requirement is around 0.5 ppm.

In five of six nondietary tumor-promotion experiments, sodium selenide significantly reduced the number of mice with tumors induced by 7,12-dimethyl-benzanthracene (DMBA)-croton oil (1).   In these experiments, sodium selenide was applied concomitantly along with croton oil to female Swiss albino mice initiated with DMBA. Riley has also observed a reduction in DMBA-phorbol ester carcinogenesis by sodium selenide (2).   The effect of selenium-deficient and selenium-adequate diets on DMBA-croton oil and benzopyrene skin carcinogenesis has also been studied. Supplemental dietary selenium inhibited both types of carcinogenesis.

Dietary selenium has also reduced carcinogen induced liver carcinogenesis. Clayton and Baumann have reported that the inclusion of 5 ppm of dietary selenium reduced the incidence of liver tumors in rats induced by 3-methyl-4-dimethylaminoazobenzene (DAB) (3).   Similar results were observed by Griffin and Jacobs (4). Dzhioev has observed a marked reduction of liver tumors induced by diethylnitrosamine (DEN) in the animals fed selenium diets (5). Marked reduction of liver tumors induced by acetyaminoflourene have been observed in rats fed dietary selenium (6) or given selenium in the drinking water (7).   Dietary selenium has also been shown to reduce the development of L-azaserine-induced preneoplastic abnormal acinar cell modules in male Wistar rats (8), the formation of aflatoxin B_1 induced gamma-glutamyltransferase (GGTP) positive foci in rat liver (9) and the formation of GGTP positive foci induced by DEN (10).

Even though dietary selenium has an effect on skin and liver carcinogenesis, even greater dietary effects have been observed on carcinogen and virally induced breast cancer and carcinogen-induced colon cancer in animals.   It may be of interest that breast and colon cancer have been shown to be enhanced by dietary fat in both man and animals. Perhaps this enhancement is due to an increase of fat peroxidation which can be reduced by antioxidants.   Schrauzer and Ishmael have fed 2 ppm of selenium in the form of SeO_2 in the drinking water for 15 months to virgin C3H female mice which are especially susceptible to virally induced spontaneous mammary tumors induced by the Bittner milk virus (11).   The incidence of spontaneous mammary tumors was 82% in the untreated controls and 10% in the selenium treated mice.   Thompson and Tagliaferro have observed that selenium supplemented diets have reduced the numbers of DMBA-induced mammary tumors per rat (12).   The fact that selenium-supplemented diets have reduced both virally and chemically induced cancer in animals indicates that both the virally and chemically induced carcinogenesis may have the same mechanism of induction.   Ip has studied the effect of selenium supplementation in the

initiation and promotion phase of DMBA-induced mammary carcinogenesis in rats fed a high-fat diet (13). In this experiment, rats
were fed 5 ppm of sodium selenite for various periods of time before and after treatment with DMBA. From this experiment the following conclusions were made: (1) both the initiation and promotion
phase of carcinogenesis can be inhibited by selenium; (2) in order
to achieve maximal inhibition of tumorigenesis, a continuous intake
of selenium is necessary; (3) the inhibitory effect of selenium in
the early promotion phase is probably reversible; (4) the usefulness of selenium is decreased when it is given long after carcinogenic injury.

Two types of epidemiological relationships have been found in
two different populations. Both relationships were inverse to selenium bioavailability and paralleled the results from animal studies. In one type of study, selenium bioavailability has been inversely related to human cancer mortality in American cities and
states (14-15). Schrauzer et.al. correlated the age-adjusted mortality from cancer at 17 major body sites with the apparent dietary
selenium intakes estimated from food consumption data in 27 countries (16). Significant inverse correlations were observed for
cancers of the large intestine, rectum, prostate, breast, ovary,
lung, and leukemia. In addition, weaker inverse associations were
found for cancers of the pancreas, skin, and bladder.

Vitamin E

Vitamin E may prevent mouse skin tumorigenesis through its known
antioxidant effect (1). Rats fed a diet containing large amounts
of vitamin E had fewer mammary tumors induced by DMBA than did the
controls (17). Shklar has observed that Syrian golden hamsters
given oral vitamin E had fewer smaller buccal pouch cancers induced
by DMBA (18). Konings and Trieling have observed an enhanced inhibition of [^{3}H] thymidine incorporation into the DNA of vitamin E-
depleted lymphosarcoma cells (19). Weisburger et.al. have observed
a greater incidence of stomach cancer in populations consuming low
levels of vitamin E and other selected micronutrients.

Vitamin C

Vitamin C may prevent tumorigenesis through its antioxidant action.
Vitamin C is water soluble and complements the antioxidant action
of vitamin E which is lipid soluble. When vitamin C was applied
concomitantly with croton oil to mouse skin previously treated with
DMBA, the total number of mouse skin papillomas was reduced (20).
Similarly, Slaga and Bracken observed a decrease in the number of
skin tumors induced by DMBA-phorbol carcinogenesis in mice treated
with vitamin C (21). Tumor inhibition by ascorbic acid has also
been observed on toad skin treated with DMBA (22). Schlegel et.
al. have observed that vitamin C reduces uroepithelial carcinoma in
mice and also suggested a similar mechanism in humans (23). The
tryptophan metabolite 3-hydroxyanthranilic acid (3-HOA) is thought
to be stabilized by ascorbic acid, thereby preventing carcinogenicity when 3-HOA is implanted in the bladder. Vitamin C is also
known to prevent tumorigenesis through its ability to block the in

vitro formation of N-nitroso compounds by the reaction between nitrous acid and oxytetracycline, morpholine, piperazine, N-methyl-
aniline, methylurea, and dimethylamine. The amount of blocking depends on the compounds nitrosated and the experimental conditions
(24). The species formed from nitrous acid responsible for the
oxidation of ascorbic acid is the same species affecting nitrosation of secondary amines (25). Between pH 1.5 and 5.0, the nitrosation of secondary amines in the presence of ascorbic acid and the
absence of oxygen can be summarized by the following two competi-
tive parallel second-order reactions:

$$\text{Amine} + N_2O_3 \quad k_1 \rightarrow \quad \text{nitrosamine} + NO_2^- + H^+ \qquad (3)$$

$$\text{Ascorbate} + N_2O_3 \quad k_2 \rightarrow \quad \text{dehydroascorbate} + 2NO + 2H_2O \qquad (4)$$

If $k_2 \gg k_1$, then reaction (4) is mostly complete before (3)
starts. Large doses of vitamin C have been observed to protect
rats from liver tumors induced by aminopyrine and sodium nitrite
(26). This inhibition is thought to result, in part, from block-
age of in vivo nitrosation, which forms dimethylnitrosamine.
There have been several epidemiological and several case reports inversely relating ascorbic acid intake from food to human
cancer mortality. These studies are interesting, but may be confounded with the fact that the same ascorbic acid containing foods,
namely fruits and vegetables, also contain large amounts of vitamin
A and fiber. Both vitamin A and fiber have been inversely related
to human cancer mortality and have been shown to inhibit several
types of chemically-induced carcinogenesis in animals. Therefore,
the possible anticancer effect of ascorbic acid may be due to other
factors.

BHA and BHT

Even though BHA (butylated hydroxyanisole) and BHT (butylated hydroxytoluene) are not naturally occurring antioxidants, various
amounts of these compounds are added to food as food preservatives
in order to reduce oxidative rancidity. Both BHA and BHT are included in the FDA list of substances generally accepted as safe
(GRAS) and many acute and chronic tests have been done. Based on
the evidence from these studies, the FDA in 1977 recommended that
BHT be removed from the GRAS list and proposed interim studies.
BHA has been demonstrated to be an important inhibitor of carcinogenesis and has been extensively studied for its ability to inhibit carcinogen-induced neoplasia. Table I lists several experiments in which BHA was administered before or during carcinogen
exposure (27).

Table I. **Inhibition of Carcinogen-Induced Neoplasia by BHA**

Carcinogen inhibited	Species	Site of Neoplasm
Benzo(a)pyrene	Mouse	Lung
Benzo(a)pyrene	Mouse	Forestomach
Benzo(a)pyrene-7,8-dehydrodiol	Mouse	Forestomach, lung and lymphoid tissue
7,12-Dimethylbenz(a)anthracene	Mouse	Lung
7,12-Dimethylbenz(a)anthracene	Mouse	Forestomach
7,12-Dimethylbenz(a)anthracene	Mouse	Skin
7,12-Dimethylbenz(a)anthracene	Rat	Breast
7-Hydroxymethyl-12-methyl-benz(a)anthracene	Mouse	Lung
Dibenz(a)anthracene	Mouse	Lung
Nitrosodiethylamine	Mouse	Lung
4-Nitroquinoline-N-oxide	Mouse	Lung
Uracil mustard	Mouse	Lung
Urethan	Mouse	Lung
Methylazoxymethanol acetate	Mouse	Large intestine
trans-5-Amino-3[2-(5-nitro-2-furyl)vinyl]-1,2,4-oxadiazole	Mouse	Forestomach, lung and lymphoid tissue

It is believed that BHA inhibits chemically induced carcinogenesis by producing a coordinated enzyme response that may be interpreted as causing a greater rate of detoxification (28). In addition, increased glutathione s-transferase and glutathione levels have been observed in mice that have been fed BHA for 1-2 weeks in carcinogen inhibition experiments (29). Glutathione s-transferase is known to be an important enzyme for detoxifying chemical carcinogens (28-29). The anticarcinogenicity of BHA and BHT in many experiments seems to depend on the relationship of the time of administration of the carcinogen and BHA or BHT administration. If BHT was given before carcinogen administration, then inhibition of carcinogenesis occurs. However, if BHT was given after the carcinogen, then enhancement of carcinogenesis occurs. Three groups of A/J mice were injected with urethan, 3-methylcholanthrene, or nitrosodimethylamine and then repeated doses of BHT. With all three carcinogens BHT treatment after carcinogen treatment significantly increased the numbers of lung tumors (30).

Malonaldehyde

Malonaldehyde, a three-carbon dialdehyde ($OHC-CH_2-CHO$), is produced during lipid peroxidation by the oxidative decomposition of arachidonic and other unsaturated fatty acids. Malonaldehyde is present in a number of food products and its concentration is increased by irradiation of cellular amino acids, carbohydrates, deoxyribose, and DNA. Recent surveys (31-32) have confirmed the presence of malonaldehyde in supermarket samples of meat, poultry, and fish,

which constitute the main sources of malonaldehyde in the North
American diet. Fruits and vegetables, in general, do not contain
detectable amounts of malonaldehyde. There is also evidence that
malonaldehyde is produced in vivo when there is an inadequate intake of vitamine E (33), which serves as a lipid antioxidant.
Evidence has been reported on the formation of malonaldehyde in
vivo during prostaglandin synthesis. Malonaldehyde is also formed
on cellular exposure to ozone, carbon tetrachloride, ethanol and
hydrocarbon compounds. Malonaldehyde (34-36) and the sodium form
(37-38) have been shown to be mutagenic in the Salmonella test system, in L 5178 lymphoma cells (39), in rat skin fibroblasts (40),
Drosophilia (41), and the Muller-5 sex-linked recessive lethal mutation system (41). Malonaldehyde also has some weak carcinogenic
activity under some circumstances. Shamberger et. al. have found
malonaldehyde to be an initiator in a malonaldehyde-croton oil test
system (42). However, Fischer et. al. have found the sodium form
of malonaldehyde to have neither initiating nor promoting activity
(43). The sodium form of malonaldehyde also has been shown to increase the number of liver lesions in mice (44). Whether or not
malonaldehyde is an important factor in the cancer process is not
known. However, malonaldehyde is known to cross-link both protein
and DNA. In general, unsaturated fat has more tumor-enhancing properties in many systems. However, there is no certain mechanism by
which the breakdown of cell membrane unsaturated fatty acids might
damage genetic material. In humans, about 50-60% of the ingested
malonaldehyde from meat is excreted in the urine (45). It is not
known how the remainder of the malonaldehyde is metabolized. The
relative importance of the mutagenicity of malonaldehyde in human
food is unknown. Certainly pyrolyzed food contains complete carcinogens such as benzopyrene and mutagenic substances such as tryptophan pyrolysates (Trp-P-1 and Trp-P-2), glutamic acid pyrolysates
(Glu-P-1 and Glu-P-2), lysine pyrolysate (Lys-P-1), phenylalanine
pyrolysate (Phe-P-1), and protein pyrolysates from broiled sardines
(IQ and MeIQ) and from broiled beef (MeIQx). It is likely that
antioxidants such as selenium and vitamins C and E also reduce the
carcinogenic and mutagenic effect of these substances formed from
pyrolyzed food in the same way that these antioxidants reduce the
mutagenicity of malonaldehyde (46). Certainly more research is
needed in this area.

Literature Cited

1. Shamberger, R.J., J. Nat. Cancer Inst. 1970, 44, 931-936.
2. Riley, J.F., Experientia 1968, 15, 1237-1238.
3. Clayton, C.C. and Baumann, C.A., Cancer Res. 1949, 9, 575-582.
4. Griffin, A.C. and Jacobs, M.M., Cancer Lett. 1977, 3, 177-181.
5. Dzhoiev, F.D., In Kantserog N-Nitrozosoedin: Deistvie, Obraz.,
   Mater Simp., 3rd Tallinn, USSR, 1978; pp 51-53.
6. Harr, J.R., Exon, J.H., Weswig, P.H., and Whanger, P.D. Clin.
   Toxicol. 1973, 8, 487-495.
7. Marshall, M.V., Arnott, M.S., Jacobs, M.M., and Griffin, A.C.,
   Cancer Lett. 1979, 7, 331-338.
8. O'Conner, T.P., Youngman, L.D., and Campbell, T.C., Fed. Proc.
   1983, 42, 670.

9. Baldwin, S., Parker, R.S., and Misslbeck., Fed. Proc. 1983, 42, 1312.
10. LeBoeuf, R.A., Laishes, B.A., and Hoekstra, W.G., Fed. Proc. 1983, 42, 669.
11. Schrauzer, G.N., and Ishmael, D., Ann. Clin. Lab. Sci. 1974, 4, 411-467.
12. Thompson, H.J., and Tagliaferro, A.R., Fed. Proc. 1980, 39, 1117.
13. Ip, C., Cancer Res. 1981, 41, 4386-4390.
14. Shamberger, R.J. and Willis, C.E. CRC Crit. Rev. Clin. Lab. Sci. 1971, 2, 211-221.
15. Shamberger, R.J., Tytko, S.A., and Willis, C.E., Arch. Environ. Health 1976, 31, 231-235.
16. Schrauzer, G.N., White, D.A., and Schneider, C.J., Bioinorg. Chem. 1977, 7, 23-24.
17. Ip, C., Carcinogenesis 1982, 3, 1453-1456.
18. Shklar, G.J., Natl. Cancer Inst. 1982, 68, 791-797.
19. Konings, A.W.T. and Trieling, W.B., Int. J. Radiat. Biol. 1977, 31, 397-400.
20. Shamberger, R.J., J. Natl. Cancer Inst. 1972, 48, 1491-1497.
21. Slaga, T.J. and Bracken, W.M., Cancer Res. 1977, 37, 1631-1635.
22. Sadek, I.A. and Abdelmegid, N., Oncology 1982, 39, 399-400.
23. Schlegel, J.U., Pipkin, G.E., Nishumura, R., and Schultz, G.N., Trans. Am. Assoc. Genitourinary Surg. 1969, 61, 85-89.
24. Mirvish, S.S., Wallace, L., Eagen, M. and Shubik, P., Science 1972, 177, 65-68.
25. Archer, M.C., Tannenbaum, S.R., Tan, T., and Weisman, M., J. Natl. Cancer Inst. 1975, 54, 1203-1205.
26. Chan, W.C. and Fong, Y.Y., Int. J. Cancer 1970, 20, 268-270.
27. Wattenberg, L.W. "In Environmental Carcinogenesis", Emmelot, P. and Kriek, E. Elsevier/North Holland Biomedical Press, Amsterdam, 1979, pp. 241-263.
28. Wattenberg, L.W., "In Cancer: Achievements, Challenges, and Prospects for the 1980's", Burchenol, J.H. and Oettgen Eds. Vol 1. Grune and Stratton, New York, 1981, pp. 517-539.
29. Benson, S.M., Cha, Y.N., Bueding, E., Heine, H.S., and Talalay, P., Cancer Res. 1979, 39, 2971-2977.
30. National Cancer Institute. Technical Report Series number 150. NIH Publ. No. 79-1706, Bethesda, Maryland: Carcinogenesis Testing Program, National Cancer Institute.
31. Shamberger, R.J., Shamberger, B.A., and Willis, C.E., J. Nutr. 1977, 107, 1404-1409.
32. Siu, G.M., and Draper, H.H., J. Food Sci. 1978, 43, 1147-1149.
33. Trostler, N., Brady, P.S., Romsos, D.R., and Leveille, G.A., J. Nutr. 1979, 109, 345-352.
34. Mukai, F.H. and Goldstein, B.D., Science, 1976, 191, 868-869.
35. Muchielli, A., 1975, Thesis, Univ. of Lille, CNRS, AO 11792.
36. Lawrence, M.J. and Tuttle, M.R., Cancer Res. 1980, 40, 276-282.
37. Marnett, L.J. and Tuttle, M.A., Cancer Res. 1980, 40, 276-282.
38. Basu, A.K. and Marnett, L.J., Carcinogenesis, 1983, 4, 331-334.
39. Yau, T.M., Mech Aging Dev., 1979, 11, 137-144.
40. Bird, R.P. and Draper, H.H., J. Toxicol. Environ. Hlth, 1980, 6, 811-823.

41. Szabad, J., Soos, I., Polgar, G., Heijja, G., Mutation Research
    1983, 113, 117-133.
42. Shamberger, R.J., Andreone, T.L., and Willis, C.E., J. Nat.
    Cancer Inst. 1974, 53, 1771-1773.
43. Fischer, S.M., Cancer Letters, 1983, 19, 61-66.
44. Bird, R.P., Draper, H.H., and Valli, V.E.O., J. Toxicol. and
    Environ. Hlth, 1982, 10, 897-905.
45. Jacobson, E.A., Newmark, H.L., Bird, R.P., and Bruce, W.R.,
    Nutr. Rep. Int., 1983, 28, 509-517.
46. Shamberger, R.J., Corlett, C.L., Beaman, K.D. and Kasten, B.L.,
    Mutat. Res. 1979, 66, 349-356.

RECEIVED September 5, 1984

Influence of Types and Levels of Dietary Fat on Colon Cancer

BANDARU S. REDDY

Division of Nutrition and Endocrinology, Naylor Dana Institute for Disease Prevention, American Health Foundation, Valhalla, NY 10595

Epidemiologic studies indicate that diets high in total fat and saturated fat and low in certain fibers are associated with an increased risk for colon cancer. In addition, certain dietary fibers and cruciferous vegetables have been associated with a reduced risk in several populations consuming the diets high in total fat. In animal models, high dietary fat (corn oil, safflower oil, beef fat and lard) increased the development of chemically-induced colon tumors; at high dietary fat levels, the types of fat (corn oil, safflower oil, lard and beef tallow) had no effect. However, diets high in saturated and monounsaturated fats of vegetable origin (coconut oil and olive oil) induced fewer colon tumors than the diets high in polyunsaturated fats (corn oil and safflower oil). Thus, the fatty acid composition is one of the important factors in colon tumor promotion. The effect of dietary fat in colon cancer has been shown to be primarily during the post-initiation phase of carcinogenesis.

Colon cancer is one of the most common tumors observed in the western population, exhibiting more than a tenfold excess when compared to the rural populations in Africa, Asia and South America. (1-3). During the past several years, epidemiologic studies have revealed that our lifestyles, including dietary and nutritional practices, are important variables. These studies also suggested that not only the diets particularly high in total fat and low in certain dietary fibers, vegetables, and micronutrients are generally associated with an increased incidence of colon cancer in man, but dietary fat may be a risk factor in the absence of factors that are protective, such as use of high fibrous foods and fiber (4-11). However, the conduct and interpretation of epidemiologic studies is complicated by inherent problems in testing the dietary practices for their reliability, validity and sensitivity to reveal narrow but biologically significant differences, and to achieve some degree of dose stratification. When another line of evidence based on experimental studies,

which have consistently supported human epidemiologic studies
supports that diet plays an important role in the etiology of colon
cancer, the relationship between diet and colon cancer deserves
immediate attention (7).

Nutritional Epidemiologic Studies

Cancer of the colon has been the subject of several epidemiologic
reviews.(2,3,12).   The variability in colon cancer incidence between countries has directed research toward specific environmental
dietary factors that are characteristic of high-risk population.
While some of these differences may be due to genetic factors or
local environmental factors, further evidence for the role of dietary environmental factors in colon cancer has been provided by
migrant studies which demonstrate a higher colon cancer incidence
rate in the first and second generation Japanese immigrants to the
United States and in Polish immigrants to Australia than in Japanese
(13).   Furthermore, time-trend in Japan showing that colon cancer
seems to be increasing is consistent with the increasing westernization of the Japanese diet (14).   These studies led several investigators to accept diet as a major etiologic factor in colon cancer.
        Wynder and Shigematsu (15) were the first to suggest that nut-
ritional factors in general and specifically differences in fat intake may be responsible for the international variation in colon
cancer incidence. Subsequent descriptive epidemiologic studies have
found a strong positive association between colon cancer mortality
or incidence in different countries and per capita availability in
national diets of total fat (4,16) and of animal fat, estimated from
food balance sheets.   Such international correlations may be
supportive of a hypothesis, but they should be interpreted with caution because the dietary data were based not on actual intake information but on food disappearance data.
        The nutritional epidemiologic studies turned to case-control
comparisons and prospective studies in order to accurately define
the etiologic factors. Wynder et al. (9) conducted a large-scale
retrospective study on colon cancer patients in Japan, which
suggested a correlation between the westernization of the Japanese
diet and dietary fat and colon cancer. A recent case-control study
in Athens, Greece, demonstrated a positive association between colon
cancer and consumption of meat, but not olive oil (17).   In another
study, no association was found within countries of regional or
ethnic colon cancer rates in relation to meat (18).   These conflicting results could be explained on the basis that several of these
studies neglected to take into consideration the other confounding
factors such as consumption of cruciferous vegetables, dietary fiber
and other food items that have been shown to reduce the risk of
colon cancer. Failure to find consistent strong relationships does
not necessarily mediate against a dietary etiology of colon cancer,
however, because certain findings may have arisen, at least in part,
from methodological limitation of these studies. Finally, some of
these studies may have been hampered by the possibility that diets
within communities have been too uniform to permit associations between diet and disease to be detected (19).

A case-control study in Canada indicated an elevated risk for those with an increased intake of calories, total fat, and saturated fat (20,21). This study estimated levels of fat consumption by combining information from diet histories with information on the fat content of foods. A recent case-control study in Utah Mormons indicated a positive association between dietary fat and colon cancer (10).

On the other hand, in several populations consuming the diets high in total fat, dietary fiber acts as a protective factor for colon cancer risk. Recent studies comparing rural and urban populations in Finland, Denmark and Sweden and urban populations in New York indicated that one of the factors contributing to the low risk of colon cancer in rural Scandinavia appears to be high-dietary fiber intake, mainly whole-grain cereals, although all populations are on a high-fat diet (3,22-24). A strong negative association was reported between regional colon cancer mortality within the United Kingdom and consumption of fiber foods containing high amount of pentose (25).

The bulk of nutritional epidemiologic evidence suggests that diets high in total fat and low in fiber are associated with an increased risk of colon cancer in man. In several populations consuming a high amount of total fat, certain dietary fibers and cruciferous vegetables act as protective factors. Moreover, laboratory animal studies discussed elsewhere have clearly demonstrated that high-fat intake promotes the development of colon cancer. Concurrence between the nutritional epidemiologic and laboratory evidence offered the strength to the concept that diet is a major etiologic factor in colon cancer.

Mechanisms of dietary fat in colon cancer

Food contains a large number of inhibitors of carcinogenesis, including fibers, phenols, indoles, aromatic isothiocyanates, plant sterols, selenium salts, ascorbic acid, tocopherols and carotenes (26). These compounds have been shown to inhibit neoplasms in animal models (26,27). Since the principal sources of these compounds in the diet are plant constituents, the type and quantity of the plant material in the diet will be of great importance in determining the activity of the protective system. Thus, the humans consuming relatively large amounts of vegetables, both cruciferous and non-cruciferous type, and fruits would have greater defenses against carcinogens than do individuals consuming a lesser amount of these foods.

Currently, much of our knowledge on the mechanism of dietary fat on colon carcinogenesis is based on experiments conducted in humans (metabolic epidemiology) and animal models (27). The major significance of these studies is that the primary effect of dietary fat appears to be during the promotional phase of carcinogenesis rather than during initiation phase (28). The amount of dietary fat modulates the concentration of intestinal bile acids as well as the metabolic activity of gut microflora, which, in turn, metabolize these sterols and other substances into tumorigenic compounds in the colon (29,30,31). These studies have demonstrated that high fat diets increase the excretion of bile acids into the gut. These bile

acids have been shown to act as colon tumor promoters but do not
have the properties of genotoxic carcinogens (31). This is important since current views on properties of promoters note that the
effect of such agents is highly dependent on dose and on length of
exposure, and thus provides an opportunity of reducing the risk of
colon cancer development by lowering the concentration of bile acids
by dietary means.

Metabolic (Biochemical) Epidemiologic Studies on Dietary Fat

The concept that dietary fat and certain fibers distinct from chemical contaminants of diet and from other environmental and genetic
factors are important determinants of colon cancer risk is reinforced by biochemical epidemiologic studies in humans and laboratory
animal studies. A key insight gained from studies in man is that
the concentration of total bile acids and individual bile acids,
namely deoxycholic acid and lithocholic acid, is much lower in
stools from low-risk populations such as Japanese and other Asians
and Africans consuming a low-fat diet when compared to high-risk
populations such as North Americans and western Europeans consuming
a high-fat diet (29,31,32). People on a high-fat diet appear to
have higher levels of fecal secondary bile acids compared to those
on a low-fat diet. In general, there are no major differences in
the fecal microflora profiles of these different risk groups although the metabolic activity of some of the constituent microflora,
particularly the nuclear dehydrogenating Clostridia and bacterial
enzymes such as β-glucuronidase and 7α-dehydroxylase, may be associated with the risk for the development of colon cancer. It may,
therefore, be concluded that the concentration of colonic bile acids
has a major role in determining the risk of developing colon cancer.

Evidence from Laboratory Animal Studies

A number of distinct animal models of colon cancer, induced by chemicals and operating by different metabolic and biochemical mechanisms, are available for studying the pathogenesis of colon cancer
and comparing it to similar stages of the disease seen in man (33).
Additionally, these animal models have been used as unique tools for
systematic studies of the risk factors observed in human setting.
Thus, as is described here, a number of major elements observed in
humans, such as the enhancing effect on colon carcinogenesis due to
fat could not have been established without careful, deliberate investigations carried out in laboratory animals.

    The possible role of dietary fat on colon carcinogenesis has
received support from studies in animal models. In several earlier
studies on dietary fat and colon cancer, interpretation of results
between high- and low-fat diets was complicated by the use of diets
of varying caloric density and confounded by different intakes of
other nutrients. However, recent studies in which the intake of all
nutrients and total calories were controlled between the high-fat
and low-fat groups, indicated that the amount of dietary fat is an
important factor in colon carcinogenesis (27).

    The stage of carcinogenesis at which the effect of dietary fat
is exerted appears to be during the promotional phase of carcino-

genesis, rather than during initiation phase (28). Ingestion of high beef fat increased the intestinal tumor incidence when fed after azoxymethane (AOM) treatment, but not during or before the carcinogen administration (34). A recent study indicates that the dietary unsaturated fat alters the metabolism of 1,2-dimethylhydrazine (DMH) and thus influences the carcinogenic process during the initiation phase of carcinogenesis (35). However, in this study, the rats were fed the experimental high-fat diet before, during and after the carcinogen treatment, making it difficult to distinguish whether the effect of fat is at the initiation or during the post-initiation stage of carcinogenesis.

Amount of Dietary Fat. Investigations were also carried out to determine the effect of high dietary fat on colon tumor induction by a variety of carcinogens, DMH, MAM acetate, 3,2'-dimethyl-4-amino-biphenyl (DMAB) or methylnitrosourea (MNU), which not only differ in metabolic activation, but also represent a broad spectrum of exogenous carcinogens (36,37). Male F344 weanling rats were fed semipurified diets containing 20 or 5% beef fat. At 7 weeks of age, animals were given DMH (subcutaneous, 150 mg/kg body wt., one dose), MAM acetate (intraperitoneal, 35 mg/kg body wt., one dose), DMAB (subcutaneous, 50 mg/kg body wt., weekly for 20 weeks) or MNU (intrarectal, 2.5 mg/rat weekly for 2 weeks) and autopsied 30-35 weeks later. Irrespective of the colon carcinogens that differed in metabolic activation, animals fed a diet containing 20% beef fat had a greater incidence of colon tumors than did rats fed a diet containing 5% beef fat (Table I).

Nigro et al. (38) induced intestinal tumors in male Sprague-Dawley rats by subcutaneous administration of AOM and compared animals fed Purina chow with 35% beef fat to those fed Purina chow containing 5% fat. Animals fed the high fat developed more intestinal tumors and more metastasis into abdominal cavity, lungs and liver than the rats fed the low-fat diet. Rogers et al. (39) found that a diet marginally deficient in lipotropes but high in fat, enhanced DMH-induced colon carcinogenesis in Sprague-Dawley rats. Diets containing 20% corn oil or 20% safflower oil markedly increased the AOM-induced colon tumors in F344 rats as compared with diets containing 5% corn oil or 5% safflower oil (40). However, a recent study indicates that a high-fat diet containing 24% corn oil, 24% beef fat or 24% Crisco had no effect on colon tumors induced by oral doses of DMH in Sprague-Dawley rats (41). However, in this study (41), all diets were prepared in a 1:1 ratio into a 5% agar solution and contained slightly higher levels of minerals and vitamins over recommended levels because it is difficult to interpret the results. It has been shown that dietary agar and a related compound, carrageenan, enhance colon tumor evoked by DMH, AOM, or MNU (42,43). These results thus suggest that total dietary fat may have a function in the pathogenesis of colon cancer.

Type of Dietary Fat. Reddy et al. (44) designed experiments to study the effect of a particular type and amount of dietary fat for two generations before animals were exposed to treatment with a carcinogen. F344 rats fed 20% lard or 20% corn oil were more susceptible to colon tumor induction by DMH than those fed 5% lard or 5%

TABLE I. EFFECT OF TYPE AND AMOUNT OF DIETARY FAT ON COLON TUMORS
IN F344 RATS

Experiment No.	Type of fat	% Dietary fat	Carcinogen	% rats with colon tumors
1	Lard			
		5	DMH[a]	17
		20	DMH	67
1	Corn oil			
		5	DMH[a]	36
		20	DMH	64
2	Beef fat			
		5	DMH[b]	27
		20	DMH	60
		5	MNU[c]	33
		20	MNU	73
		5	MAM acetate[d]	45
		20	MAM acetate	80
3	Beef fat			
		5	DMAB[e]	26
		20	DMAB	74

[a] Female F344 rats, at 7 weeks of age, were given DMH s.c. at a
weekly dose rate of 10 mg per kg body wt for 20 weeks and autopsied
10 wks later.
[b] Male F344 rats, at 7 weeks of age, were given a single s.c. dose
of DMH, 150 mg per kg body weight, and autopsied 30 weeks later.
[c] Male F344 rats, at 7 weeks of age, were given MNU i.r., 2.5 mg
per rat, twice a week for 2 weeks and autopsied 30 weeks later
[d] Male F344 rats, at 7 weeks of age, were given a single i.p. dose
of MAM acetate, 35 mg per kg body wt and autopsied 30 weeks later.
[e] Male F344 rats, at 7 weeks of age, were given DMAB s.c. at a
weekly dose rate of 50 mg per kg body wt for 20 weeks, and autopsied 20 wks later.

corn oil (Table I).   The type of fat appears to be immaterial at the 20% level, although at the 5% fat level there is a suggestion that unsaturated fat (corn oil) predisposes to more DMH-induced colon tumors than saturated fat (lard).   Sprague-Dawley rats fed a 20% safflower oil diet (45) or 10% corn oil diet (35) had more DMH-in- duced colon tumors than did those fed a 20% coconut oil or a 9% coconut oil + 1% linoleic acid diet, respectively.   Donrye rats fed semipurified diet containing 5% linoleic acid demonstrated a signi- ficantly higher incidence of colon tumors, more tumors per rat, and greater malignant differentiation than did those 4.7% stearic acid + 0.3% essential fatty acid (46).

A recent study from our laboratory in which intake of all nutrients and calories except fat calories were controlled provides some evidence for the effect of type of fat on colon carcinogenesis (40).   AOM-induced colon tumor incidence was increased in F344 rats fed 20% corn oil or 20% safflower oil diets compared to those fed 5% corn oil or 5% safflower oil diets (Table II).   However, diets con- taining 20% coconut oil or 20% olive oil had no enhancing effect on colon tumor promotion; rats fed the 20% olive oil diet or a 20% coconut oil diet had a colon tumor incidence the same as that in rats fed the diets containing 5% olive oil, 5% corn oil or 5% safflower oil.   In summary, these and other results indicate that diets high in saturated fat of vegetable origin (coconut oil) or monounsaturated fat of vegetable origin (olive oil), polyunsaturated fats (corn oil or safflower oil) and saturated fats of animal origin (lard or beef tallow) differ in colon tumor promotion.   The varied effects of different types of fat on colon cancer suggest that the fatty acid composition is one of the important factors in determin- ing the modifying effect of various fats in colon tumor promotion.

TABLE II.   AOM-INDUCED COLON TUMOR INCIDENCES IN FEMALE F344 RATS FED THE DIETS CONTAINING CORN OIL, SAFFLOWER OIL, OLIVE OIL, AND COCONUT OIL

Diet group	% Animals with colon tumors		
	Total	Adenoma	Adenocarcinoma
5% corn oil(30)[a]	17	10	7
20% corn oil(28)	46[c]	14	32
5% safflower oil(30)	13	7	6
20% safflower oil(28)	36[c]	14	22
5% olive oil(29)	10	7	3
20% olive oil(30)	13	10	3
20% coconut oil	13	10	3

[a]   Effective number of animals are shown in parenthesis.
[b]   Values are expressed as means.
[c]   Significantly different from their respective 5% fat diet at p<0.05.

Dietary Fat and Fiber and Bile Acid Excretion.   In order to under- stand the specifics of the mechanisms whereby dietary fat influences colon cancer, the effect of type and amount of dietary fat on bili- ary and fecal bile acids was studied in rats (40,47,48).   These

studies indicate that the effect of dietary fat on colon carcinogenesis is mediated through a concomitant change in the concentration of colonic bile acids. Biliary excretion of cholic acid,
β-muricholic acid and deoxycholic acid was higher in rats fed diets
containing 20% corn oil or 20% lard than in rats fed diets containing 5% corn oil or 5% lard. High-fat (corn oil or lard) intake was
associated with an increased excretion of fecal secondary bile acids
-- deoxycholic acid and lithocholic acid. Type of fat (corn oil vs
lard) had no effect on biliary and fecal bile acid excretion. In
another study, there was a significant increase in the concentration
of colonic deoxycholic acid and lithocholic acid in rats fed diets
containing 20% corn oil or 20% safflower oil when compared to rats
fed diets containing 5% corn oil or 5% safflower oil (40). In contrast, there was no difference in the concentrations of deoxycholic
acid and lithocholic acid between animals fed the 20% olive oil
diet, 5% olive oil diet or 20% coconut oil diet.

    Thus, the excretory pattern of fecal secondary bile acids ob-
served in these studies correlated with colon tumor incidences in
animal models. These studies also suggest that high dietary intake
of certain types of fat may be necessary for the full expression of
risk for colon cancer.

Bile Acids and Colon Tumor Promotion. The evidence of the importance of bile acids as colon tumor promoters came from our studies
(49,52). Lithocholic acid or deoxycholic acid applied topically to
the colon increased MNNG-induced colon adenocarcinomas in rats. The
bile acids themselves did not produce any tumors. Cohen et al.
(52) reported that cholic acid in the diet increased MNNG-induced
colon carcinogenesis in rats. Total fecal bile acids, particularly
deoxycholic acid output, were elevated in animals fed cholic acid as
compared with controls. This increase in fecal deoxycholic acid was
due to bacterial 7α-dehydroxylation of cholic acid in the colonic
contents. These studies demonstrate that the secondary bile acids
have a promoting effect in colon carcinogenesis.

    Although the molecular mechanisms of tumor-promoting action of
bile acids are incompletely understood, recent studies of Takano et
al (53) suggest that the induction of colonic epithelial ornithine
decarboxylase activity and bile acid administration may play a role
in these mechanisms. Although the classical tumor promoter, TPA,
showed more potent induction of ornithine decarboxylase activity
than the deoxycholate, the maximal induction was greater in the case
of deoxycholate treatment. The studies reported indicate that the
colonic epithelial responses of the polyamine biosynthetic enzymes
to applications of bile acids are among the earliest changes to
occur in this tissue in response to promoting agents. This study
also indicates that a specific bile acid structure with a definite
spatial relationship of the hydroxyl groups (lithocholate, cheno-
deoxycholate, deoxycholate, apocholate, etc.) is required for induction of ornithine decarboxylase activity.

Conclusion

During the last decade, a substantial amount of progress has been
made in the understanding of the relationship between the dietary

constituents and the development of colon cancer in man. The information base is sufficiently convincing with respect to an enhancing effect as a function of total fat intake and a protective effect of certain dietary fibers in colon cancer. The populations with high incidence of colon cancer are characterized by consumption of high-dietary fat which may be a risk factor in the absence of factors that are protective, such as use of whole-grain cereals, high fibrous foods and vegetables mainly of cruciferous type. Application of the findings made thus far in colon cancer research for the general public is, therefore, to have a far-reaching impact on the major premature, killing diseases in the western world.

Current research in animal models which suggests that the carcinogenic response to a variety of colon carcinogens is enhanced by the dietary fat and inhibited by several dietary fibers, indicates that these nutritional factors may operate during the promotional phase of carcinogenesis. The carcinogenic process in humans may have similar characteristics. The fact that ubiquitous environmental carcinogens are present at very low concentrations and the extent of the carcinogenic stress from this source is probably rather weak suggests that promoting factors may have a preponderant influence on the eventual outcome of the neoplastic process in humans. The understanding of post-initiating events appears to offer some promise that intervention in the cancer process in man prior to the occurence of overt tumors may be an achievable and realistic goal. Because promotion or post-initiating events are a reversable process, in contrast to the rapid irreversible or long-lasting process of initiation by carcinogens, manipulation of promotion would seem to be the ideal method of colon cancer prevention. However, in prevention, it makes little difference by what mechanism an agent operates, provided that its partial or total elimination can be shown to lead to a decline in cancer incidence. In this regard, advice to the public at large assumes particular importance because several decades may span the gap between initiating and clinical manifestation of cancer, and, therefore, steps taken today may have a major impact on the nature of future events (54,55).

Literature Cited

1. Waterhouse, J.; Muir, C.; Correa, P.; Powel, J. Cancer Incidence in Five Continents, Vol. 3, I.A.R.C. Sci. Publ. No. 15. International Agency for Research on Cancer, Lyon, France, 1976.
2. Correa, P.; Haenszel, W. Adv. Cancer Res. 1978, 26, 1.
3. Jensen, O.M. In "Experimental Colon Carcinogenesis", Autrup, H.; Williams, G.M., Eds., CRC Press: Boca Raton, 1983; 3.
4. Armstrong, D.; Doll, R. Int. J. Cancer 1975, 15, 617.
5. National Research Council, "Diet, Nutrition and Cancer", Assembly of Life Sciences, National Research Council, National Academy Press, Washington, D.C., 1982.
6. Burkitt, D.P. Am. J. Clin. Nutr. 1978, 31, S58.
7. Reddy, B.S.; Cohen, L.A.; McCoy, G.D.; Hill, P.; Weisburger, J.H.; Wynder, E.L. Adv. Cancer Res. 1980, 32, 237.

8.   Graham, S.; Dayal, H.; Swanson, M.; Mittleman, A.;
     Wilkinson, G. J. Natl. Cancer Inst. 1978, 51, 709.
9.   Jensen, O. M.; MacLennan, R.; Wahrendorf, J. Nutr. Cancer
     1982, 4, 5.
10. West, D. W.; Lyon, J. L.; Gardner, J. W.; Schuman, K.;
     Stanish, W.; Mahoney, A.; Sorenson, A.; Avlon, E. In
     "1983 Workshop: A Decade of Achievements and Challenges in
     Large Bowel Carcinogenesis". National Large Bowel Cancer
     Project, Houston, Tx.; p. 3, 1983.
11. Wynder, E. L.; Reddy, B. S. Seminars in Oncology 1983, 10, 264.
12. McKeown-Eyssen, G. E.; Bright-See, E. Nutr. Cancer 1984, 6, 160.
13. Haenszel, W.; Berg, J.W.; Segi, M.; Kurihara, M.; Locke, F.B.
     J. Natl. Cancer Inst. 1973, 51, 1765.
14. Hirayama, T. Nutr. Cancer 1979, 1, 67.
15. Wynder, E.L.; Shigematsu, T. Cancer 1967, 20, 1520.
16. Carroll, K.K.; Khor, H.T. Prog. Biochem. Pharmacol. 1975, 10,
     308.
17. Manousos, O.; Day, N.E; Trichopoulous, D.; Gervassilis, E.;
     Tzonow, A.; Polychronopoulous, A. Int. J. Cancer, 1983, 32,
     1.
18. Kolonel, L.N.; Hankin, J.H.; Lee, J.; Chu, S.Y.; Nomura,
     A.M.Y.; Ward, H.M. Br. J. Cancer 1981, 44, 332.
19. McKeown-Eyssen, G. In "Diet, Nutrition, and Cancer: From
     Basic Research", Roe, D.A., Ed.; Alan R. Liss, Inc., New York,
     1983, 243.
20. Jain, M.; Cook, G.M.; Davis, F.G.; Grace, M.G.; Howe, G.R.;
     Miller, A.B. Int. J. Cancer 1980, 26, 757.
21. Miller, A.B.; Howe, G.R.; Jain, M.; Craib, K.J.P.; Harrison,
     L. Int. J. Cancer 1983, 32, 155.
22. Reddy, B.S.; Hedges, A.R.; Laakso, K.; Wynder, E.L. Cancer
     1978, 42, 2832.
23. Domellof, L.; Darby, L.; Hanson, D.; Simi, B.; Reddy, B.S.
     Nutr. Cancer 1982, 4, 120.
24. Reddy, B.S.; Ekelund, G.; Bohe, M.; Engle, A.; Domellof, L.
     Nutr. Cancer 1983, 5, 34,
25. Bingham, S.; Williams, D.R.R.; Cole, T.J.; James. W.P.T. Br.
     J. Cancer 1979, 40, 456.
26. Wattenberg, L.W. Cancer Res. 1983, 43, 2448 S.
27. Reddy, B.S. In "Diet, Nutrition, and Cancer: From Basic Re-
     search to Policy Implications", Roe, D.A., Ed.; Alan R. Liss,
     Inc., New York.
28.   Reddy, B.S.   In "Mechanisms of Tumor Promotion", Vol. 1;
     Slaga, T., Ed.; CRC Press, Boca Raton; 1983, 107.
29. Hill, M.J.; Drasar, B.S.; Aries, V.C.; Crowther, J.S.;
     Hawksworth, G.B.; Williams, R.E.O. Lancet 1971, 1, 95.
30. Aries, V.; Crowther, J.S.; Drasar, B.S.; Hill, M.J.; Williams,
     R.E.O. Gut 1969, 10, 334.
31. Reddy, B.S. Cancer Res. 1981, 41, 3700.
32. Reddy, B.S.; Wynder, E.L. J. Natl. Cancer Inst. 1973, 50,
     1437.
33. Shamsuddin, A.K.   In "Experimental Colon Carcinogenesis",
     Autrup, H.; Williams, G.M., Eds.; CRC Press, Boca Raton, FL;
     1983, 51.
34. Bull, A.W.; Soullier, B.K.; Wilson, P.S.; Haydon, M.T.; Nigro,
     N.D. Cancer Res. 1979, 39, 4956.

35.   Wargovich, M.J.; Felkner, I.C.   Nutr. Cancer 1982, 4, 146.
36.   Reddy, B.S.; Watanabe, K.; Weisburger, J.H.   Cancer Res. 1977, 37, 416.
37.   Reddy, B.S.; Ohmori, T.   Cancer Res. 1981, 41, 1363.
38.   Nigro, N.D.; Singh, D.V.; Campbell, R.L.; Pak, M.S.   J. Natl. Cancer Inst. 1975, 54, 429.
39.   Rogers, A.E.; Newberne, P.M.   Cancer Res. 1975, 35, 3427.
40.   Reddy, B.S.; Maeura, Y.   J. Natl. Cancer Inst. 1984, 72, 745.
41.   Nauss, K.M.; Locniskoor, M.; Newberne, P.M.   Cancer Res. 1983, 43, 4083.
42.   Watanabe, K.; Reddy, B.S.; Wong, C.Q.; Weisburger, J.H.   Cancer Res. 1978, 38, 4427.
43.   Glauert, H.P.; Bennink, M.R.; Sander, C.H..   Fd. Cosmet. Toxicol. 1981, 19, 281.
44.   Reddy, B.S.; Narisawa, T.; Vukusich, D.; Weisburger, J.H; Wynder, E.L.   Proc. Soc. Exp. Biol. Med. 1976, 151, 237.
45.   Broitman, S.A.; Vitale, J.J.; Vavrousek-Jakuba, E.; Gottlieb, L.S.   Cancer 1977, 40, 2455.
46.   Sakaguchi, M.; Hiramatsu, Y.; Takada, H.; Yamamura, M.; Hioki, K.; Saito, K.; Yamamoto, M.   Cancer Res. 1984, 44, 1472.
47.   Reddy, B.S.; Mangat, S.; Sheinfil, A.; Weisburger, J.H.; Wynder, E.L.   Cancer Res. 1977, 37, 2132.
48.   Nigro, N.D.; Bull, A.W.   In "Experimental Colon Carcinogenesis", Autrup, H.; Williams, G.M., Eds.; CRC Press, Boca Raton, FL; 1983, 215.
49.   Narisawa, T.; Magadia, N.E.; Weisburger, J.H.; Wynder, E.L.   J. Natl. Cancer Inst. 1974, 53, 1093.
50.   Reddy, B.S.; Narisawa, T.; Weisburger, J.H; Wynder, E.L.   J. Natl. Cancer Inst. 1976, 56, 441.
51.   Reddy, B.S.; Watanabe, K.; Weisburger,J.H.; Wynder, E.L.   Cancer Res. 1977, 37, 3238.
52.   Cohen, B.I.; Raicht, R.F.; Deschner, E.E.; Takahashi, M.; Sarwal, A.N.; Fazini, E.   J. Natl. Cancer Inst. 1980, 64, 573.
53.   Takano, S.; Akagi, M.; and Bryan, G.T.   Gann 1984, 75, 29.
54.   Wynder, E.L.   Cancer 1983, 43, 3024.
55.   Palmer, S.   Cancer Res. 1983, 43, 2509 S.

RECEIVED January 18, 1985

Modulation of Mammary Tumor Incidence by Dietary Fat and Antioxidants

A Mechanistic Approach

M. MARGARET KING[1], JUNJI TERAO[1,3], GEMMA BRUEGGEMANN[1], PAUL B. McCAY[1], and ROBERT A. MAGARIAN[2]

[1]Biomembrane Research Program, Oklahoma Medical Research Foundation, Oklahoma City, OK 73104

[2]Division of Medicinal Chemistry and Pharmacodynamics, College of Pharmacy, University of Oklahoma Health Sciences Center, Oklahoma City, OK 73190

Investigations on the effect of dietary fats and anti-oxidant compounds on the incidence of mammary tumors in female rats have provided clear evidence for modification of the tumorigenic process by these dietary components. High fat diets, particularly diets rich in polyunsaturated fats, markedly enhance the incidence of DMBA-induced mammary tumors in comparison with rats fed diets which are low in fat. Polyunsaturated fats easily undergo peroxidation unless the latter is prevented by the presence of antioxidant substances. Because antioxidant substances had been reported to inhibit carcenogenesis in some tumor models, we undertook to investigate the effect of antioxidants with little or no known toxicity supplemented in the diets of animals fed the different types of fat. The purpose was to determine if the antioxidants were exerting their protective effect on tumorigenesis primarily in animals fed diets rich in polyunsaturated fat. The results tend to support this concept excepting that some antioxidants are effective tumor inhibitors and some are not under these experimental conditions. Experiments were performed to determine if a differential uptake and turnover of antioxidant by the mammary gland could explain this inconsistency. The results presented in this report suggest that the most effective inhibitor of DMBA-induced mammary tumor is one that accumulated in mammary gland in the largest amount for the longest time.

Over the past ten years the role of various levels and types of dietary fat and dietary antioxidants in modifying chemically induced cancer has been actively investigated in this laboratory with most of the work centering on mammary cancer.

[3]Current address: Research Institute for Food Science, Kyoto University, Uji, Kyoto 611, Japan

0097–6156/85/0277–0131$06.00/0

It has become very well-established that the intake of elevated
levels of dietary fat, especially polyunsaturated fat, must be
accompanied by an elevated level of antioxidant if tissue damage is
to be avoided (1). In the absence of an antioxidant, animals consuming a high polyunsaturated fat diet develop various pathological and
somewhat species-specific tissue damage (2). The higher the polyunsaturated fatty acid intake, the higher the anti oxidant requirement
becomes in order to prevent this damage. It was demonstrated by
Bieri et al. that some species fed very low levels of dietary fat had
no apparent requirement for an antioxidant (3). From such studies it
was found that α-tocopherol as vitamin E was an effective naturally-
occurring antioxidant which provided protection to tissues from the
damaging effect of polyunsaturated fat-feeding (4). It was soon
found that other structurally unrelated, naturally occurring and even
synthetic antioxidants could provide similar protection against the
injurious effects of unsaturated fat consumption (5).

A low level of dietary polyunsaturated fat is essential for life
in higher organisms since the total polyunsaturated fatty acid
structure required for prostaglandin production cannot be synthesized
in these animals. Thus, the requirement for linoleic acid to be
provided in the diet (6). Linoleic acid is found in the food chain
in a variety of plant sources (7). An intake of linoleic acid at the
average dietary level of most Americans would cause significant
tissue damage to certain organs of various laboratory animals,
especially young rapidly growing animals, unless it was accompanied
by an adequate intake of dietary antioxidant. In spite of extensive
investigations to determine the mechanism of this specific and
reproducible effect, the exact mechanism of tissue injury is still
unknown. Peroxidative alterations of membrane lipids have been
strongly implicated (8).

Many investigations have indicated that dietary fat, especially
polyunsaturated fat, enhances tumorigenesis in both humans and
laboratory animals. The importance of understanding the role of
these dietary factors in carcinogenesis is perhaps best indicated by
world-wide epidemiological surveys which have generated data showing
a strong correlation between dietary fat intake and breast cancer in
women (9) (Figure 1). A similar high degree of correlation was found
for epidemiological evidence of colon cancer in both men and women
(9). The United States has one of the highest per capita consumption
levels of fat in the world and also ranks among the highest in the
incidence of cancer of the colon and breast.

In laboratory animals, it is well-established that higher levels
of dietary fat, especially polyunsaturated fat, increase tumor incidence in those treated with certain carcinogens. The early studies
of Tannenbaum in the 1940's (11) demonstrated that dietary fat
enhances mammary tumor incidence. This point has now been shown by.
many investigators, including ourselves (11, 12, 13). That this is a
specific dietary fat effect and separate from a general influence of
a high caloric intake, has been shown many times as early as the
1940's (14-18) and extending through our own work being presented
here.

Similarly, it has been demonstrated that various antioxidants
inhibit carcinogenesis induced by a wide variety of compounds and in
several organ sites (19, review). The antagonism between dietary
fats and antioxidants on carcinogenesis suggests that a common factor

may be involved in the balance between dietary unsaturated fat and the antioxidant content required to maintain tissue integrity.

Experimental Design

Initially a model was established and tested many times to insure that reproducible results were obtained.

Diets. Three basic diets were utilized (Table I), a 2% low fat diet (2% linoleic acid methyl esters), a 20% polyunsaturated fat diet containing 20% stripped corn oil, and a high saturated fat diet containing 18% coconut oil and 2% linoleic acid methyl esters to prevent an essential fatty acid deficiency (6). All diets were prepared to our specifications by ICN Life Sciences (Cleveland, OH) and analyzed both by ICN and our laboratory for fatty acids, antioxidants and some trace minerals. They are routinely stored in sealed plastic containers at 4°. Antioxidants when added (see Figure 2) were supplemented just prior to feeding and at 0.2% or 0.3% of the diet by weight as specified in each experiment.

Table I. Diets

	High Polyunsaturated Fat Diet	High Saturated Fat Diet	Low Fat Diet
	%	%	%
Casein	23	23	23
Fat	20[a]	20[b]	2[c]
Sucrose	46	46	64
Salt mixture[d]	4	4	6
Alphacel (non-nutrient bulk)	6	6	6
Vitamin mixture[e]	1	1	1

[a]Stripped corn oil.
[b]Stripped, hydrogenated coconut oil, 18% + linoleic acid, 2%.
[c]Linoleic acid.
[d]Salt mixture: Hubbell et al., J. Nutr. 14: 273-285, 1937 (modified to contain 0.03% zinc chloride).
[e]Vitamin mixture (vitamin fortification mixture (tocopherol deleted) of ICN Life Sciences Co., Cleveland, OH 44128).

A modification of the Huggins model was utilized in which 50 day-old female Sprague-Dawley rats (Sasco Inc., Omaha, NE) receiving 10 mg 7,12-dimethylbenz(α)anthracene (Sigma Chemical Co., St. Louis, MO) i.g. in 1 ml stripped corn oil at 50 ±1 day of age following a 24 hr fast. Unless otherwise noted, all animals were started on their respective diets at weaning (21 days old), the time they were received into the Facility. They were weighed upon arrival and randomly divided into experimental groups of 30 and housed 5, 10 or 15 per cage. At 5-6 wks of age, each animal was given a stainless

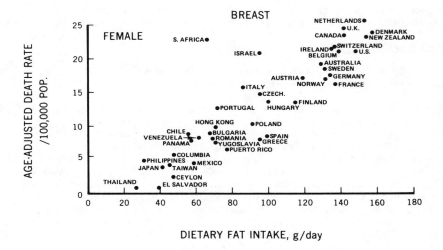

Figure 1.   Incidence of dietary fat in relation to tumorigenesis.

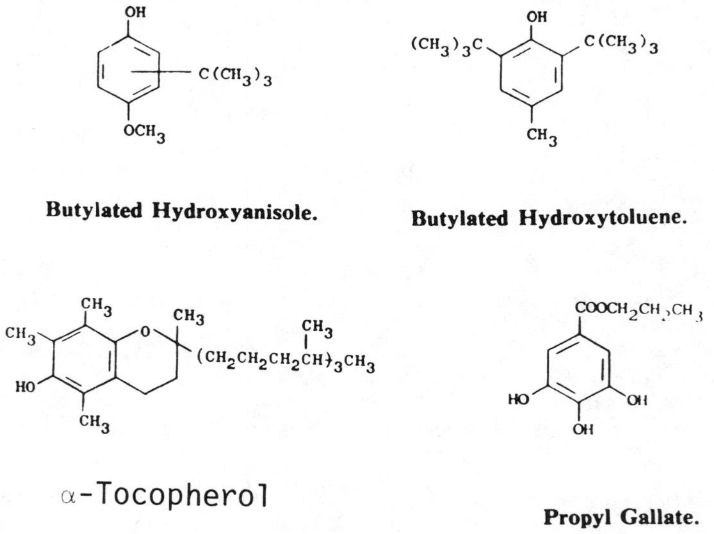

Butylated Hydroxyanisole.

Butylated Hydroxytoluene.

α-Tocopherol

Propyl Gallate.

Figure 2.   Structures of antioxidant compounds used in these investigations.

steel ear tag with a distinctive and sequential number for identification. All animals were housed in an AAALAC-accredited animal care
facility with a controlled temperature (68–72°) and humidity (50–60%)
and a 12 hr light/dark cycle. All experimental animals were weighed
weekly from the time of arrival and palpated weekly for tumors
beginning three weeks after carcinogen treatment. Only tumors
verified histologically as mammary adenocarcinomas were included in
incidence data.

      Animals used for studying drug metabolism and measuring various
microsomal parameters were placed on diets, weighed and treated in
exactly the same manner as those being used for mammary tumor
incidence studies, except that they were killed at 50 days of age,
the time for exposure of rats in the other experimental group to the
carcinogen. Livers and/or mammary glands were harvested for preparation of subcellular fractions and drug metabolism studies as previously described (28). Antioxidant measurements in tissues were made
using similar animals that had been fed the basic diets supplemented
with antioxidants for the specific times as indicated for each
experiment.

Results and Discussion

Over the past several years the DMBA-induced rat mammary tumor model
has been tested many times with various specific changes in the
experimental parameters being tested. The very first incidence study
utilized the same three basic diets (incorporating the Hubbell salt
mix) with and without 0.7% BHT supplementation (13). It was found in
this study that BHT given at this level, although an effective tumor
inhibitor, was also slightly toxic, resulting in a slight decrease in
weight gain and occasional and intermittent hair loss. This study
was repeated using the same diets, but with only 0.3% BHT supplementation. Almost identical tumor incidence and tumor numbers were
obtained using this level of BHT, but weight gains were now the same
as in non-BHT-supplemented animals and no evidence was seen of any
toxic side effects. The same protocol was employed for testing each
of the following: BHA, α-tocopherol (as α-tocopheryl acetate) and
propyl gallate (PrG) as mammary tumor inhibitors. Weight gains in
all groups ± antioxidants were essentially identical and no toxic
side effects were observed.

      Figure 3 demonstrates the tumor incidence results obtained in
these studies when just the three dietary regimens were compared,
i.e. LF (2%), HPF (20% stripped corn oil) and HSF (18% stripped corn
oil ± 2% linoleic acid). As can be seen in this figure, the animals
consuming the HPF diet routinely develop a 97–100% tumor incidence.
Those on the HSF diet develop a 55–70% incidence and those on the LF
develop only a 20–30% incidence of mammary tumors. These values
represent three sets of experiments with 30 rats per group or 90
total rats per each diet represented. There is a 10–15% variability
in the incidence rates between experiments performed under identical
conditions whether done concurrently or in a sequence of times.
These results have been used as the standard for comparison of additional experiments, and those being performed most recently compare
well with the earlier experiments. Thus, this seems to be a satis-
factorily reproducible model.

For various reasons over the past ten years, primarily in attempt to improve the biological design, changes have been made in the original basic diets. One of the first changes was from the use of Hubbell Salt Mix to the AIN 76 Salt Mix. The changes caused no detectable difference in the results with regard to tumor incidence or tumor numbers per tumor-bearing rat. In some experiments, diets have been isocalorically pair-fed to the LF diet, and more recently, adjusted so that all diets have equivalent nutrient-to-calorie ratios. The last adjustment was made (Table II) to compensate for the fact that the animals which are fed the LF diets consume more diet (in g) to obtain the same number calories availabe to the HSF and HPF-fed animals in a much smaller amount of diet. Through this adjustment, all animals in the various dietary groups will receive essentially the same amount of trace elements and vitamins. Our more recent studies have been carried out using these adjusted diets (Table II). When the BHT and BHA studies were repeated with the various diets, similar results were obtained compared to the earlier diets (Table I and reference 13). These results, along with the companion results that similar tumor number and incidence were obtained, support the hypothesis that the influence of diet on this tumor model is an effect of the type and quantity of fat fed, and does not appear to be a caloric effect. This point has been repeatedly stressed in both formal and informal scientific exchanges of views, and our work as well as the work of others continues to show that caloric density per se is not responsible for the enhancement of tumorigenesis seen in this model.

Table II. Experimental Diets
(Equivalent Nutrient:Calorie Ratios)

	High Polyunsaturated Fat Diet	High Saturated Fat Diet	Low Fat Diet
	% by wt.	% by wt.	% by wt.
Casein	28.20	28.20	23.0
Fat	20.00[a]	20.00[b]	2.0[c]
Sucrose	38.77	38.77	64.0
Salt Mixture[d]	4.90	4.90	4.0
Alphacel (Non-Nutrient Bulk)	6.93	6.93	6.0
Vitamin Mixture[e]	1.20	1.20	1.0

[a]Stripped corn oil.
[b]18% coconut oil + 2% linoleic acid methyl esters.
[c]2% linoleic acid methyl esters.
[d]AIN-76 mineral mixture.
[e]AIN-76 vitamin mixture.

With the addition of the different antioxidants to the basic semipurified diets differing in fat content, varied results have been obtained. Both BHT and PrG have routinely given good protection when added to the diet at a level of 0.3% (w/w). BHA and α-tocopherol have shown only marginal or no significant protection against mammary adenocarcinomas (Figure 4). The fact that BHA showed no significant protection against mammary tumorigenesis in this model was of particular interest because of its similarity to BHT, and because it had been reported to be an effective tumor inhibitor in other models of carcinogenesis (19). Quite a variety of antioxidants have been tested and found to be effective in several different models and the effect is far from consistent. All antioxidants do not inhibit any one tumor model and some tumor models do not appear to be inhibited by any antioxidant (20-22). Implicit in many of these studies has been the assumption that it is the antioxidant properties of this class of phenolic compounds that is responsible for their tumor inhibitory capabilities. Certainly insufficient information is available presently to make a decision one way or another in this regard. This research area requires further investigation in order to gain insights which may suggest the mechanisms involved in regulating tumor growth rather than approach the problem to find actual and practical means of cancer prevention.

More recently, we have focused on the strategy of investigating the mechanism of inhibition of carcinogenesis by BHT in terms of the alterations in specific organ biochemistry that result from feeding this and other antioxidants. In this vein, we have been focusing on the following experiments designed to provide information as to the mechanisms of tumor incidence/growth modification by dietary fat and antioxidants: 1) investigations to determine how the level of unsaturation per se influences the effectiveness of antioxidants as inhibitors of mammary gland tumorigenesis; 2) investigations to determine the effect of time during which the antioxidant to be tested was supplied to the animal with respect to the time of exposure to the carcinogen, DMBA; and 3) determinations of the actual tissue concentrations of the various antioxidants with respect to time of feeding, and amount and type dietary fat being fed.

The degree of unsaturation of animal tissues is a function of the level of unsaturated fat consumed in the diet. Hence, a balance between dietary factors which either facilitates or inhibits carcinogen metabolism may have an important effect on the eventual outcome of chronic carcinogen exposure. One possible effect of dietary lipids and antioxidants on chemical carcinogenesis that must be considered is the influence of these dietary components on the metabolism of chemical carcinogens. After PAH's enter the body, they are oxidized in the endoplasmic reticulum of many tissues (liver, skin, mammary, etc.) to hydroxylated products which, being water-soluble, are more readily excreted (Figure 5). Unfortunately, in this process which usually results in detoxification, some compounds are converted to reactive alkylating agents which are carcinogenic. Benson observed that mammary tissue from animals on a high fat diet appeared more metabolically active when compared to tissue from animals being fed a low fat diet (28). More recently, Dao's laboratory has demonstrated that mammary gland tissue per se is capable of metabolizing DMBA, and that this metabolism can be affected by known inducers of the hepatic monooxygenase system such as 3-methylcholanthrene (30, 31). Virgin mammary glands from female Sprague-Dawley rats have been shown to contain an inducible cytochrome P-450 in the microsomal monooxygenase system (29). It is reasonable to assume that dietary

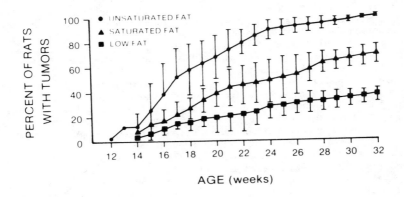

Figure 3. Incidence of mammary tumors in female Sprague-Dawley rats fed diets containing different amounts and types of fat. [●] 20% corn oil fat; [▲] 20% coconut oil; [■] 2% methyl linoleate. See Experimental Design for details of these diets.

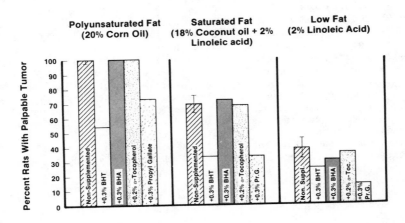

Figure 4. Dietary fat and antioxidant influences on DMBA-induced mammary carcinogenesis.

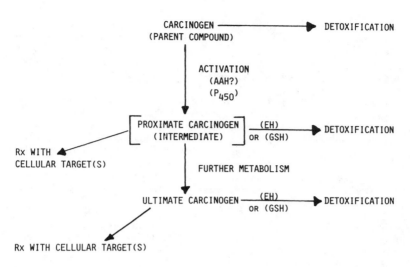

Figure 5. Scheme of carcinogen metabolism in mammalian target tissues.

fat can affect carcinogen metabolism in the mammary gland, since it has been shown to affect microsomal metabolic activities in other extra-hepatic tissues. For example, AHH activity has been shown to increase in the rat kidney as dietary fat is increased above 4% in the diet, reaching a maximum after the diets have been fed for seven days (23).

Another parameter of the metabolic process which could potentially be affected by dietary fats and antioxidants is a major component of the endoplasmic reticular monooxygenase system, cytochrome(s) P-450. These cytochromes along with their associated enzyme NADPH-cytochrome P-450 reductase, are also likely to be involved in the oxidation of potentially carcinogenic substrates. This reductase is a flavoprotein which transfers electrons from NADPH to cytochrome P-450 in two steps. The selective induction of several liver monooxygenases by BHT is well-established (25, 34). Dietary BHT in male rats fed a chow diet apparently produces a change in the relative proportion of individual forms of cytochrome P-450 without altering the total concentration of cytochromes (26). Similarly, in male rats fed either the HPF or HSF diets, the specific content of cytochrome P-450 is significantly higher in liver microsomes from rats fed these diets compared to the low-fat fed animals (29). Whether the fat was saturated or polyunsaturated did not affect these microsomal components. With female rats, however, BHT produces an induction of liver microsomal cytochrome P-450 content (Table III) in animals consuming semipurified diets high in either polyunsaturated or saturated fat (27).

Marked decreases in NADPH cytochrome P-450 reductase activity were consistently seen when BHT was included in the diet of male rats (24) but no significant effects were noted in female rats (27).

Reductase activities were only 30-35% of those in microsomes from unsupplemented male animals, the most profound decrease occurring in the low-fat-fed animals. Reductase is generally considered to be the rate-limiting component of the microsomal monooxygenase system and this decrease in activity could have profound effects on the metabolism of these foreign compounds.

Mammary AHH has been shown in virgin rats and found to vary as a function of the age of the animal, being highest in younger animals (30-60 days old) (32, 33). Induction of this enzyme is also age-dependent, being highly inducible between 40 and 60 days of age. AHH activity is important from the standpoint that this type of activity results in the formation of highly reactive electropholic intermediates, arene oxides, from relatively inert precursors. Preliminary data from our laboratory suggests that AHH activity is specifically influenced by both the level and type of dietary fat. As can be seen from Table IV, hepatic AHH activity measured as benz(α)pyrene hydroxylase and read against standard 3-OH-benzpyrene, is highest in the HPF dietary group followed by the HSF and lowest in the LF-fed group, and the lowest value for LF is significantly induced by HPF ($P < 0.05$). Addition of BHT to the diet at a level of 0.3% as before, resulted in approximately a four- to fivefold increase in AHH activity (Table IV). Thus, diet also influences the AHH level with the HPF value significantly ($P < 0.05$) induced above LF (student's t-test).

Table III. Effects of Dietary Fat and Antioxidants on Hepatic Microsomal Cytochrome P_{450} Levels in Female Sprague-Dawley Rats

Diet	Total Cytochrome P_{450} (n moles/mg MS Protein)
High Polyunsaturated Fat	0.79 ± 0.04†
• BHT	1.18 ± 0.05*
• BHA	0.87 ± 0.06
• α-Toc	0.79 ± 0.05
• PrG	0.80 ± 0.04
High Saturated Fat	0.85 ± 0.06
• BHT	1.10 ± 0.08*
• BHA	0.73 ± 0.07
• α-Toc	0.74 ± 0.06
• PrG	0.77 ± 0.03
Low Fat	0.81 ± 0.04
• BHT	0.92 ± 0.07
• BHA	0.76 ± 0.06
• α-Toc	0.78 ± 0.06
• PrG	0.74 ± 0.03

†Mean ± SEM.
*Differ significantly from that for the group on the corresponding non-supplemented diet ($P < 0.05$ by student's t test).
   BHT = butylated hydroxytoluene (0.3% by weight)
   BHA = butylated hydroxyanisole (0.3%)
   α-Toc = α-tocopheryl acetate (0.2%)
   PrG = propyl gallate (0.3%)

Table IV.   Aryl Hydrocarbon Hydroxylase Activity in Hepatic
Microsomes from Animals Consuming Various Levels
and Types of Fat ± 0.3% BHT

	Polyunsaturated Fat	Saturated Fat	Low Fat
-BHT	6.3 ± 0.4*†	4.0 ± 0.2	3.4 ± 0.1
+BHT	26.5 ± 1.5	21.6 ± 1.0	17.3 ± 0.9

†Mean ± S.E. of 10-12 determinations.
*AHH activity measured as $\Delta OD/min/mg$ microsomal protein.

   Thus, it can be easily theorized that the shift seen in the
microsomal enzyme and cytochrome patterns caused by dietary fat and
antioxidants may be related to the inhibitory and enhancing effects
of these compounds on chemical carcinogenesis. Further studies are
indicated to look at specific carcinogen metabolites produced by the
drug metabolizing systems of animals consuming the various diets, and
to attempt to correlate the corresponding cytochrome and enzyme
levels with these metabolites and ultimately with resultant tumor
incidences and tumor numbers.

Critical Time of BHT Exposure. Two complimentary studies were performed with the specific objective of determining the critical time
during which BHT must be fed to realize protection against DMBA-
induced mammary carcinogenesis. These studies have been reported
elsewhere (35) and will only be briefly summarized here. The results
were comparable in both the HPF and HSF-supplemented groups. In the
first study 0.3% BHT was added to the HPF and HSF diets at various
times from weaning (21 days of age) to one week before carcinogen
administration (42 days of age), at 50 days of age, the time of DMBA
treatment, or one, two or three weeks after DMBA, and included in the
diet from that time throughout the experimental period of 30 weeks.
In a similar experiment, BHT was added to the diet for only short
periods of time, one week starting at weaning (21 days old) then
removed from the diet, or added for two, three. four, five or six
weeks from weaning and then removed. This encompasses the time from
weaning up to and including three weeks post-carcinogen treatment
after each of the respective BHT feeding periods, the antioxidant was
removed from the diets and the animals continued for the remainder of
the experimental period on their respective HPF or HSF diets. When
mammary tumor incidence rates were compared with non-BHT treated
animals it was found from the first experiment that BHT was most
effective if added to the diet at the time of weaning or up to the
time of carcinogen treatment. If one waited until three weeks post-
carcinogen to supplement the diets with BHT, essentially no protection was seen, i.e. the results were comparable to those when no BHT
was added to the diet throughout the experimental feeding time.
   In the short-term BHT supplementation experiment, it was found
that no protection was obtained if BHT was added for only 1 or 2
weeks and then removed from the diet (2 weeks pre-carcinogen treatment). If it was continued for three weeks (to 1 week pre-carcinogen), only minimal protection was seen. If fed up to the time of
DMBA-treatment or for one, two or three weeks post-carcinogen then
removed, maximal protection was seen, comparable to the group that
consumed BHT throughout the entire experimental period. These two

studies indicate that BHT needs to be present in the diet for two-three weeks before and after the time of carcinogen exposure to be effective. Stopping it too soon or starting it too late after DMBA exposure does not allow it to be effective as a tumor inhibitor. These results implicate BHT as having a role in the activation, initiation or early promotional phase of DMBA-induced chemical carcinogenesis. A definite possibility is that it may require this period of time to allow for the induction of specific metabolic enzymes involved in the handling of DMBA. This time may be required for the attainment of sufficient levels in the tissues to allow effectiveness as an inhibitor. Further studies are certainly needed to narrow the wide range of possibilities.

Many questions in the investigation of a possible mechanism for antioxidant inhibition of mammary carcinogenesis have led us to the need to be able to measure actual tissue concentrations of these compounds. Since BHT was found to be a very effective mammary tumor inhibitor in this model, and BHA to have no measurable effect under the same experimental conditions, one has to ask the question as to whether or not both are absorbed and taken up by the tissues, specifically mammary tissue, since this is the target tissue. BHT was not effective as an inhibitor when fed for three weeks from weaning, then stopped one week prior to carcinogen treatment (35). BHT was effective in reducing tumor development when added to the diet two-three weeks before and up to the time of carcinogen exposure, and maintained in the diet from that time on through the 30 week experimental time. The effectiveness of BHT in inhibiting tumorigenesis decreased as the time of initiating BHT feeding after carcinogen treatment increased, with similar results being obtained in both HPF and HSF-fed animals. It was of interest to study how BHT protects against mammary tumors, while BHA does not (13, 36). All these observations lead one to ask "what are the actual tissue concentrations of BHT and BHA after being consumed at 0.3% of the diet by weight for various periods of time?" Are they taken up equally well, or at all by the mammary tissue and/or the liver?

Initially, a sensitive and reproducible method of detection had to be developed. A high performance liquid chromatographic (HPLC) procedure was found to be a very sensitive and exacting way of measuring these antioxidants allowing for detection of as little as 0.1 µg/ml of antioxidant. Standard curves were established relating concentration of antioxidant to peak height for both BHA and BHT and the results were found to be both linear and reproducible. A typical chromatogram is shown for BHT (Figure 6) and BHA (Figure 7) with absorbance being measured at λ_{max} = 280 nm.

Samples of mammary gland, serum and liver from 50 day-old female Sprague-Dawley rats consuming non-antioxidant-containing semipurified diets were obtained. To each of these was added a known amount of an antioxidant and an extraction procedure developed. Prior to this time, no simple method has been reported for determining tissue concentrations of these compounds, short of steam distillations (37, 38). A modification of the Bligh and Dyer (39) method for extracting lipids was utilized for the first step. Details of this procedure are reported in Terao et al. (40). A brief summary is given for BHA from mammary gland in Figure 8 (the same procedure is used for BHT but varies slightly for serum and liver [40]). When standard curves for each of these compounds were plotted following extraction, it was found that average recoveries for three known amounts of antioxidants

in samples of mammary tissue were 98.7% and 99.7% for BHT (Figure 9)
and BHA (Figure 10), respectively. The standard curves indicated a
good correlation between peak height and antioxidant concentration,
and it was felt that an accurate and reproducible method for measuring tissue and serum concentrations had been defined.

The actual experiments began by feeding female Sprague-Dawley
rats 0.3% BHT in a low fat diet for various periods of time. At the
end of the feeding period, the animals were euthanized in a N_2 chamber, mammary tissue removed, placed in an ice bath, and trimmed free
of extraneous fat and lymph glands. The tissue was extracted and
analyzed by HPLC as described.

It was found that BHT is not retained in any detectable amount
(< 0.1 µg/ml) in the serum or serum lipids of animals fed the antioxidant for two or three weeks, or for seventeen weeks. The total
mean lipid content in the serum of six animals fed BHT for two and
three weeks was found to be 2.0 ± 0.7 mg/ml and 1.7 ± 0.1 mg/ml,
respectively.

Co-chromatograms of a BHT standard and extracts of liver and
mammary tissue confirmed the presence of BHT in both (Figure 6;
mammary, liver not shown). Other than the presence of the BHT peak,

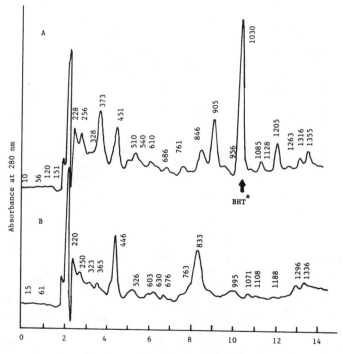

Figure 6. HPLC analysis of mammary tissue extracts. (A) Rat fed
low fat diet containing 0.3% BHT for 2 weeks. (B) Control rat fed
low fat diet only. * The arrow shows the position of the BHT
peak.

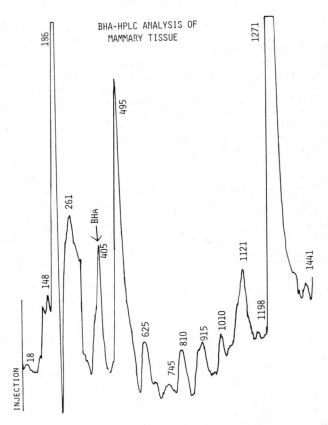

Figure 7. HPLC analysis of mammary tissue extracts from rats fed
a diet containing butylated hydroxyanisole (BHA).

there were no differences in the chromatograms between the control
and experimental. Animals fed BHT for two weeks had greater concentrations (0.64 ± 0.26 µg/g) than those fed the antioxidant for three
weeks (0.35 ± 0.09 µg/g of liver). BHT levels found in the liver
lipid (33.3 ± 9.7 µg/g) of animals fed the antioxidant for two weeks
was 15.22 ± 2.10 µg/g lipid compared to the amount from livers of
animals on BHT for three weeks of 10.80 ± 2.71 µg/g lipid.
     BHT levels found in mammary tissue and mammary lipid are shown
in Table V. A high concentration of BHT was found in mammary tissue,
along with several suspected metabolite peaks. The BHT peak was
collected, analyzed by gas chromatography/mass spectroscopy and confirmed by comparison with an authentic sample.

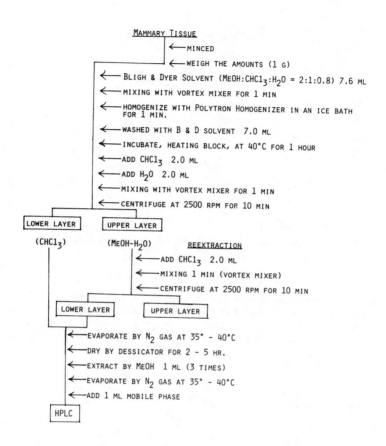

MAMMARY TISSUE
←— MINCED
←— WEIGH THE AMOUNTS (1 G)
←— BLIGH & DYER SOLVENT (MEOH:CHCl$_3$:H$_2$O = 2:1:0.8) 7.6 ML
←— MIXING WITH VORTEX MIXER FOR 1 MIN
←— HOMOGENIZE WITH POLYTRON HOMOGENIZER IN AN ICE BATH FOR 1 MIN.
←— WASHED WITH B & D SOLVENT 7.0 ML
←— INCUBATE, HEATING BLOCK, AT 40°C FOR 1 HOUR
←— ADD CHCl$_3$ 2.0 ML
←— ADD H$_2$O 2.0 ML
←— MIXING WITH VORTEX MIXER FOR 1 MIN
←— CENTRIFUGE AT 2500 RPM FOR 10 MIN

LOWER LAYER   UPPER LAYER
(CHCl$_3$)   (MEOH-H$_2$O)   REEXTRACTION
←— ADD CHCl$_3$ 2.0 ML
←— MIXING 1 MIN (VORTEX MIXER)
←— CENTRIFUGE AT 2500 RPM FOR 10 MIN

LOWER LAYER   UPPER LAYER
←— EVAPORATE BY N$_2$ GAS AT 35° - 40°C
←— DRY BY DESSICATOR FOR 2 - 5 HR.
←— EXTRACT BY MEOH 1 ML (3 TIMES)
←— EVAPORATE BY N$_2$ GAS AT 35° - 40°C
←— ADD 1 ML MOBILE PHASE
HPLC

Figure 8. Extraction procedure used in the determination of BHA in mammary gland in rats fed a diet containing this antioxidant.

BHT levels in mammary tissue and mammary lipids of animals placed on dietary BHT at different ages are shown in Table V. Group I animals at 91 days of age were divided into three groups (10/group) and fed 0.3% BHT in a LF diet for 1, 2 and 3 weeks. Group II animals were fed BHT as above beginning at 35 days of age, but for 2 or 17 weeks. BHT was significantly increased in mammary tissue of Group I fed this antioxidant for 2 weeks compared to 1 week, and this increase was seen on a per tissue weight or a per lipid weight basis. In the Group II animals, BHT levels were significantly lower than those in Group I animals fed BHT for 2 weeks indicating a definite difference in tissue uptake in animals of different ages. One factor that might be responsible is that the whole mammary tissue weight in younger rats (Group II) was only about one-half (1.10 ± 0.19 g) that of the older rats in Group I (2.45 ± 0.67 g).

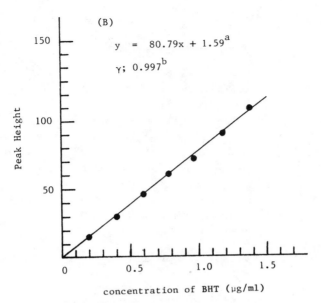

Figure 9.   Standard curve for analysis of BHT.   Sensitivity
increased 8 times higher for the concentration range of 0.1 to 1.0
µg/ml of BHT.   [a]Regression line y = mx + b, where y = peak
height and x = concentration of BHT.   [b]Correlation coefficient.

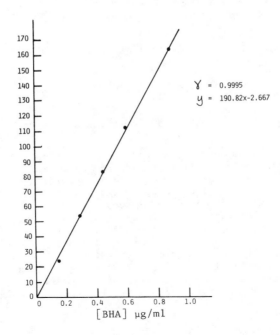

Figure 10.   Standard curve for the determination of BHA by HPLC.

Table V. BHT Levels in Mammary Tissue[a]

Period of 0.3% BHT Feeding	BHT Levels in Mammary Tissue (µg/g tissue)	BHT Concentration in Mammary Lipid (µg/g lipid)
Group I: 91 days of age[b,c]		
1 week	2.82 ± 0.92^{d}	9.13 ± 2.04^{d}
2 weeks	6.37 ± 1.37^{d}	20.08 ± 7.94^{d}
3 weeks	4.52 ± 1.77	14.40 ± 5.48
Group II: 35 days of age[b,c]		
2 weeks	1.42 ± 0.35	6.81 ± 2.56
17 weeks	3.04 ± 0.43	6.35 ± 1.03

[a] Average value ± S.D. for six rats.
[b] Ages when animals were placed on the BHT diet.
[c] The lipid content in the mammary tissue of rats in Group I were found to be: 1 week → 328 ± 74 mg/g; 2 weeks → 341 ± 77 mg/g; and 3 weeks → 316 ± 34 mg/g. In Group II, the lipid content for animals fed BHT for 2 weeks and 17 weeks were 227 ± 32 mg/g and 534 ± 98 mg/g, respectively.
[d] Significant difference (P < 0.0005), Student's t-test.

In Group II, the animals fed BHT for seventeen weeks showed a significantly higher level of antioxidant than those fed for only two weeks, although both had approximately the same BHT concentration in mammary lipids.

Much higher levels of BHT were detected in mammary than in liver and serum. The difference appears to be due to the lipid content of the tissue which is ten times greater in mammary than in liver. BHT would be expected to be distributed equally in all lipid areas due to its lipophilic character. Its tissue concentration should then be dependent upon the level of lipids in any specific tissue. The lipid content could certainly account for the greater amounts of BHT found in mammary compared to liver tissues.

In similar studies, much lesser amounts of BHA were found in the mammary tissue of rats fed 0.3% BHA in their diets for 2 and 3 weeks (Table VI). This may be due to an apparent rapid formation of a BHA metabolite as detected by HPLC (40). Other workers have also reported the rapid metabolism of BHA (41, 42). This definite difference found in the levels of BHA and BHT in the target tissue, i.e. mammary gland, may help explain the lack of significant protection against mammary adenocarcinoma seen with BHA supplementation in this model and using these semipurified diets. Further studies using this methodology and testing the time factor of uptake and retention of these antioxidants by mammary gland are in progress to test this hypothesis.

Table VI. BHA Content in Mammary Tissue

Period of Feeding	Tissue Weight (g)	BHT Content (µg/g tissue)	Lipid Content (mg/g tissue)	BHA Content in Lipid (µg/g lipid)
2 weeks	3.26 0.34	0.27 0.02	219.7 87.3	1.44 0.60
3 weeks	6.40 0.84	0.77 0.10	496.6 20.7	1.55 0.15

[a] 86-day-old female Sprague-Dawley rats were fed a low fat diet containing 0.3% BHA.
[b] Mean level S.D. for 6 rats (2 weeks) or 4 rats (3 weeks).

Acknowledgments

The authors wish to thank Ms. Kay Wallace and Ms. Lisa Gropf for
their attention to detail and their excellent skills in the preparation of this manuscript.
   This work was supported in part by NIH/NCI Grant No. CA34143 to
Dr. King.

Literature Cited

1. Horwitt, M. K. In "International Symposium on Vitamin E"
    Shimazono, N.; Takagi, Y., Eds.; Kyoritsu Chippan Co. Ltd.:
    Japan, 1970; p. 45.
2. Dam, H. Pharmacol. Rev. 1957, 9, 1-16.
3. Bieri, J. G.; Briggs, G. M.; Pollard, C. J.; Spivey-Fox, M.R.
    J. Nutri. 1960, 70, 47-52.
4. Witting, L. A. Arch. Biochem. Biophys. 1969, 129, 142-151.
5. Vasington, F. D.; Reichard, S. M.; Nason, A. Vitam. Horm. 1960,
    18, 43-87.
6. Mohrhauer, H.; Holman, R. T. J. Lipid Res. 1963, 4, 151-9.
7. Aaes-Jorgensen, E. Physiol. Rev. 1961, 41, 1-51.
8. Witting, L. A. Am. J. Clin. Nutr. 1979, 27, 952-9.
9. Wynder, E. L. Fed. Proc. 1976, 35, 1309-15.
10. Carroll, K. K.; Khor, H. T. Cancer Res. 1970, 30, 2260-4.
11. Tannenbaum, A.; Silverstone, H. Cancer Res. 1949, 9, 162-73.
12. Carroll, K. K.; Khor, H. T. Lipids 1971, 6, 415-20.
13. King, M. M.; Bailey, D. M.; Gibson, D. D.; Pitha, J. V.; McCay,
    P. B. J. Natl. Cancer Inst. 1979, 63, 657-63.
14. Tannenbaum, A. Cancer Res. 1945, 5, 616-25.
15. Silverstone, H.; Tannenbaum, A. Cancer Res. 1950, 10, 448-53.
16. Tannenbaum, A.; Silverstone, H. In "Cancer"; Raven, R. W., Ed.;
    Butterworth: London, 1957; Vol. 1, pp. 306-34.
17. Engel, R. W.; Copeland, D. H. Cancer Res. 1951, 11, 180-3.
18. Chan, P. C.; Dao, T. L. Cancer Res. 1981, 41, 164-7.
19. Wattenberg, L. W. J. Natl. Cancer Inst. 1978, 60, 11-18.
20. Clapp, N. K.; Tyndall, R. L.; Satterfield, L. C.; Klima, W. C.;
    Bowles, N. W. J. Natl. Cancer Inst. 1978, 61, 177-82.
21. Clapp, N. K.; Bowles, N. D.; Satterfield, L. C.; Klima, W. C.
    J. Natl. Cancer Inst. 1979, 63, 1081-5.
22. Witschi, H. P. Toxicology 1981, 21, 95-104.
23. Paine, A. J.; McLean, A. E. M. Biochem. Pharmacol. 1973, 22,
    2875-80.
24. Rikans, L. E.; Gibson, D. D.; McCay, P. B.; King, M. M. Food
    Cosmet. Toxicol. 1981, 19, 89-92.
25. Allen, J. R.; Engblom, J. F. Food Cosmet. Toxicol. 1972, 10,
    769-79.
26. Kahl, R.; Wulff, U. Toxicol. Appl. Pharmacol. 1979, 47, 217-27.
27. King, M. M.; McCay, P. B. Food Cosmet. Toxicol. 1981, 19, 13-
    18.
28. Benson, T.; Lev, M. Cancer 1956, 16, 135-7.
29. Rikans, L. E.; Gibson, D. D.; McCay, P. B. Biochem. Pharmacol.
    1979, 28, 3039-42.
30. Tamulski, T. S.; Morreal, C. E.; Dao, T. L. Cancer Res. 1973,
    33, 3117-22.

31. Dao, T. L.; Sinha, O. K. J. Natl. Cancer Inst. 1972, 49, 591-3.
32. Fysh, J. M.; Okey, A. B. Biochem. Pharmacol. 1978, 27, 2968-72.
33. Greiner, J. A.; Bryan, A. H.; Malan-Shibley, L. B.; Janss, D. H. J. Natl. Cancer Inst. 1980, 64, 1127-33.
34. Creaver, P. J.; Davies, W. H.; Williams, R. T. J. Pharm. Pharmacol. 1966, 18, 485-9.
35. King, M. M.; McCay, P. B.; Russo, I. H. "Diet Nutrition and Cancer: From Basic Research to Policy Implications"; Alan R. Liss Inc.: New York, 1983; pp. 61-90.
36. McCay, P. B.; King, M. M.; Pitha, J. V. Cancer Res. 1981, 41, 3745-8.
37. Black, H. S.; Kleinhaus, C. M.; Hudson, H. T.; Sayre, R. M.; Agen, P. P. Photochem. Photobiophys. 1980, 1, 119-23.
38. Collins, A. J.; Sharratt, M. Food Cosmet. Toxicol. 1970, 8, 409-12.
39. Bligh, E. G.; Dyer, W. J. Can. J. Biochem. Physiol. 1959, 37, 911-17.
40. Terao, J.; Magarian, R. A.; Brueggemann, G.; King, M. M. Anal. Biochem. 1984, in press.
41. Golder, W. S.; Ryan, A. J.; Wright, S. E. J. Pharm. Pharmacol. 1962, 14, 268-71.
42. Astill, B. D.; Fassett, D. W.; Roundabush, R. L. Biochem. J. 1960, 75, 543-51.

RECEIVED March 15, 1985

Modulation of Benzo[a]pyrene Metabolism by Dietary Sulfur Amino Acids

EDWARD L. WHEELER, DANIEL E. SCHWASS, LADELL CRAWFORD, and DAVID L. BERRY

Western Regional Research Center, Agricultural Research Service, U.S. Department of Agriculture, Albany, CA 94710

Nutritional and nutritional status markedly influence xenobiotic metabolism in laboratory animals. Microsomes were prepared from the livers of rats which had been fed chow or modified AIN-76 diets with or without oxidized or unoxidized sulfur amino acids for 7 days. The pattern of benzo(a)pyrene (BaP) metabolites formed by each microsomal preparation in the presence of a NADPH-generating system was determined using high performance liquid chromatography (HPLC). The results indicate that oxidized sulfur amino acids induce different forms of cytochromes P-450 in rat liver which are reflected by different BaP metabolic profiles.

It is well established that diet can play a part in the cancer process (1,2,3). Food-borne chemicals, either additives or "natural", can induce profound changes in monooxygenase systems of the liver and gastrointestional tract, especially (but not exclusively), in the various cytochrome P-450 isoenzymes responsible for the initial oxidation steps in xenobiotic metabolism (4,5,6,7,8). Constitutive forms of cytochrome P-450 may be repressed while other forms are induced. It is the induced forms, particularly cytochrome P-448 or aryl hydrocarbon hydroxylase, that are primarily responsible for converting aromatic hydrocarbons such as benzo(a)pyrene (BaP), a compound prevalent in fried and broiled meats and cigarette smoke, into highly carcinogenic metabolites (9,10,11).

In addition to cytochrome P-450 induction, other diet induced metabolic effects are likely to be involved in carcinogenesis. High temperature processing or long-term storage of foods with attendant exposure to oxygen can lead to the formation of lipid peroxides and oxidized sulfur amino acids in the food. The partially oxidized S-amino acids cystine monoxide (CMO) and methionine sulfoxide (MSO) are nutritionally available, but require in vivo conversion to the reduced amino acids at the

expense of NADH and NADPH (11, 12, 13). Lipid peroxides promote
the oxidation of S-amino acids and many other cellular
components, and are detoxified in vivo at the expense of reduced
glutathione (GSH) (14,15). This information leads to the
hypothesis that diversion of cellular reducing equivalents to the
reduction of oxidized dietary protein or lipid may effect a
nutritional stress on the animal that detracts from or alters its
ability to metabolize xenobiotics such as BaP via NADPH dependent
cytochromes P-450 reactions.

This preliminary work demonstrates that dietary oxidized
S-amino acids do lead to altered BaP metabolism by liver
microsomes under in vitro conditions of excess NADPH and O_2.

Materials and Methods

Male Sprague Dawley rats, seven days post weanling (Bantin and
Kingman, Inc., Fremont, CA) were fed pelleted rodent chow (5001,
Ralston Purina Co., St. Louis, MO) or modified AIN-76 diets
(BioServ, Inc., Frenchtown, NJ) with or without added sulfur
amino acids . Chow, diets, and water were supplied to the rats
ad libitum. The AIN-76 diet (16) was modified to contain 12%
casein (normally 20% casein), and the weight difference made up
with cornstarch. The normal methionine supplement was not
included. The cornstarch and sucrose portions were held
separately from the casein/vitamin/mineral (CVM) mixture for the
purpose of mixing amino acids with the cornstarch and sucrose
(CsS). Methionine (MET), methionine sulfoxide (MSO) and cysteine
sulfinic acid (CSA) were obtained from Sigma Chemical Co., St.
Louis, MO. Cysteine monoxide (CMO) was prepared by the method of
Savige et al., (17).

Amino acid additions to the diets (if any) were accomplished
by progressively mixing small amounts of the amino acid and CsS
in a mortar until all of the amino acid was added. The CsS/amino
acid mixture was transferred to a Hobart N-50 mixer (Troy, OH)
and the remainder of the CsS and CVM were added and mixed. The
level of supplementation of sulfur amino acids to the diets was
equivalent to 3.63 mmoles amino acid/100 gm diet. Six animals
were held on each diet for seven days before they were sacrificed
by cervical dislocation. The livers were immediately removed,
pooled with others in the group, weighed, minced and homogenized
in 3 x w/v buffer (pH 7.2, 0.05 M potassium phosphate, 0.025 M
potassium chloride, 0.0025 M magnesium chloride,0.25 M sucrose).
Microsomes were prepared by the method of Mazel (18) as modified
by Wheeler (19), and cytochrome P-450 levels determined by the
method of Omura and Sato using an absorptivity constant of 91
$mM^{-1}cm^{-1}$. Protein was determined by the method of Lowry using
bovine serum albumin (Fraction V, Sigma Chemical Co., St. Louis,
MO) as a standard. A Perkin-Elmer Model 320 (Norwalk, CT) was
used for spectrophotometric measurements.

BaP (Sigma Chemical Co., St. Louis, MO) was oxidized at $37^{\circ}C$
under a blanket of O_2 by microsomal cytochrome P-450 in a
reaction mixture containing 0.03 M Mg^{++}, 30 mg
glucose-6-phosphate (Sigma), 1 mg NADPH (P-L Biochemicals,
Milwaulkee, WI), 8 units glucose-6-phosphate dehydrogenase

(Sigma) and 1 nmole cytochrome P-450. These components were diluted to a total volume of 2.0 ml with 0.05 potassium phosphate, pH 7.4. The reaction was started by adding 60 nmole BaP (15 μl of a 1 mg/ml solution in acetonitrile). After 15 min, the mixture was saturated with sodium chloride and extracted three times with 4.0 ml cold ethyl acetate: acetone (2.5:1). The aqueous and organic layers were separated by centrifugation and the combined organic fractions evaporated under a stream of nitrogen. The residue was dissolved in 300 μl methanol and 25 μl of this solution was separated using a Spectra-Physics SP8700 liquid chromatograph (Santa Clara, CA) fitted with a 25 cm., 5 micron C-18 column (Rainin Inst. Co., Woburn, MA) and equipped with a variable wavelength detector (Spectro-monitor III, Laboratory Data Control, Riviera Beach, FL) and a fluorescence detector (Model 420-C, Waters Assoc., Inc., Milford, MA). Samples were not filtered before injection because certain metabolites, especially the diols and an unknown compound eluting just before the 7,8- diol, absorbed to both nylon 66 and PTFE filters .

A methanol-water rate gradient was developed which separated the standard BaP metabolites (received from the National Cancer Institute Chemical Carcinogen Reference Standard Repository, a function of the Division of Cancer Cause and Prevention, NCI, Bethesda, MD 20205) and re-equilibrated the column in about 30 min. A diagram of the gradient is shown in Figure 1. A mixture of BaP metabolite standards was separated using this system and eluted in the following order: 7,8-diol-9,10-epoxide and 9,10-diol (overlapping peaks); 4,5-diol; 7,8-diol; 1,6-dione; 3,6-dione; 4,5-epoxide; 6,12- dione; 9-hydroxy; 6-hydroxy and 1-hydroxy (overlapping peaks); 3-hydroxy; and unchanged BaP. The 4,5-diol and 4,5-epoxide were quantified by UV absorbance at 255 nm, and the other compounds by fluorescence intensity at 450 nm. Metabolites from extracted reaction mixtures were identified and quantified by comparison with standard mixtures of known concentration.

Organic solvents used for liquid chromatography were from OmniSolv (MCB Manufacturing Chemists, Inc., Cincinnati, OH) and water was distilled, deionized and filtered through a 0.2μ nylon 66 membrane (Rainin). All chemicals with no source identified were of reagent grade.

RESULTS AND DISCUSSION

Microsomes from rats fed diets deficient in methionine and containing added methionine have the lowest levels of cytochrome P-450, the modified AIN-76 (methionine deficient) diet apparently causing a depression in the level of cytochrome P-450 compared to the control (AIN/MET) diet (Table I). The other diets induced cytochrome P-450 in the livers, including the chow diet which induced cytochrome P-450 approximately twice as much as any of the other diets. In addition, chow and AIN/CSA shifted the cytochrome P-450-CO reduced difference-spectra peak to 449.3 nm, indicating that a significant amount of cytochrome P-448 was induced by these diets. In the case of the rodent chow, oxidized lipids as well as oxidized sulfur amino acids could be

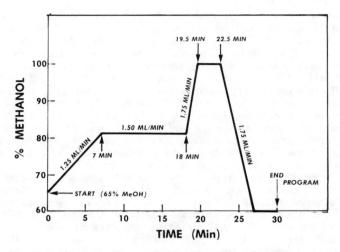

Fig. 1. Solvent program (methanol-H$_2$O) for HPLC separation
of BaP metabolites at 21°C.

TABLE I

DIFFERENCES IN CYTOCHROMES P-450 INDUCTION AS A FUNCTION OF DIET

DIET	REDUCED CO ABS MAX (NM)	µM P-450	NMOLE P-450 PER MG P
CHOW	449.3	5.30	0.64
*AIN	450	1.25	0.31
**AIN/MET	450	1.60	0.38
AIN/MSO	450	2.34	0.40
AIN/CMO	450	3.00	0.45
AIN/CSA	449.3	2.31	0.40

*The modified AIN-76 diet described under "Methods"

**AIN/MET as the "control" diet throughout the work

responsible for the induction and peak shift. One implication of this result is that investigators studying cytochrome P-450 induction should be wary of using commercial chow as a control diet.

A typical fluorescence chromatogram of BaP metabolites is shown in Figure 2. The non-fluorescing (thus not shown) 4,5-diol elutes at 10.2 min between the unknown compound (C) and the 7,8-diol (D). If any 6-hydroxy BaP had been found, it would have eluted just before the 1-hydroxy peak (K). Two of the metabolites that are particularly interesting are the tetrols (A) and the unidentified peak (C), in that there are major differences among the various microsomes in the quantities of these compounds which were formed (Table II). The tetrols, which arise from the unstable, highly carcinogenic 7,8 diol, 9,10 epoxide (20), were conspicuously absent from reaction mixtures from the AIN/MET and AIN/MSO microsomes. The tetrols were always present in the other four cases, however, and were highest from the chow microsome reaction mixtures. The implication is that dietary stress such as may be incurred by the presence of oxidized lipids (chow) or the absence of essential amino acids (methionine), may play a role in the oncogenic process by the induction of different forms of cytochrome P-450 and/or the supression of constitutive forms. The unknown peak (C) in Figure 1 may also prove to be important. The BaP metabolism catalyzed by the control (AIN/MET) microsomes yielded no more than a trace of peak C, while the diet not supplemented with methionine (AIN) and the cysteine sulfinic acid-supplemented diet (AIN/CSA) had measurable amounts. Levels of peak C were highest in the cases of the other three diets (chow, AIN/MSO and AIN/CMO), especially for AIN/MSO and AIN/CMO. In this case, the dietary stress may have arisen from the need for CMO and MSO to be reduced back to the free amino acid forms for use by the rat. This unknown compound may have been overlooked by other investigators using UV absorption for the detection of metabolites because it has a very low absorptivity constant at 255 nm. and is unstable. Most of the fluorescence at this retention time disappears after overnight sample storage at -10°C.

The microsomes from the CMO-fed rats produced the most striking differences in metabolic profile compared to the control microsomes. The data shown in Table III and Fig 3 (for clarity) demonstrate that microsomes from animals fed the cysteine monoxide diet (AIN/CMO) are far more efficient at metabolizing BaP (more BaP oxidized per mole cytochrome P-450/unit time) than are microsomes from rats fed the control diet (AIN/MET). Lower recovery of BaP and metabolites was obtained from the microsomes of the AIN/CMO-fed rats compared to the AIN/M-fed rats (87 to 91%) and a control run containing no NADPH (94% recovery). This result is probably due to the fact that the tetrols and the unknown metabolite, both present in much greater amounts in the CMO case than in the MET (control) case, are not quantifiable, and thus have not been considered in the calculations. Microsomes from the chow-fed rats behaved similarly to the microsomes from AIN/CMO-fed rats, while the other cases showed intermediate values of recovery (data not shown). In every case,

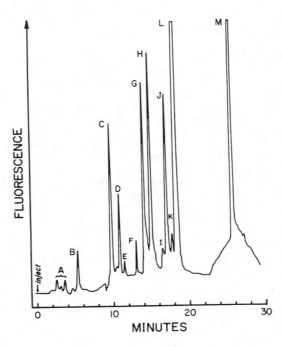

Figure 2. Fluorescence chromatogram of BaP metabolites formed
by microsomes from livers of rats fed the diets described in
"Methods". Key: A, various tetrols; B, 9,10 dihydrodiol;
C, unknown; D, 7,8 dihydrodiol; E, unkown; F, extraneous microsomal
material; G, 1,6 quinone; H, 3,6 quinone; I, 6,12 quinone;
J, 9 hydroxy; K, 1 hydroxy; L, 3 hydroxy; M, unchanged BaP.

TABLE II

Relative Differences in the Amounts of Tetrols and a Major
Unknown Metabolite Formed by Microsomes from Livers of
Rats Fed Various Diets

	CHOW	AIN	AIN/M	AIN/MSTO	AIN/CMO	AIN/CSA
Total* Tetrols	3700	2150	trace	trace	3000	3500
Unkown* Peak D	8865	1483	trace	10,170	10,070	2860

*Arbitrary Integration units

TABLE III

Dietary Influence on Microsomal BaP Metabolism

METABOLITE OF BaP	Diet AIN/M		AIN/CMO		CONTROL*
	nmoles	% of Total	nmoles	% of Total	
9,10 Diol	.039	0.84	.065	1.50	----
4,5 Diol	.048	1.06	.050	1.16	----
7,8 Diol	.007	0.16	.016	0.37	----
1,6 Quinone	.053	1.18	.093	2.15	----
3,6 Quinone	.071	1.57	.169	3.91	----
9-OH	.013	0.30	.021	0.49	----
1-OH	.015	0.33	.029	0.67	----
3-OH	.152	3.37	.251	5.80	----
Parent BaP	4.11	91.1	3.63	84	4.66
Totals	4.51		4.32		4.66
% Recovery**	91		87		94

*No NADPH added to the original reaction mixture.

**nmoles of unchanged BaP plus all metabolites = 4.96 nmoles if 100% recovery

the major metabolite was 3-OH BaP, followed by the 3,6 and the 1,6 quinones.

The results depicted in figures 4, 5, and 6 perhaps best demonstrate the differences in BaP metabolism among the microsomes from rats fed the various diets. The nmoles of the listed metabolites in each case are compared with the nmoles of metabolites found for the AIN/MET control diet, which were arbitrarily assigned a value of 1.0. The most notable differences appear to be: CSA and CMO supplemented diets led to more of all the metabolites than the MET supplemented diet, as did MSO and chow to a lesser extent; and the highly reactive (on a cellular level) 7, 8-diol and 1,6 and 3,6 quinones were found at much higher levels in the CSA and CMO cases (and chow also) than in the MET case . The variation among the various diets in the amounts of the primary metabolic product 3-OH BaP formed (Figure 6) is not large compared to variations in the other secondary products such as the 7,8 diol (Figure 4), quinones (Figure 5), and tetrols (shown in Table II). Therefore it is the secondary oxidation reactions that are significantly altered by diets containing oxidized S-amino acids.

The major point shown by this preliminary study is that various oxidized sulfur amino acids in the diet induce different forms of cytochrome P-450 in rat livers which, in equimolar amounts, have different efficiencies and yield different BaP metabolite profiles _in vitro_. An illation that may be drawn from these results is that eating partially oxidized foods may lead to carcinogen activation via the dietary induction or alteration of various forms and relative quantities of cytochromes P-450 and related activities.

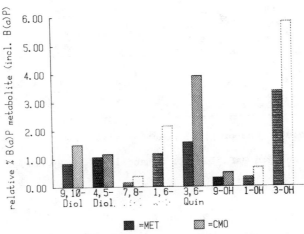

Fig. 3.   Relative % of BaP metabolites (including unreacted BaP) formed by microsomes from rats fed AIN/MET and AIN/CMO diets.

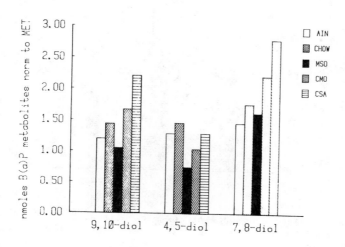

Figure 4.   Relative amounts of BaP metabolites, 9,10-diol, 4,5-diol, and 7,8-diol, formed by the five test diets normalized to the control AIN/MET diet.

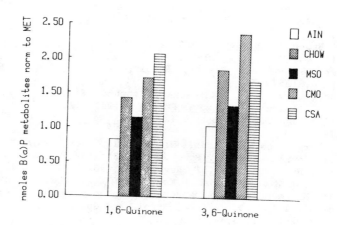

Figure 5.   Relative amounts of BaP metabolites, 1,6-quinone and 3,6-quinone, formed by the five test diets normalized to the control AIN/MET diet.

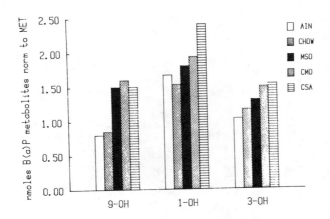

Figure 6. Relative amounts of BaP metabolites, 9-OH, 1-OH, and 3-OH, formed by the five test diets normalized to the control AIN/MET diet.

LITERATURE CITED

1. Ames, Bruce N., _Science_, 1983; 221: 1256.
2. Newell, Guy R., _Cancer_, 1983; 51: 2420.
3. Palmer, Sushma and Bakshi, Kulbir, _J. Natl Cancer Inst._, 1983; 70: 1153.
4. Pascoe, Gary A., Sakai-Wong, Joanne, Soliven, Eva and Correia, Almira M., _Biochem. Pharma._, 1983, 32: 3207.
5. Hendrich, S. and Bjeldanes, L.F., _Fd. Chem. Toxicol._, 1983; 21:479.
6. Wattenberg, Lee W., Loub, William D., Lam, Luke K., and Speier, Jennine L., _Fed. Proc._, 1976; 35: 1327.
7. Gelboin, Harry V., _Physiol. Rev._, 1980; 60:1107.
8. Hennig, Eva E., Dobrzanski, Krzysztof K., Sawicki, Jozef T., Mojska, Hanna and Kujawa, Marek, _Carcinogenesis_, 1983; 4:1243.
9. Robertson, Iain G.C., Zeiger, Errol, and Goldstein, Joyce A., _Carcinogenesis_, 1983; 4: 93.
10. Parke, Dennis V., _Biochem Soc. Trans_, 1983; 11:457.
11. Levin, W., Wood, A.W., Lu, A.Y.H., Ryan, D., West, S., Conney, A.H., Thakker, D.R., Yagi, H., and Jerina, D.M., _A.C.S. Symp. Series_, 1977; 44:99.
12. Aymard, C., Seyer, L., and Cheftel, J.C., _Agric. Biol. Chem._, 1979; 43:1869.
13. Crawford, L., Finley, J.W., and Robbins, K., _Nutr. Reports International_ 1984; 29:791

14. Plummer, J.L., Smith, B.R., Sies, H., and Bend, J.R., <u>Methods in Enzymology</u>, 1981; 77:50.
15. Sies, H., Akerboom, T.P.M., and Cadenas, E., <u>Biochem. Soc. Trans</u>., 1982; 10;79.
16. Second Report of Ad Hoc Committee on Standards for Nutritional Studies. <u>J. Nutrition</u>, 1980; 110:1726.
17. Savige, W.E., Eager, J., Maclaren, J.A., Rexburgh, C.M., <u>Tetrahedron Letters</u>, 1964; 44, 3389.
18. Mazel, P., in "Fundamentals of Drug Metabolism and Drug Disposition", B.N., LaDu, G.H., Mandel, E.L. Way, eds., Williams and Wilkins Co., Baltimore, MD., 1972; 546.
19. Wheeler, E.L., <u>Biochem. Biophys. Res. Comm</u>., 1983; 110:646.
20. Phillips, D.H., Sims, Peter, in "Chemical Carcinogens and DNA", Philip L. Grover, ed., CRC Press, Inc., Boca Raton, Fla., 1979.

RECEIVED October 8, 1984

Dietary Factors Affecting Biological Responses to Esophageal and Colon Chemical Carcinogenesis

PAUL M. NEWBERNE

Massachusetts Institute of Technology, Cambridge, MA 02139

Cancer of the esophagus and colon are frequent in populations of the western world and are associated with diet and lifestyle. There is also a high incidence of esophageal cancer in some areas of developing countries; these areas are restricted to relatively small geographic locations within countries and support the concept that the etiology is related to the environment. In the United States and in other western countries esophageal cancer is correlated with alcohol and tobacco consumption. In developing countries correlations exist between malnutrition and environmental contaminants. The incidence of colon cancer is high in western populations except for Japan and low in most developing nations. The high incidence is associated with high dietary fat. Low fiber intake has also been associated with the high colon cancer incidence in some populations. The epidemiologic data, relative to dietary fiber, has been supported by animal studies but experiments with dietary fat have been conflicting and generally do not indicate a fat effect. Other dietary factors which associate with colon cancer in animal studies are deficits of lipotropes and of vitamin A.

Cancer of the esophagus is not amenable to satisfactory surgical or chemical intervention and must therefore be addressed by searching for preventative measures. This type of neoplasm provides a unique epidemiologic model for the study of cancer causation and offers a means to learn more about initiation and promotion of this unique tumor.

The incidence of esophageal cancer varies widely in different areas of the world (1). There is as much as 300-fold variation from areas of low incidence to that of the highest rates in places such as the southern Caspian littoral in Iran, the Transkei in South Africa and in some parts of China. These epidemiological observations provide opportunities to identify environmental factors and to test these real or potential factors in appropriate animal models (2).

0097–6156/85/0277–0163$06.00/0

A number of investigators have found a consistent relationship between mortality from esophageal cancer and ethanol consumption (3-5). These observations have been supported by case-control studies (6-8) which have shown strong correlations between alcohol consumption and esophageal cancer but without consistent association with any specific type of beverage (9,10).

Alcohol consumption cannot account for the pattern of esophageal cancer in Asia and Africa, however (11-13). Correlation studies in Iran suggest that the intakes of pulses, green vegetables, fresh fruit, animal protein, vitamin A, vitamin C and riboflavin are lower in areas of high risk (14,15). Similar studies in China have implicated low intakes of trace elements (molybdenum), animal products, fruits and vegetables, fat, calcium, and riboflavin (13). There was also a reported concomitant intake of foods contaminated with N-nitroso compounds and fungal toxins. Marasas et al (16) have also reported mycotoxin contamination of foods in areas of South Africa where a high incidence of esophageal cancer is found.

Lin et al (17) observed low concentrations of zinc in serum, hair, and esophageal tissue in patients with other types of cancer or with other diseases (Table I).

Table I. Zinc Levels in Serum, Hair and Esophageal Tissues From Esophageal Cancer Patients

| | Zinc Concentrations (g/100 ml or g) | | | |
| | | | Esophageal | |
	Serum	Hair	Tumor	Esophagus
Normal Subjects	102.7±18.5	195.0±29.0	110.0±22.4	160.0±28.7
Patients With:				
Esophageal Cancer	78.0±14.9	162.0±33.0	---	---
Other Cancers	114.4±31.8	169.0±37.0	---	---
Other Disorders[a]	96.2±15.0	212.0±48.0	149.0±18	248.0±17.0

[a]Taken from data on accidental deaths, unrelated to the esophageal cancer study. Lin et al., 1977, abridged.

In summary, alcohol, tobacco, and a number of dietary nutrients and contaminants have been implicated in esophageal cancer by epidemiological studies in several different geographic areas of the world where this type tumor is found in high incidence in human populations. Currently, there are no convincing data available for specific etiologic factors but some are suggested from epidemiologic observations; these are now being tested in animal models. Results of some of these studies will be briefly described below.

Studies have been designed to test the suggestions of Lin et al (17) that zinc deficiency, which alone damages the esophagus, enhances chemically-induced esophageal cancer. In a series of studies in rats, using methylbenzylnitrosamine (MBN) as the carcinogen we have clearly shown that dietary zinc deficiency lowers the concentration of zinc in serum, hair and esophageal tissues, and markedly enhances the induced esophageal cancer (18-20). Table II lists data typical of results from our earlier studies. Zinc levels were significantly lower in the serum, hair and esophagus of zinc-deficient rats, with or without treatment with MBN. Zinc deficiency alone or MBN alone resulted in lowered esophageal zinc concentration. Both dietary deficiency and treatment with MBN severely depleted esophageal zinc content.

Table II. Zinc Levels in Rats Fed a Zinc Deficient Diet and Treated With Methylbenzylnitrosamine (MBN)[a]

	Serum (µg/100 ml)	Hair (ppm)	Esophagus (ppm)
Control	101.9 ± 12.7	223.7 ± 25.5	211.3 ± 38.8
Control + MBN	124.4 ± 12.9	202.8 ± 11.4	156.2 ± 12.3
Zinc Deficient	38.3 ± 11.6	165.2 ± 15.2	136.6 ± 16.8
Zinc Deficient + MBN	46.8 ± 15.5	160.8 ± 15.6	126.0 ± 37.2

[a]Differences in zinc concentrations of serum and hair of control and zinc deficient groups significant p < 0.01. Data expressed as mean ± S.D.

Table III lists results of carcinogenicity studies associated with zinc deficiency. These rats were given 17 doses of MBN, beginning at seven weeks of age. Fifty eight days after the first dose of MBN, all zinc-deficient rats had developed tumors of the esophagus, 83% of which were invasive carcinomas. Five weeks later, all deficient rats had tumors, 33% of which were invasive, clearly, a marked enhancement of carcinogenesis by zinc deficiency.

Table III. Esophageal Tumor Incidence in Control and Zinc Deficient Rats Exposed to Methylbenzylnitrosamine

Diet	MBN, mg/kg Body Wt.	Time, 1st Dose MBN to Sacrifice	Tumor Incidence No./% Carcinoma	Papilloma
Zinc Deficient ad libitum	34	58	5/6(83)	6/6(100)
Control, Pair-fed	34	58	0/6(0)	2/6(33)
Zinc Deficient ad libitum	34	93	4/12(33)	12/12(100)
Control, Pair-fed	34	93	0/12	8/12(66)

From Fong et al., 1978, by permission. Consult reference for details.

In follow-up studies (19) with an additional risk factor (alcohol) the results confirmed earlier observations and additional significant findings. Table IV lists the salient features of the study. Zinc deficiency significantly enhanced carcinogenesis. Alcohol tended to further enhance cancer incidence and 13-cis retinoic acid offered no protection. Switching the zinc deficient group from deficient (7 ppm Zn) to the control diet (60 ppm) after exposure to the carcinogen afforded significant protection, indicating protective effects during both the initiation and the promotion stages of carcinogenesis.

A partial explanation for the effects of alcohol on zinc status may reside in the observations that: 1) alcohol increases zinc excretion (21), and 2) the increased zinc excretion precipitates a crisis resulting in a conditioned deficiency in the esophagus and greater susceptibility to carcinogenesis.

Table IV. Tumor Incidence Induced by MBN in Rats Deficient in Zinc
           and Given Ethyl Alcohol and 13-cis Retinoic Acid

Treatment, Zinc Content	MBN	4% Alcohol in Drinking Water	13-cis Retinoic Acid	No. Rats With Tumors, %	
Control, 60 ppm	-	-	-	0/12	0
Control, 60 ppm	+	-	-	14/35	40.0
Deficient, 7 ppm	+	-	-	25/33	75.7
60 ppm Control, Deficient 7 ppm to Post Dosing	+	-	-	18/35	51.4
Deficient	+	+	-	29/34	85.3
Deficient	+	+	+	33/35	94.3

From Gabrial et al., 1982, abridged.

In comparing the tissue zinc concentration in rats fed either a
marginally zinc-deficient diet or a zinc-deficient diet plus alcohol
we have observed that the simple addition of alcohol precipitated an
acute deficiency with accompanying esophageal lesions (Table V) (22).
There is also clinical evidence in human patients (21) for an enhanced excretion of zinc following consumption of alcohol, which has
been supported by studies in rats (23)(Table VI). A marginal deficiency of zinc, when interacting with alcohol consumption quickly
progressed to an acute deficiency with the typical histologic lesion
of parakeratosis occurring; this did not appear with the marginal
deficiency alone.

Table V. Comparison of Tissue Zinc Concentration and Esophageal
          Epithelium Changes in Zinc Deficient Alcohol (ZDA) Diet
          Fed Rats and Their Corresponding Zinc Deficient (ZD)
          Fed Controls

	Tissue Zinc Concentration (μg/gm Wet Wt.)		Esophageal Histologic Findings Parakeratosis
	Liver	Hair	
Baseline Animals	25.5±2.9	212.4±23.8	
ZD Diet Fed Animals	11.6±0.5	146.4±09.0	1 (11%)
ZDA Diet Fed Animals	9.0±0.5	110.0±18.3	7 (78%)

From Mobarhan et al., 1984 .

Table VI. Fecal Zinc Excretion (μg/day) in Zinc Deficient Ethanol
          (ZDE) Fed Animals and Their Corresponding Pair-Fed Zinc
          Deficient (ZD) Controls*

	ZDE (μg/day)	ZD (μg/day)	P Value
Day 0	51.3 ± 5.6	51.3 ± 5.6	NS
Day 7	31.7 ± 11.9	17.9 ± 9.5	< .001
Day 14	29.1 ± 17.6	12.3 ± 7.2	< .003
Day 21	24.4 ± 9.6	12.9 ± 3.8	< .002
Day 28	36.9 ± 18.3	15.7 ± 10.7	< .007

*Seven pairs of animals were studied. Numbers are expressed as mean
± S.D. and P values are derived from a paired T-test comparison.
Each data point consists of an average of 3 days; e.g. day 7 repre-
sents an average excretion from days 6, 7, and 8. (23).

Additional studies have further supported a role for zinc in the etiology of cancer of the esophagus (24,25). In the presence of a zinc deficit, the precursors of methylbenzylnitrosamine (MBN) more readily induced both esophageal and forestomach tumors in rats, compared to zinc-supplemented control rats. Table VII illustrates these effects.

Table VII. Incidence of Tumors in the Esophagus and Forestomach in Zinc-Deficient and Zinc-Sufficient Rats Fed Concurrently MBA and NaNO$_2$ in Drinking Water for 37 Weeks

Group	Diet	Weight (g)	Tumor Incidence	
			Carcinoma	Papilloma
IIa 0.05% MBA + 0.5% NaNO$_2$	Zn-Deficient ad libitum	209 ± 62	4/18	12/18
	Zn-Sufficient ad libitum	290 ± 73	2/6	5/6

From Fong et al., 1984, abridged.

Further studies with zinc deficiency have demonstrated that the deficiency state not only enhances esophageal carcinogenicity of MBN but can also change the target site for carcinogenesis by another carcinogen. N-nitrosodimethylamine (DMN), an accepted carcinogen for the liver and the kidney, depending on the dose schedule (26) will induce tumors of the esophagus and the forestomach in zinc deficient rats (27,28).

We have fed control and zinc-deficient rats their respective diets and administered N-nitrosodimethylamine (DMN) at a dose level of 2 mg/kg twice weekly for 3 weeks followed by 4 mg/kg of the same carcinogen for another 5 weeks, a total of 52 mg/kg. After 45 weeks none of the control rats had developed esophageal or forestomach lesions but, as shown in Table VIII, most of the zinc-deficient rats developed forestomach lesions or tumors (28). Mechanisms for this interesting observation are unclear but the underlying toxicology probably resides in metabolism affecting the site of tumor occurrence and type of activation of DMN.

Table VIII. Histopathology of Forestomach of Zn-Deficient Rats Fed DMN

Lesion	Number of Rats (%)
1. Epithelial Changes	
Hyperkeratosis	51(100)
Acanthosis	45 (88)
Focal Parakeratosis, Dyskeratosis, and/or Erosion/Ulceration	23 (45)
2. Tumors	
Junctional	19 (37)
Junctional and Other Areas	13 (25)

From Fong et al., 1984, abridged.

Esophageal cancer can also be influenced by other nutrients. Riboflavin (B_2) deficiency results in severe changes in the epithelium of the oral tissues and esophagus in rats and primates. The effects of riboflavin deficiency in human populations are well known (29,30) but animal models for investigation of consequences of the deficiency have been used very little.

Dr. Henry Foy (personal communication) has drawn attention to the severe effects of riboflavin deficiency in the baboon, with particular attention to the dysplasia of the epithelium of the oral cavity and esophagus. Dr. Foy has pursued these studies for many years at the Wellcome Research Laboratories in Nairobi. We have observed similar lesions in the Rhesus monkey, and have further pursued the effects of riboflavin deficiency in the rat. We have superimposed an esophageal carcinogen (MBN) on the deprived, damaged oral cavity and esophageal epithelium. Table IX lists results of a five month study, emphasizing the profound enhancement the deficiency can have on the esophagus (31).

Table IX. Riboflavin (B_2) Deficiency in the Rat: Enhanced
           Esophageal Carcinogenesis

Treatment	Incidence of Neoplasms	
	No.	%
Control Diet	0/10	0.0
Control Diet + MBN*	8/20	40.0
B_2 Deficiency	0/20	0.0
B_2 Deficiency + MBN	23/26	88.0

*Methylbenzylnitrosamine. Newberne, 1984.

We have not pursued mechanisms but suggest that the enhancement of carcinogenesis may be related to a role for riboflavin in the activation of enzymatic processes involved with metabolic detoxification of MBN, similar to azo reductase and its role in the detoxification of 4-dimethylaminoazobenzene (32). In this case riboflavin activates azo reductase in the liver and this, in turn, is associated with decreased carcinogenicity. Conversely, when animals are deprived of riboflavin, there is less active enzyme present to detoxify the chemical and the induction of liver cancer is enhanced. A similar process may be functioning in our MBN, riboflavin deprived model but the exact nature of the mechanism requires additional research.

Colon Cancer

Studies of the incidence of and mortality from colon cancer at the international level suggest an association of this neoplasm with total dietary fat (33,34). Lui et al (35), studying the disappearance rate of food and mortality from colon cancer between the years 1967-1973 in 20 industrialized countries, concluded that there was a direct correlation of this tumor type and the per capita intake of total fat, saturated and monounsaturated fat and cholesterol. Furthermore, fiber intake was inversely correlated with colon cancer in these studies.

Berg and Howell (36) and Howell (37) reported a high correlation for meat intake and colon cancer, particularly beef. Enstrom, on the other hand (38) suggested that trends in per capita intake of beef and fat in the United States do not correlate with trends in incidence of and mortality from colon cancer. An examination of the crude data support this suggestion since beef consumption (and accompanying fat) have increased about 2-fold during the last 20-30 years but age-adjusted death rates from colon cancer have remained about the same.

Bingham et al (39)   related foods, nutrients and dietary fiber to the regional pattern of death from colon cancer and suggested that the pentosan fraction of dietary fiber was most significant as a protective fiber component. Further to the point of fiber relationships to colon cancer, Malhotra (40) has suggested that the absence of colon cancer among the Punjabis of Northern India is a result of a diet rich in roughage including cellulose and vegetable fiber. There was also a suggestion that short-chain fatty acids in fermented milk products offered some protection.

MacLennan et al (41) reviewed the diets of adult males from Kuopio, Finland and from Copenhagan, Denmark, the latter where the incidence of colon cancer is four times higher than Kuopio. Among other findings they noted that the estimated fat consumption was similar but fiber intake was higher in Kuopio men, associated with lower colon cancer rates.

Selenium has been reported to have a positive, enhancing effect (42) or an inverse correlation between the intake of selenium and colon cancer (43,44). Birt et al (45) have reported inhibition of colon cancer in rats by dietary selenium.

The work of Phillips et al (46-48), Lyon and Sorenson (49), Lyon et al (50) and Kolonel et al (51) have provided convincing arguments for a role of a number of dietary factors in colon cancer in man. The data of Phillips and Snowdon (48) illustrate as well as any the relation of diet to colon cancer in subsets of an American population; the California Adventists. Table X shows the comparable mortality from large bowel cancer in California Adventists comparable to non-Adventists, and all USA whites. Despite a very wide variation in meat use, there is no apparent relationship between meat use and fatal colon cancer. The definitive studies are yet to be done however, and, as noted below, animal studies are also inserting conflicting data into the already confused literature of dietary effects on colon cancer. In terms of epidemiologic data perhaps the NAS document (1) has made the appropriate suggestions to which this investigator would add a disclaimer. The points made by the NAS document are: 1) there may be a causal association of human colon cancer with total, perhaps saturated fat; 2) there may be a protective effect of dietary fiber; and 3) cruciferous vegetables may afford some protection against human colon cancer. All of these presuppositions require confirmation.

In the case of animal studies with colon carcinogenesis, there are equally disquieting hypotheses, none of which have been adequately tested. For example, there are those (52,53) who suggest that dietary fat and fiber, and the consequences of these on such parameters as bile acids and other contributory factors are the key to colon carcinogenesis. These hypotheses are still being tested and preliminary results should be regarded with caution. The animal data, detailed below, will point out both encouraging and discouraging aspects of state of the art experimentation.

Table X.   Large Bowel Age-Adjusted Cancer Mortality/100,000 for
           California Adventists, Non-Adventists and All USA Whites,
           Compared to Their Meat Consumption

Group	Large Bowel Mortality Per 100,000	Meat and Poultry Use Days/Week and Mortality/100,000	
California Adventists	32.6	None	22.7
Comparable Non-Adventists	50.6	1-3 Times Per Week	27.2
All Use Whites	57.5	4 or More	19.1

Compiled from Phillips and Snowdon, 1983, abridged, see reference for
details.

Lipids and Fiber

Some of the earlier, significant publications on the role of dietary
fat in experimental colon cancer are those of Reddy et al (53-57).
These investigators have reported that rats fed 5% corn oil diets had
a higher tumor incidence and a larger number of tumors per animal
than those fed a 5% lard diet.   Tumor incidence and multiplicity increased with higher (20%) fat levels but the incidence and multiplicity of tumors were comparable with corn oil or lard.   Table XI illustrates some of their observations.

Table XI.   Colon Tumor Incidence With Two Levels and Types of
            Dietary Fat

Diet	Colon Tumors(%)	Total Tumors Per Rat
Corn oil, 5%	36	0.77
Lard, 5%	17	0.22
Corn oil, 20%	64	1.55
Lard, 20%	67	1.50
Purina Chow	25	0.25

From Reddy et al., 1976, modified.

One hypothesis linking dietary fat to colon cancer is that cholesterol is converted to bile acids which act as promoters of carcinogenesis (58).   Epidemiological studies have shown however, (38)
that when beef consumption in the United States doubled (between 1940-
1970) the incidence of colon cancer mortality was virtually unchanged.
In addition, the incidence of colon cancer is the same in Seventh Day
Adventists, who eat meat sparingly (59) and Mormons, who consume a
conventional diet (60).
        These epidemiological observations have suggested a metabolic
clue to the effect of fats which may be through fecal steroid metabolism and excretion.   These have been measured in populations at
high and at low risk for colon cancer.   Table XII lists results of
one such investigation.   The absolute amount of steroids excreted is
much lower in control subjects but this could reflect the health
status of the individuals.   In the neutral sterol fraction the ratio
of cholesterol to its metabolites is higher in colon cancer patients,
perhaps indicating inability to metabolize cholesterol.   Comparisons
of fecal steriods in populations of varying susceptibility to colon
cancer have also given variable results.

Table XII.   Fecal Steroids in Three Groups of Subjects
             mg/g Dry Feces

Steroid	Control (40)*	Adenomatous Polyps (15)*	Colon Cancer (35)*
Neutral			
Cholesterol	3.2	6.4	12.6
Coprostanol	12.9	19.6	18.7
Coprostanone	1.9	4.0	3.9
Acidic			
Cholic	0.4	0.4	0.5
Chenodeoxycholic	0.2	0.3	0.5
Deoxycholic	3.7	0.3	7.0
Lithocholic	3.1	5.4	6.5

From Reddy, 1979, abridged.   *Number subjects.

If bile acids are indeed a risk factor in colon carcinogenesis, substances which enhance excretion of bile acids should inhibit the development of colon tumors. This has been tested in experimental animals. Bran and cellulose inhibit DMH-induced colon tumors in rats (61,62). Despite tumor inhibition, neither of these fibers bind bile acids to any appreciable extent (63). Moreover, Nigro et al (64) have shown that cholestyramine, a bile acid-binding resin, when added to the diet of rats given one of three carcinogens significantly increased tumor incidence (Table XIII). These data argue against any direct effect of bile acids on colon tumorigenesis.

Table XIII.   Cholestyramine and Colon Cancer

Carcinogen	Diet	Number of Colon Tumors Proximal	Distal
1,2-Dimethylhydrazine	Normal Diet (ND)	15	1
	Normal Diet + Cholestyramine (NDC)	31	29
Azoxymethane	ND	19	8
	NDC	33	36
Methylazoxymethanol	ND	4	2
	NDC	18	15

From Nigro et al., 1973, abridged

The influence of dietary fiber on colon cancer has been the subject of extensive investigations by epidemiologists and experimental oncologists (65). The results from human populations have been variable; animal investigations have been variable as well but, in general, point to an effect of fiber on induced colon tumors. Table XIV taken from the work of Watanabe et al (66) illustrates results characteristic of many studies. These authors suggest that the effects are related to bile acid binding capacity and that this correlates with severity of mucosal damage. Thus, the bile acid and fiber effects may be mechanical rather than because of metabolic aberrations.

In contrast to some of the results referred to above where increased dietary fat enhanced experimentally induced colon cancer in rats, we have failed to observe an effect of either quality or quantity of fat on induced tumor incidence (67,68). Table XV lists results of studies with three different fats and two different colon carcinogens. The negative nature of these two carefully conducted studies, one of which (DMH) has been repeated with similar results, casts doubt on the significance of dietary fat on colon carcinogenesis. The conflicting data between epidemiological and experimental studies might be explained in a number of ways. Most logical would be the diversity of exposures of humans to environmental factors, compared to a single variable in animal studies.

Table XIV. Dietary Fiber and Colon Cancer in Rats Induced by Two Carcinogens

Fiber (15% of Diet)	Carcinogen and Tumor Incidence (%)	
	Azoxymethanol (AOM)	Methylnitrosourea (NMU)
Control	57.7	69.0
Alfalfa	53.3	83.3
Pectin	10.0	58.6
Bran	33.0	60.0

From Watanabe et al., 1979, abridged.

Table XV. Quality and Quantity of Dietary Fat and Colon Carcino-Genesis With Two Colon Carcinogens

Dietary Fat % (Wt)	Type	Carcinogen/% Colon Tumors	
		DMH	NMU
5	Mixed	77	55
24	Beef Tallow	68	63
24	Corn Oil	63	55
24	Crisco	55	38

From Nauss et al., 1983; 1984, abridged. Each group comprised of 40 rats each.

Lipotropes and Colon Cancer

While there are no epidemiologic data available on lipotropic factors and colon cancer in human populations, results of animal studies suggest a possible role for this class of nutrients (choline, methionine, vitamin B_{12} and folate) in colon carcinogenesis (69). Table XVI lists results typical of those observed when rats are fed a diet high in fat, low in lipotropes and exposed to a colon carcinogen. The lipotropic agents are intimately involved with methylation and it is perhaps through this mechanism that they exert their effects. Aberrant methylation of nucleic acids and a relation to carcinogenesis under a variety of conditions, is currently under intensive investigation in several laboratories (70,71).

Table XVI. Dietary Fat and Rat Colon Tumors Induced by DMH

Diet	Dimethylhydrazine Dose ,mg/kg	Rats With Colon Carcinoma, %	No. of Tumors/Tumor-Bearing Rat
Control	300	86	2.0
High-Fat	300	100	3.7
Control	150	56	1.1
High-Fat	150	85	2.6

From Rogers and Newberne, 1975, abridged.

Vitamin A and Colon Cancer

There is little in the literature relative to vitamin A and colon
cancer in human populations. Experimental animal studies, however,
strongly suggest that vitamin A deficiency may have a role in this
type of cancer. We have shown that a deficiency of vitamin A increased DMH-induced tumors and shortened the lag time for induction,
compared to normally supplemented controls (72). More recently (73)
we have confirmed a protective role for vitamin A in colon carcinogenesis (Table XVII). Furthermore, we have shown (74) that vitamin A
deficiency can result in colon tumors in rats given aflatoxin B_1
(AFB_1) which is normally a liver carcinogen (Table XVIII). The colon
tumors associated with the hepatocarcinogen AFB_1 appear to be a result of differences in metabolism and binding of AFB_1 or its metabo-
lite(s) to colon DNA under conditions of vitamin A deficiency (75).

Table XVII.   Effects of 13-cis Retinoic Acid on DMH-Induced Tumors
in The Rat

Treatment	No. Animals At Risk	No. Animals With Colon Tumors	% With Tumors	Average No. Tumors/ Animal
Control Diet 3.0 µg Retinyl Acetate	20	20	100	3.1
Control Diet 3.0 µg Retinyl Acetate + 67 µg/g 13-cis Retinoic Acid	20	8	40	2.3

From Newberne and Suphakarn, 1977.

Table XVIII.   Vitamin A Status, Aflatoxin B_1, and Liver and Colon
Tumors in Rats

Dietary Retinyl Acetate (µg/g)	AFB_1	No. Rats at Risk	Sex	Tumor Incidence (%)		
				Liver	Colon	Both
Control						
3.0	0	24	M	0.0	0.0	0.0
3.0	0	26	F	0.0	0.0	0.0
3.0	+	24	M	87.5	4.1	4.1
3.0	+	24	F	79.1	8.3	8.3
Low						
0.3	0	10	M	0.0	0.0	0.0
0.3	0	12	F	0.0	0.0	0.0
0.3	+	66	M	89.4	28.8	25.7
0.3	+	42	F	76.2	28.6	11.9
High						
30.0	0	23	M	0.0	0	0
30.0	0	20	F	0	0	0
30.0	+	26	M	92.3	7.7	7.7
30.0	+	31	F	83.9	9.7	6.4

From Newberne and Rogers, 1976.

Literature Cited

1. "Diet, Nutrition and Cancer," National Academy of Sciences, 1982, p. 17-1.
2. Doll, R. Brit J. Cancer 1969, 23, 1-8.
3. Chilvers, C.; Fraser, P.; Beral, V. J. Epidemiol. Community Health 1979, 33, 127-133.
4. Lipworth, L.L.; Rice, C.A. Cancer 1979, 43, 1927-1933.
5. Tuyns, A.J.; Pequignot, G.; Abbatucci, J.S. Int. J. Cancer 1979, 23, 443-447.
6. Keller, A.Z. Prev. Med. 1980, 9, 607-612.
7. Pottern, L.M.; Morris, L.E.; Blot, W.J.; Zeigler, R.G.; Fraumeni, Jr., J.F. J. Natl. Cancer Inst. 1981, 67, 777-783.
8. Schmidt, W.; Popham, R.E. Cancer 1981, 47, 1031-1041
9. Williams, R.R.; Horm, J.W. J. Natl. Cancer Inst. 1977, 58, 525-547.
10. Mettlin, C.; Graham, S.; Priore, R.; Marshall, J.; Swanson, M. Nutr. Cancer 1980, 2, 143-147.
11. Bradshaw, E.; Schonland, M. Br. J. Cancer 1974, 30, 157-163.
12. Gatei, D.G.; Odhiambo, P.A.; Orinda, D.A.O.; Muruka, F.J.; Wasuma, A. Cancer Res. 1978, 38, 303-307.
13. Yang, C.S. Cancer Res. 1980, 40, 2633-2644.
14. Hormozdiari, H.; Day, N.E.; Aramesh, B.; Mahboubi, E. Cancer Res. 1975, 35, 3493-3498.
15. Joint Iran-IARC Study Group. J. Natl. Cancer Inst. 1977, 59, 1127-1138.
16. Marasas, W.F.O.; Van Rensburg, S.J.; Mirocha, C.J. J. Agric. Food Chem. 1979, 27, 1108-1112.
17. Lin, H.J.; Chan, W.C.; Fong, Y.Y.; Newberne, P.M. Nutr. Rpts. Internat. 1977, 15, 635-643.
18. Fong, L.Y.Y.; Sivak, A.; Newberne, P.M. J. Natl. Cancer Inst. 1978, 61, 145-150.
19. Gabrial, G.N.; Schrager, T.F.; Newberne, P.M. J. Natl. Cancer Inst. 1982, 68, 785-789.
20. Newberne, P.M.; Schrager, T.F. Environmental Health Perspectives 1983, 50, 71-83.
21. Russell, R.M. Am. J. Clin. Nutr. 1980, 33, 2741-2745.
22. Mobarhan, S.; Russell, R.M.; Newberne, P.M.; Ahmed, S.B. Nutr. Rpts. Internat. 1984, 29, 639-645.
23. Ahmed, S.B.; Russell, R.M. J. Lab. Clin. Med. 1982, 100, 211-217.
24. Fong, L.Y.Y.; Lee, J.S.K.; Chan, W.C.; Newberne, P.M. In Bartsch, H.; Castegnaro, M.; O'Neill, I.K.; Okada, M., Eds.; IARC SCIENTIFIC PUBLICATIONS No. 41, 1982, pp. 679-683.
25. Fong, L.Y.Y.; Lee, J.S.K.; Chan, W.C.; Newberne, P.M. J. Natl. Cancer Inst. 1984, 72, 419-425.
26. Magee, P.N.; Montesano, R.; Preussmann, R. In "Chemical Carcinogens"; Searle, C.E., Ed.; ACS Monograph No. 173, American Chemical Society: Washington, D.C., 1976.
27. Fong, L.Y.Y.; Ng, W.L.; Newberne, P.M. In "N-Nitroso Compounds"; IARC PROCEEDINGS: Banff, Canada, 1983.
28. Fong, L.Y.Y.; Ng, W.L.; Newberne, P.M. Cancer Letters, 1984, in press.

29. Chandra, R.K.; Newberne, P.M. In "Nutrition, Immunity and Infection: Mechanisms of Interactions"; Chandra, R.K.; Newberne, P.M., Eds.; Raven Press: New York, 1977; p. 246.
30. Greene, H. In "Textbook of Pediatric Nutrition"; Suskind, R.M., Ed.; Raven Press: New York, 1981; pp. 119-120.
31. Newberne, P.M. In "The Toxicologist"; The Society of Toxicology: Akron, 1984.
32. Miller, J.A.; Miller, E.C. Advances in Cancer Res. 1953, 1, 339-396.
33. Armstrong, B.; Doll, R. Internat. J. Cancer 1975, 15, 617-631.
34. Wynder, E.L. Cancer Res. 1975, 35, 3388-3394.
35. Lui, K.; Moss, D.; Persky, V.; Staniler, J.; Garside, D.; Soltero, I. Lancet 1979, 2, 782-785.
36. Berg, J.W.; Howell, M.A. Cancer 1974, 34, 804-814.
37. Howell, M.A. J. Chronic Disease 1975, 28, 67-80.
38. Enstrom, J.E. Brit. J. Cancer 1975, 32, 432-439.
39. Bingham, S.; Williams, D.R.R.; Cole, T.J.; James, W.P.T. Br. J. Cancer 1979, 40, 456-463.
40. Malhotra, S.L. Med. Hypotheses 1977, 3, 122-126.
41. MacLennan, R.; Jensen, O.M.; Mosbech, J.; Vuori, H. Am. J. Clin. Nutr. 1978, 31, 5239-5242.
42. Jansson, B.; Jacobs, M.M.; Griffin, A.C. Adv. Exp. Med. Biol. 1978, 91, 305-322.
43. Schrauzer, G.N.; White, D.A.; Schneider, C.J. Bioinorg. Chem. 1977a, 7, 23-34.
44. Schrauzer, G.N.; White, D.A.; Schneider, C.J. Bioinorg. Chem. 1977b, 7, 35-36.
45. Birt, D.F.; Lawson, T.A.; Julius, A.D.; Runice, C.E.; Salmasi, S. Cancer Res. 1982, 42, 4455-4459.
46. Phillips, R.L.; Kuzma, J.W.; Lotz, T.M. In Banbury Report No. 4, Cold Spring Harbor Lab: New York, 1980a.
47. Phillips, R.L.; Kuzma, J.W.; Beeson, W.L.; Lotz, T. Am. J. Epidemiol. 1980b, 112, 296-314.
48. Phillips, R.L.; Snowdon, D.A. Cancer Res. (Suppl.) 1983, 43, 2403s-2408s.
49. Lyon, J.L.; Sorenson, A.W. Am. J. Clin. Nutr. 1978, 31, 5227-5230.
50. Lyon, J.L.; Gardner, J.W.; West, D.W.; Mahoney, A.M. Cancer Res. (Suppl.) 1983, 43, 2392s-2396s.
51. Kolonel, L.N.; Abraham, M.Y.; Nomura, M.; Ward, H.; Hirohata, T.; Hankin, J.H.; Lee, J. Cancer Res. (Suppl.) 1983, 43, 2397s-2402s.
52. Reddy, B.S.; Hedges, A.R.; Laakso, K.; Wynder, E.L. Cancer 1978, 42, 2832-2838.
53. Reddy, B.S.; Sharma, C.; Darby, L.; Laakso, K.; Wynder, E.L. Mutation Res. 1980, 72, 511-522.
54. Reddy, B.S.; Weisburger, J.H.; Wynder, E.L. J. Natl. Cancer Inst. 1974, 52, 507-511.
55. Reddy, B.S.; Watanabe, K.; Weisburger, J.H. Cancer Res. 1977. 37, 4156-4159.
56. Reddy, B.S. Advances Nutr. Res. 1979, 2, 199-218.
57. Reddy, B.S.; Mangat, S.; Sheinfil, A.; Weisburger, J.H.; Wynder E.L. Cancer Res. 1977, 37, 2132-2137.

58. Kritchevsky, D. In "Molecular Interrelations of Nutrition and Cancer"; Arnott, M.S.; VanEys, J.; Yang, Y.M.; Eds.; Raven Press: New York, 1982; pp. 209-217.
59. Phillips, R.L. Cancer Res. 1975, 35, 3513-3522.
60. Lyon, J.L.; Klauber, M.R.; Gardner, J.W.; Smart, C.R. N. Eng. J. Med. 1976, 294, 129-133.
61. Barbolt, T.A.; Abraham, R. Proc. Soc. Exp. Biol. Med. 1978, 157, 656-659.
62. Freeman, H.J.; Spiller, G.A.; Kim, Y.S. Cancer Res. 1980, 40, 2661-2665.
63. Story, J.A.; Kritchevsky, D. J. Nutr. 1976, 106, 1292-1294.
64. Nigro, N.D.; Bhadrachari, N.; Chomchai, C. Dis. Colon Rectum 1973, 16, 438-443.
65. Doll, R.; Peto, R. J. Natl. Cancer Inst. 1981, 66, 1191-1308.
66. Watanabe, E.; Reddy, B.S.; Weisburger, J.H.; Kritchevsky, D. J. Natl. Cancer Inst. 1979, 63, 141-145.
67. Nauss, K.M.; Locniskar, M.; Newberne, P.M. Cancer Res. 1983, 43, 4083-4090.
68. Nauss, K.M.; Locniskar, M.; Sondergaard ,D.; Newberne, P.M. Carcinogenesis 1984, 5, 225-260.
69. Rogers, A.E.; Newberne, P.M. Cancer Res. 1975, 35, 3427-3431.
70. Newberne, P.M.; deCamargo, J.L.V.; Clark, A.J. Toxicologic Path. 1982, 10, 95-109.
71. Bosan, W.S.; Shank, R.C. Tox. and Appl. Pharm. 1983, 70, 324-334.
72. Rogers, A.E.; Herndon, B.J.; Newberne, P.M. Cancer Res. 1973, 33, 1003-1009.
73. Newberne, P.M.; Suphakarn, V. Cancer 1977, 40, 2553-2556.
74. Newberne, P.M.; Rogers, A.E. In "Fundamentals in Cancer Prevention"; Magee, P.N.; Takayama, S.; Sugimura, T.; Matsushima, T., Eds.; Tokyo University Press: Tokyo, 1976; pp. 15-40.
75. Suphakarn, V.; Newberne, P.M.; Goldman, M. Nutrition and Cancer 1983, 5, 41-50.

RECEIVED January 23, 1985

Influence of Diet on Hormone-Dependent Cancers

KENNETH K. CARROLL

Department of Biochemistry, University of Western Ontario, London, Ontario, N6A 5C1 Canada

Evidence that diet affects hormone-dependent cancers comes from epidemiological data and from studies on tumorigenesis in experimental animals. Breast cancer incidence and mortality are positively correlated with the amounts of fat, animal protein and total calories available for consumption in different countries. Of these variables, experiments with animals have provided the strongest support for the correlation with dietary fat. Cancers of the prostate, ovary and uterus also show positive correlations with dietary fat but as yet there is little evidence from animal experiments to support these correlations. Polyunsaturated fats enhance the yield of mammary tumors in animals more effectively than saturated fats, apparently because of a requirement for essential fatty acids, but breast cancer mortality in humans seems to correlate best with the amount rather than the type of dietary fat. Dietary fat appears to act as a promoter rather than an initiator of mammary carcinogenesis in animals. The mechanism is not known but various possibilities are being actively investigated. Promotion of carcinogenesis involves continuing exposure to the promoting agent over a period of time. It is potentially reversible, and experiments with animals have shown that tumorigenesis can be inhibited by reducing the level of dietary fat after a period of promotion with a high-fat diet. Low-fat diets may therefore be useful in prevention and treatment of cancer in humans.

My interest in the influence of diet on hormone-dependent cancers was first stimulated about 20 years ago by studies carried out in collaboration with colleagues at the Collip Medical Research Laboratory of the University of Western Ontario. They were involved in studies on the role of hormones in mammary cancer and for this purpose were inducing tumors in rats with 7,12-dimethylbenz(α)-anthracene (DMBA) as described by Huggins et al (1). They were concerned to know whether hormonal treatment might affect tumorigenesis by altering the degree and time of exposure of mammary

0097-6156/85/0277-0177$06.00/0
© 1985 American Chemical Society

tissues to the DMBA. In order to investigate this, I assisted them in developing a method for analyzing DMBA in tissues by gas-liquid chromatography (2).

Much of my previous research experience had been in lipid biochemistry and DMBA, a polycyclic hydrocarbon, is essentially a lipid xenobiotic. The suggestion had been made by Dao et al (3) that the specific induction of mammary tumors by DMBA and other polycyclic hydrocarbons might be due to their tendency, as lipids, to accumulate and persist in the adipose tissue of the mammary gland, thereby increasing the exposure to the susceptible mammary epithelial tissue. If this were indeed a factor in the ability of these compounds to produce mammary tumors, it seemed to us that it might be possible to influence their effectiveness by altering fat metabolism in the body.

Effects of Dietary Fat on Mammary Carcinogenesis

One of the easiest ways of altering fat metabolism is to feed diets containing different levels and types of dietary fat. We therefore carried out an experiment in which weanling female Sprague-Dawley rats were fed semipurified diets containing 0.5% corn oil, 20% coconut oil or 20% corn oil. The rats were given a single 10 mg intragastric dose of DMBA in sesame oil at 50 days of age, since Huggins et al (1) had shown that rats were most susceptible at about that age. Because we wished to avoid any effects of dietary fat on absorption of the carcinogen from the gut, Purina Chow was substituted for the semipurified diets from two days before until one day after receiving the DMBA. They were then returned to the semipurified diets and the development of tumors was followed for a period of four months, at which time the animals were autopsied.

One of the advantages of studying mammary tumors as opposed to tumors of internal organs is that they develop just under the skin and can be palpated as hard lumps when they are still very small. This means that their development can be followed without killing the animals. Tumors begin to appear about a month after treatment with DMBA, and the numbers continue to increase with time. They may develop in any of the six pairs of mammary glands, and animals usually develop multiple tumors.

The results of our first experiment showed no significant differences between the groups fed diets containing 0.5% corn oil or 20% coconut oil, but in the group fed the 20% corn oil diet, nearly all of the animals developed tumors and there were about twice as many tumors as in either of the other two groups (Figure 1). The levels of DMBA in the mammary glands after oral administration to animals fed these diets did not show differences that seemed likely to account for the higher tumor yield in animals fed the 20% corn oil diet (5).

Our finding that dietary fat could enhance mammary tumorigenesis in animals was not in fact a new observation. Beginning with the studies of Tannenbaum (6), a number of investigators had shown that animals fed high-fat diets develop mammary tumors more readily than those fed low-fat diets. Similar observations had also been made for skin tumors, but not all types of tumors show this association with dietary fat (7). Much of this work was done in the 1940's and early 1950's, and there were few publications on the subject during the decade prior to our first experiment.

Epidemiological Data on Diet and Carcinogenesis

The results of that experiment stimulated us to look for data on dietary fat in relation to breast cancer in human populations, and we found that mortality from breast cancer in different countries showed a strong positive correlation with the level of fat in the diet (8). This correlation was noted at about the same time by Lea (9) and Wynder (10). Mortality from cancer at other sites, such as the prostate, colon, rectum, ovary and pancreas is also positively correlated with dietary fat, but there is little correlation with cancer at other sites, such as esophagus and stomach, and a negative correlation with liver cancer (7).

    More recent experiments with animals have shown that high-fat diets can also enhance tumorigenesis at sites such as the colon (11) and pancreas (12). As in the case of mammary cancer, the experimental results are supported by epidemiological data and this has stimulated much interest in the role of dietary fat in carcinogenesis.

    In human diets, other variables such as total calories and dietary protein, particularly animal protein, are positively correlated with dietary fat (Table I). It is therefore not surprising that these dietary variables have also shown a strong positive correlation with mortality from cancer at sites such as the breast (7). Although experiments with animals have shown that tumorigenesis can be inhibited by restricting caloric intake, in most cases the restriction has been rather severe and paired-feeding experiments have indicated that dietary fat can affect tumorigenesis independently of caloric intake (7). Increasing the level of protein in the diet can enhance tumorigenesis in animals, but very high levels tend to be inhibitory, and there is little evidence that the type of protein in the diet significantly affects tumor development (13,14). In general, the studies on experimental animals support the conclusion that dietary fat has a greater effect on tumorigenesis than either caloric intake or dietary protein.

Mechanism of Action of Dietary Fat

Studies on mammary tumors have shown that the effect of dietary fat can be demonstrated with spontaneous tumors and with tumors induced by a variety of chemical or physical agents (15). Furthermore, experiments in our laboratory have shown that dietary fat effectively increases the yield of mammary tumors induced in rats by DMBA, even when the high-fat diet is first instituted one to two weeks after treatment with a carcinogen (7). These observations suggest that dietary fat is not involved in tumor initiation but acts by providing a more favorable environment for proliferation of tumor cells.

    The exact mechanism of action is not known, but various possibilities have been suggested. Mammary tumorigenesis is clearly influenced by hormones, and high-fat diets may alter the hormonal pattern in ways that favor tumor growth (16,17). It seems less likely that a hormonal mechanism would be involved in effects of dietary fat

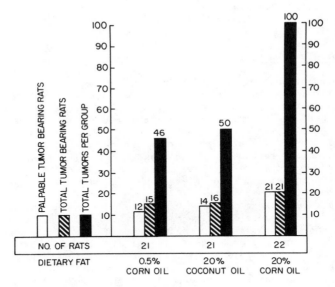

Figure 1. Influence of diet on hormone—dependent cancers. Data
from Gammal et al. (4).

Table I.   Correlation Coefficients Between Dietary
           Variables

	Total Fat	Animal Fat	Animal Protein	Total Calories	Total Protein	Vegetal Fat	Carbo- hydrate
Animal Fat	+0.951						
Animal Protein	+0.931	+0.931					
Total Calories	+0.878	+0.841	+0.827				
Total Protein	+0.801	+0.777	+0.784	+0.867			
Vegetal Fat	+0.402	-0.099	+0.224	+0.335	+0.286		
Carbohydrate	-0.078	-0.070	-0.075	+0.071	+0.182	-0.044	
Vegetal Protein	-0.268	-0.300	-0.360	+0.018	+0.264	+0.069	+0.413

————— P < 0.01

------- P < 0.05

Note: Based on food balance sheets for 132 countries (see
Reference 13).

on tumors of non-endocrine tissues. In the case of colon tumors, for example, dietary fat may act by increasing the flow of bile acids which can serve as promoters of tumorigenesis (18).

Effects of Different Types of Dietary Fat. As indicated above, our first dietary experiment on mammary carcinogenesis showed that a high-polyunsaturated fat diet greatly increased the tumor yield, while a high-saturated fat diet had no significant effect. Subsequent experiments provided further evidence that polyunsaturated fats are more effective than saturated fats in promoting mammary tumorigenesis (19). This difference appears to be related to a requirement for polyunsaturated fatty acids which is not met by the small amounts present in naturally-occurring saturated fats, such as beef tallow and coconut oil. In further experiments, diets containing 3% polyunsaturated fat and 17% saturated fat were found to promote mammary tumorigenesis as effectively as diets containing 20% polyunsaturated fat (20). Linoleic acid appeared to be capable of satisfying the requirement for polunsaturated fatty acids, but a fish oil containing polyunsaturated fatty acids derived mainly from linolenic acid was also effective, so the requirement may not be specific for n-6 fatty acids (21).

Polyunsaturated fat has also been found to be more effective than saturated fat in promoting the development of pancreatic tumors in rats (12). Similar results have been reported recently for colon cancer (22), although earlier experiments had indicated that saturated and polyunsaturated fats were about equally effective at high levels of intake (11). It thus appears that there may be a general requirement for polyunsaturated fatty acids in promotion of carcinogenesis by dietary fat.

Since polyunsaturated fats are present in substantial amounts in the phospholipids of cell membranes, and since cellular proliferation requires formation of new membranes, this might explain the requirement for polyunsaturated fatty acids in tumor promotion, but there are also other possibilities. For example, there is evidence that cell-mediated immune responses are inhibited by linoleic acid, and reduced responsiveness of the immune system could help to promote tumorigenesis (23).

Polyunsaturated fatty acids are relatively susceptible to oxidation and can give rise to many different types of oxidation products in the body as a result of both enzymatic and non-enzymatic processes. These include lipid peroxides and such biologically-active products as prostaglandins, thromboxanes and leukotrienes. There is evidence that prostaglandins can act as promoters of tumorigenesis (24), and prostaglandin synthesis inhibitors are capable of preventing the promotion of mammary tumorigenesis by high-fat diets (25-27).

If lipid oxidation is a factor in promotion of tumorigenesis by dietary fat, one might expect the process to be inhibited by dietary antioxidants. This topic is discussed in more detail elsewhere in this symposium (28), but the results have not provided clear-cut answers to the question. Some of the synthetic antioxidants such as butylated hydroxytoluene (BHT) appear to inhibit the promotion of tumorigenesis by dietary fat, but results with vitamin E, a naturally-occurring antioxidant, have been largely negative (29).

Reversal of Promoting Effect of Dietary Fat

Carcinogenesis is now generally considered to be a multistage process (30). The first stage, initiation, is thought to occur rapidly and to involve an alteration of the genome, which is essentially irreversible. Subsequent proliferation of transformed cells during the promotional phase appears to be quite susceptible to environmental factors. Promotion occurs over a much longer time period, requires repeated exposure to the promoting agent, and is potentially reversible, at least during the early stages.

Experiments in our own and other laboratories have provided evidence that the enhancement of mammary tumorigenesis by high-fat diets can be largely prevented by substituting a low-fat diet after several months of feeding a high-fat diet (31-33). This indicates that many of the sites initiated by exposure to carcinogen are prevented from developing into tumors by this procedure. Results such as this suggest the possibility that potential tumors may likewise be prevented from developing in human populations by reducing the fat content of the diet. It may also be possible to prevent or at least delay the development of metastatic lesions, which constitute the major threat in breast cancer and often in other types of cancer as well.

In this connection, it is of interest that cancer incidence decreased in England and Wales with the introduction of food rationing in 1940, and remained at a lower level for about 25 years (34). Breast cancer occurs much less frequently in Japanese women than in American women, and there is also evidence that Japanese breast cancer patients have longer survival times than those in the United States (35).

In the animal experiments referred to above, inhibition of tumorigenesis was achieved by restriction of dietary fat to a degree that would not be acceptable in human diets. Another experiment was therefore carried out in our laboratory to test the effect of a more moderate decrease in dietary fat (36). For this purpose, rats were treated with DMBA at 50 days of age and, beginning one week later, were fed a high-polyunsaturated fat diet containing 20% by weight of sunflowerseed oil to promote mammary tumor development. After seven weeks on this diet, when about one-third of the rats had developed tumors, they were divided into 5 groups of 31 rats each, with tumor-bearing rats divided equally among the different groups. One group was continued on the high-polyunsaturated fat diet, one group was given a fat-free diet, and the other three groups were fed diets containing 10% lard, 10% butter and 10% coconut oil respectively. Five months later, the group that remained on the high-poly-unsaturated fat diet had significantly more tumors than any of the other groups, and the diets containing 10% fat suppressed tumorigenesis at least as effectively as the fat-free diet (Figure 2).

In this experiment, the type of fat as well as the amount was changed because earlier studies had shown that saturated fats were less effective promoters of mammary carcinogenesis than poly-unsaturated fats. Lard, however, has a higher content of linoleic acid than either butter or coconut oil and increased the tumor yield almost as much as polyunsaturated fats when fed at the 20% level

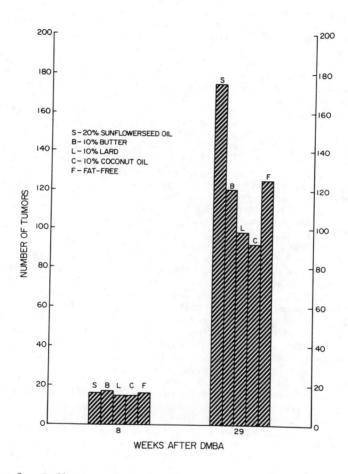

Figure 2.   Influence of diet on hormone-dependent cancers.   Data from Kalamegham and Carroll (36).

(19,20), but suppressed tumorigenesis to about the same extent as the more saturated fats when fed at the 10% level in the present experiment. This difference may be related to the lower intake of total fat, of polyunsaturated fatty acids, or both.

North American diets typically contain about 40% of energy as fat (37), corresponding to approximately 20% by weight, with a degree of unsaturation somewhat greater than that of lard (38). It would therefore be of interest to carry out an experiment similar to that described above in which tumorigenesis is first promoted by a diet containing 20% of fat having this degree of unsaturation. The effect on tumorigenesis of reducing the fat content without changing its composition could then be investigated. The results would be of interest in relation to effects of dietary fat on carcinogenesis in humans, since epidemiological data indicate that mortality from breast cancer and several other types of cancer correlates better with the amount rather than the type of dietary fat (39).

In recent years breast cancer mortality has, if anything, shown a tendency to increase (40), indicating that current methods of treatment are having relatively little impact on this disease. The epidemiological data nevertheless show large differences in the mortality rates in different countries, which are strongly correlated with dietary fat in the food supplies. It is evident that new approaches are required to reduce the death toll from breast cancer in the more affluent countries of the world, and one way might be to reduce dietary fat intake as recently recommended by the NRC-NAS Committee on Diet, Nutrition and Cancer (14).

The main source of fat in the North American diet is the visible fats and oils used as spreads, cooking fats and salad oils. Other major sources are meats and dairy products (40). Foods such as eggs and nuts are relatively high in fat but are not eaten in sufficient quantities to make a large contribution to total dietary fat. Most other dietary components, including cereal products, fruits and vegetables, are quite low in fat. It is thus relatively easy to identify high-fat foods but more difficult to achieve a substantial reduction in dietary fat because it provides qualities of taste and satiety that add to the enjoyment of eating.

A clear demonstration that reducing the level of dietary fat can decrease the risk of cancer in humans would no doubt provide much greater incentive for this type of dietary modification. It would be very difficult to obtain such evidence in a free-living population, but it might be possible with groups of high-risk individuals. A high proportion of breast cancer patients experience recurrence of the disease from metastatic cells shed from the primary tumor. Since dietary fat appears to act by stimulating the proliferation of tumor cells, it seems possible that recurrence might be delayed or even prevented by reducing fat intake. With recurrence as an end point, it may be possible to obtain definitive evidence of the potential benefits of a low-fat diet in breast cancer. Clinical trials along these lines are already being suggested (35,41).

Acknowledgment

Support by the National Cancer Institute of Canada is gratefully acknowledged.

Literature Cited

1. Huggins, C.; Grand, L.C.; Brillantes, F.P. Nature (London) 1961, 189, 204-7.
2. Gammal, E.B.; Carroll, K.K.; Muhlstock, B.H.; Plunkett, E.R. Proc. Soc. Exp. Biol. Med. 1965, 119,1086-9.
3. Dao, T.L.; Bock, F.G.; Crouch, S. Proc. Soc. Exp. Biol. Med. 1959, 102, 635-8.
4. Gammal, E.B.; Carroll, K.K.; Plunkett, E.R. Cancer Res. 1967, 27, 1737-42.
5. Gammal, E.B.; Carroll, K.K.; Plunkett, E.R. Cancer Res. 1968, 28, 384-5.
6. Tannenbaum, A. Cancer Res. 1942, 2, 468-75.
7. Carroll, K.K.; Khor, H.T. Prog. Biochem. Pharmacol. 1975, 10, 308-53.
8. Carroll, K.K.; Gammal, E.B.; Plunkett, E.R. Can. Med. Assoc. J. 1968, 98, 590-4.
9. Lea, A.J. Lancet 1966, 2, 332-3.
10. Wynder, E.L. Cancer 1969, 24, 1235-40.
11. Reddy, B.S.; Cohen, L.A.; McCoy, G.D.; Hill, P.; Weisburger, J.H.; Wynder, E.L. Adv. Cancer Res. 1980, 32, 237-345.
12. Roebuck, B.D.; Yager, J.D. Jr.; Longnecker, D.S.; Wilpone, S.A. Cancer Res. 1981, 41, 3961-6.
13. Carroll, K.K. Cancer Res. 1975, 35, 3374-83.
14. Committee on Diet, Nutrition, and Cancer, "Diet, Nutrition, and Cancer," National Academy Press: Washing-ton, D.C., 1982.
15. Carroll, K.K. In "Dietary Fats and Health"; Perkins, E.G.; Visek, W.J., Eds.; American Oil Chemists' Society; Champaign, IL, 1983, pp. 710-20.
16. Welsch, C.W.; Aylsworth, C.F. JNCI 1983, 70, 215-21.
17. Dao, T.L.; Chan, P.-C. Environ. Health Perspect. 1983, 50, 219-25.
18. Reddy, B.S. In "Dietary Fats and Health"; Perkins, E.G.; Visek, W.J. Eds.; American Oil Chemists' Society; Champaign, IL, 1983; pp. 741-60.
19. Carroll, K.K.: Khor, H.T. Lipids 1971, 6, 415-20.
20. Hopkins, G.J.; Carroll, K.K. JNCI 1979, 62, 1009-12.
21. Hopkins, G.J.; Kennedy, T.G.; Carroll, K.K. JNCI 1981, 66, 517-22.
22. Reddy, B.S.; Maeura, Y. JNCI 1984,72, 745-50.
23. Vitale, J.J.; Broitman, S.A. Cancer Res. 1981, 41, 3706-10.
24. Levine, L.; Adv. Cancer Res. 1981, 35, 49-79.
25. Abraham, S.; Hillyard, L.A. In "Dietary Fats and Health": Perkins, E.G.; Visek, W.J., Eds.; American Oil Chemists' Society: Champaign, IL, 1983; pp. 817-53.
26. Carter, C.A.; Milholland, R.J.; Shea, W.; Ip, M.M. Cancer Res. 1983, 43, 3559-62.
27. Kollmorgen, G.M.; King, M.M.; Kosanke, S.D.; Do, C. Cancer Res. 1983, 43, 4714-9.
28. King, M.M.; Terao, J.; Magarian, R.; Brueggemann, G., McCay, P.B.; This symposium (in press).
29. McCay, P.B.; King, M.M. In "Dietary Fats and Health"; Perkins, E.G.; Visek, W.J., Eds; American Oil Chemists' Society; Champaign, IL, 1983; pp. 761-89.

30. Slaga, T.J.; Sivak, A.; Boutwell, R.K. Eds. "Carcinogenesis — A Comprehensive Survey. Vol. 2. Mechanism of Tumor Promotion and Cocarcinogenesis"; Raven Press: New York, 1978.

31. Ip, C.; Ip, M.M. Cancer Lett. 1980, 11, 35–42.

32. Cohen, L.A.; Chan, P.C.; Wynder, E.L. Cancer 1981, 47, 66–71.

33. Davidson, M.B.; Carroll, K.K. Nutr. Cancer 1982, 3, 207–15.

34. Ingram, D.M. Nutr. Cancer 1981, 3, 75–80.

35. Wynder, E.L.; Cohen, L.A. Nutr. Cancer 1982, 3, 195–9.

36. Kalamegham, R.; Carroll, K.K. Nutr. Cancer 1984, 6, 22–31.

37. "The Lipid Research Clinics Population Studies Data Book, Vol. II. The Prevalence Study — Nutrient Intake"; U.S. Department of Health and Human Services, Public Health Service, National Institutes of Health, Bethesda, MD, 1982, pp. 42–3.

38. Select Committee on Nutrition and Human Needs, United States Senate. "Dietary Goals for the United States", Second Ed. U.S. Government Printing Office: Washington, DC, 1977, pp. 39–41.

39. Carroll, K.K. In "Atherosclerosis VI"; Schettler, G.; Gotto, A.M.; Middelhoff, G.; Habenicht, A.J.R.; Jurutka, K.R., Eds.; Springer–Verlag: Berlin, 1983, pp. 223–7.

40. Carroll, K.K. Cancer Res. 1981, 41, 3695–9.

41. de Waard, F. Nutr. Cancer 1982, 4, 85–9.

RECEIVED August 17, 1984

Carcinogen–DNA Binding
A Probe for Metabolic Activation In Vivo and In Vitro

C. ANITA H. BIGGER and ANTHONY DIPPLE

LBI-Basic Research Program, Chemical Carcinogenesis Program, NCI-Frederick Cancer Research
Facility, Frederick, MD 21701

Electrophilic metabolites of chemical carcinogens
are believed to be responsible for initiation of
the carcinogenic process. These metabolites are
generally too reactive to permit direct measurement
in biological systems, but their formation can be
conveniently monitored through examination of their
DNA reaction products. Using this approach, we have
found that in mouse embryo cells in vitro or in
mouse skin in vivo 7,12-dimethylbenz[a]anthracene
(DMBA) binds to deoxyadenosine and deoxyguanosine
residues in DNA through metabolically generated syn
and anti bay region dihydrodiol epoxides. However,
in subcellular systems, i.e. liver 9000 x g supernat-
ants or microsomal preparations, other reactive
metabolites, including the 5,6-epoxide, are primarily
responsible for DNA binding, indicating that these
systems are not good models for the in vivo metabolic activation of DMBA. DMBA–DNA binding was also
studied in mouse skin in the presence of inhibitors
of tumor initiation by DMBA and in mouse strains of
different susceptibiities to DMBA. Tumor inhibition
was in some cases, but not all, correlated with an
alteration in DMBA–DNA binding, suggesting that in
order to initiate the carcinogenic process, DMBA may
be required, in addition to binding covalently to
DNA, to interact in some other way with target cells.

Chemical carcinogens are not generally directly acting per se but
are metabolically activated to electrophilic derivatives which are
believed to be the actual initiators of the carcinogenic process
(1). The electrophilic derivatives are extremely reactive and it
is difficult, if not impossible, to monitor their production
directly in biological systems. However, their formation can be
monitored by analyzing the products of their reaction with DNA.
This approach was used historically very successfully in studies of

0097–6156/85/0277–0187$06.50/0

the activation of certain polycyclic aromatic hydrocarbon carcinogens. For example, in 1973, the work of Baird et al. (2) cast
doubt on the then popular theory (3) that the K-region epoxide
metabolites (Figure 1) of polycyclic aromatic hydrocarbons were
ultimate carcinogens by showing that the K-region epoxide of 7-
methylbenz[a]anthracene was not the metabolite binding to DNA in
mammalian cells. In that same year, Borgen et al. (4) demonstrated
that a dihydrodiol metabolite of benzo[a]pyrene was a precursor to
DNA-binding in an in vitro microsome-catalyzed DNA binding system.
As a consequence of these studies, Sims et al. (5) proposed that
the DNA-reactive and carcinogenic metabolite was a vicinal
dihydrodiol epoxide (Figure 1). They substantiated this by showing
that the DNA-binding products formed in cells treated with benzo[a]-
pyrene were chromatographically identical to those formed by allowing a crude preparation of the synthetic dihydrodiol epoxide of
this compound to react in vitro with DNA. The dihydrodiol epoxide
theory of activation of polycyclic aromatic hydrocarbons was
further refined by Jerina and Daly (6) who, through structure-
activity studies, proposed that the most reactive vicinal dihydrodiol epoxide would have the epoxide adjacent to a bay region, e.g.
the area between positions 1 and 12 of 7,12-dimethylbenz[a]anthra-
cene (DMBA) (Figure 1). This theory has been largely substantiated
by the carcinogenic activities of appropriate metabolites (7).

These studies demonstrated that DNA-binding can be a reliable
probe of metabolic activation. In contrast to studies of metabolites per se, which usually involve large numbers of metabolite
intermediates, DNA-binding monitors only chemically reactive metabolites. Also, if there is no selective repair of specific adducts,
DNA-binding monitors the cumulative production of metabolites
over time, while direct measurement of metabolites can show the
metabolite spectrum only at the time observed. This can be particularly critical for studies of activation of complex chemicals
such as polycyclic aromatic hydrocarbons whose primary metabolites
are subject to secondary and tertiary metabolism (8).

For these reasons, we have used DNA-binding as a probe of
metabolic activation of the polycyclic aromatic hydrocarbon carcinogen DMBA. This carcinogen has not been studied as extensively as
certain other polycyclic aromatic hydrocarbon carcinogens because
synthesis of the proposed ultimate carcinogenic metabolite, the
bay region dihydrodiol epoxide, has not been achieved. However,
we chose to study this carcinogen, and continue to do so, because
it is the most potent of the polycyclic aromatic hydrocarbons and
analysis of its activation may reveal more readily than that of
weaker carcinogens the cellular interactions specific to initiation of the carcinogenic process.

Materials and Methods

DNA was isolated from mouse skin (9,10) and cells in culture (11-
13) exposed to [^{3}H]- or [^{14}C]-DMBA, or recovered from mixtures
containing calf thymus DNA, [^{3}H]-DMBA, cofactors and either
Aroclor-induced rodent liver microsomes (14-17), S-9 fraction
(16-18) or 12 h DMBA-induced (100 nmoles in 0.1 ml benzene) mouse

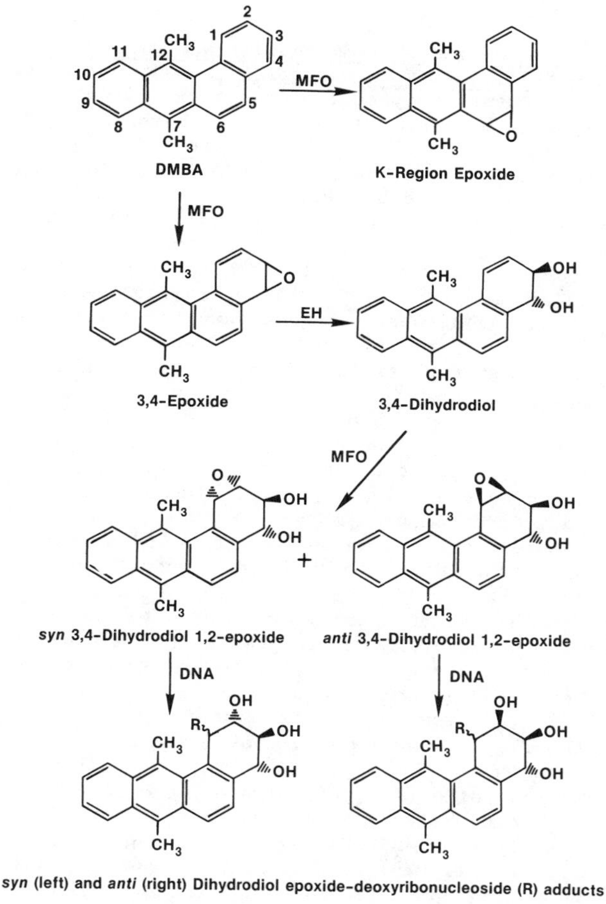

Figure 1. Metabolic pathways for activation of DMBA. MFO, mixed function oxidase; EH, epoxide hydrase.

skin epidermal homogenate (19). In some experiments, mouse skin was pretreated (5 min) with various inhibitors before [^{3}H]-DMBA treatment (10). After purification, the DNA was enzymatically hydrolyzed to DMBA-deoxyribonucleoside adducts (20) and analyzed by Sephadex LH-20 column chromatography (21), where DMBA-deoxyribonucleoside adducts elute after 250 ml of eluant has cleared the column, and by high pressure liquid chromatography (9,20).

Results and Discussion

Identification of DNA-Reactive Metabolites Generated in a Target Tissue, Mouse Skin, In Vivo. Our initial studies focused on activation of DMBA in mouse embryo cells in culture because of the ease of isolation of sufficient DNA for adduct characterization. The cells were exposed to DMBA and the isolated DNA enzymatically hydrolyzed to deoxyribonucleosides. DMBA-deoxyribonucleoside adducts were characterized by fluorescence measurements (11,22), by photosensitivity studies (12) and by column chromatography (23,24). These studies provided evidence that the DNA-reactive metabolite generated in these cells is a bay region dihydrodiol epoxide. The enzymatic steps in this activation pathway (Figure 1) involve oxidation of DMBA by mixed function oxidases to a 3,4-epoxide which is converted by epoxide hydrase to a 3,4-dihydrodiol. This is, in turn, oxidized by mixed function oxidases to the dihydrodiol epoxide.

Characterization of the mouse embryo cell DMBA-DNA adducts allowed the use of cochromatography to investigate the DMBA-DNA adducts formed in a target tissue, mouse skin. Tritium-labeled DMBA was painted on the shaved backs of mice and carbon-14-labeled DMBA was used to treat mouse embryo cells in culture. After isolation, mouse embryo cell and mouse skin DMBA-DNA were enzymatically digested and the DMBA-deoxyribonucleoside adducts analyzed by Sephadex LH-20 column chromatography (15). As can be seen in Figure 2, the mouse skin and mouse embryo cell adducts exhibit identical chromatographic behavior. This indicates that activation in mouse skin also proceeds through the bay region dihydrodiol-epoxide pathway. These results are in agreement with results obtained through different approaches in other laboratories. Vigny et al. (25) found the fluorescence spectrum of mouse skin DMBA-DNA consistent with reaction of the DNA with a bay region dihydrodiol epoxide of DMBA. The bay region dihydrodiol epoxide of DMBA has not yet been chemically synthesized, so it has not been possible to compare biologically activated DMBA-DNA adducts with an authentic standard. However, Cooper et al. (26) found that the products of reaction of the m-chloroperoxybenzoic acid-oxidized 3,4-dihydrodiol of DMBA with DNA gave DMBA-DNA adducts which cochromatographed with those obtained from DMBA-treated mouse skin. In addition, the 3,4-dihydrodiol of DMBA (precursor of the bay region dihydrodiol epoxide) is a very potent carcinogen in initiation-promotion tests on mouse skin suggesting that the DNA-reactive metabolite in mouse skin is also the ultimate carcinogen (27-29).

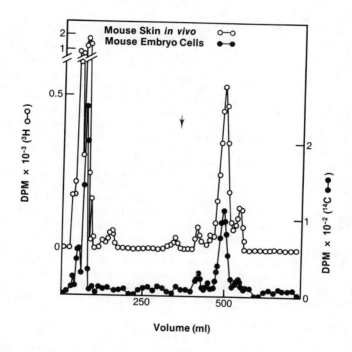

Figure 2.   Sephadex LH–20 column chromatography of DMBA-deoxyribonucleoside adducts formed by enzymatic digestion of DNA from mouse
embryo cells exposed to [^{14}C]-DMBA (0.2 μg/ml) for 24 h (●-●) and
of DNA from the skin of female NIH Swiss mice treated with [^{3}H]-DMBA
(10 μg/mouse) for 24 h (O-O).   The arrow denotes the position of
elution of an added uv-absorbing marker 4-(p-nitrobenzyl)pyridine.
"Reproduced with permission from Ref. 15.   Copyright 1980, IRL
Press".

Comparison of the Activation Provided by Tissue Homogenates, Intact Cellular Systems, and Target Tissue. Short term tests for detection of chemical carcinogens commonly rely on the inclusion of subcellular homogenates, such as a rat liver S-9 fraction, to provide metabolic activation of test chemicals (30). The justification for the use of homogenates seems to rest on an assumption that they reproduce target tissue activation. We decided to test that assumption by examining the DNA-reactive metabolites generated by homogenate in vitro metabolic activation systems. In our initial study (14), we compared the DMBA-DNA adducts formed in the presence of rat-liver microsomes and calf thymus DNA with those formed in mouse skin in vivo and with those formed by reaction of the chemically synthesized K-region epoxide (Figure 1) of DMBA with calf thymus DNA. Figure 3 shows the Sephadex LH-20 column chromatographic profiles for these DMBA-deoxyribonucleoside adducts. The microsomally-generated adducts were not chromatographically identical with the mouse skin adducts but instead eluted in coincidence with the K-region epoxide-derived adducts. This suggested that rat liver homogenates are not good models for in vivo activation. We examined activation by other subcellular in vitro metabolic activation systems under various conditions. Figure 4 shows the effect of a 10-fold difference in substrate concentration on the DMBA-DNA adducts generated by rat liver S9 fraction (18). At a high substrate concentration (Figure 4b), a large proportion of the adducts was derived from the K-region epoxide of DMBA (peaks D and E) plus adducts derived from an unidentified metabolite (peak B). However, when the concentration of substrate was lowered 10-fold, the Sephadex LH-20 column chromatographic profile changed dramatically (Figure 4a). Peaks A and C now predominated. We have shown that the elution of peak C coincides with elution of the mouse embryo cell bay region dihydrodiol epoxide adducts (18), while peak A elutes at the same position in the gradient as adducts identified as 7-hydroxymethyl-12-methylbenz[a]anthracene-bay region dihydrodiol epoxide-deoxyribonucleosides (24). Similar results were obtained when mouse liver (Figure 5) or hamster liver (Figure 6) microsomes were substituted in the assay. This suggests that the biologically active metabolites at one end of a dose response curve in a short-term test might be very different from those at the other end of the curve. In the case of polycyclic aromatic hydrocarbons, for example, this could mean that at high concentrations of substrate the K-region epoxide, though not thought to be carcinogenic, would be responsible for giving positive results in a short-term test using mutagenesis as an endpoint (31).

In contrast, we did not find these concentration-dependent qualitative changes when activation occurred in intact cellular systems (16). We examined the adducts formed in mouse embryo cells in culture and in mouse skin in vivo over 40- and 100-fold DMBA concentration ranges, respectively, and found quantitative, but no qualitative, changes in binding (16). At all concentrations, activation appeared to be through the bay region dihydrodiol epoxide pathway. The cellular systems are physically very different from the homogenate systems and it is difficult to

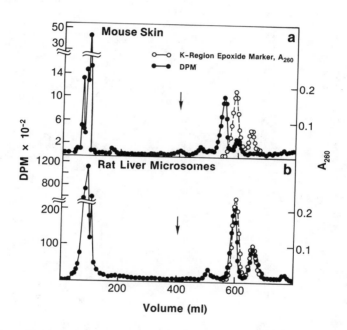

Figure 3.   Comparison of Sephadex LH-20 column chromatography of
DMBA K-region epoxide-deoxyribonucleoside products (0-0) formed by
enzymatic digestion of calf thymus DNA which had been reacted with
DMBA K-region epoxide <u>in vitro</u> with enzymatically digested DMBA-DNA
products from (a) female NIH Swiss mouse skin treated 24 h with
[³H]-DMBA (10 μg/mouse) and (b) calf thymus DNA treated with [³H]-
DMBA (320 nmol/mg microsomal protein) for 2 h in the presence of
Aroclor-induced rat liver microsomes.   The arrow is as defined in
Figure 2.

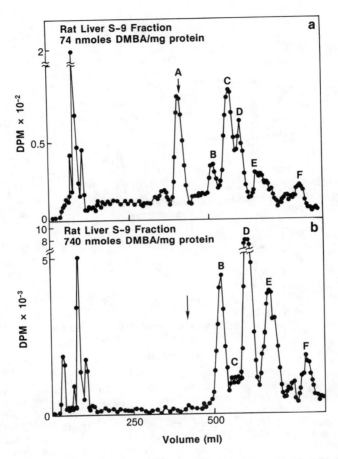

Figure 4. Comparison of Sephadex LH-20 column chromatography of DMBA-deoxyribonucleoside adducts formed by enzymatic digestion of calf thymus DNA that had been treated for 2 h in the presence of Aroclor-induced rat liver S9 fraction with (a) 74 or (b) 740 nmol [³H]-DMBA per mg S9 fraction protein. The arrow is as defined in Figure 2 and the identities of peaks A-F are discussed in the text.

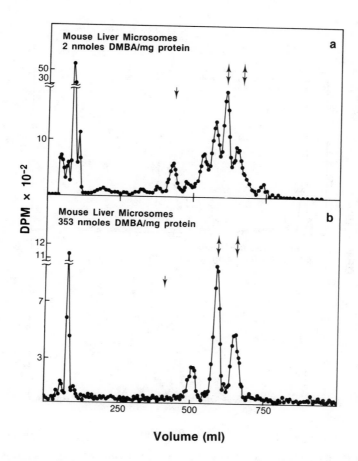

Figure 5. Comparison of Sephadex LH-20 column chromatography of DMBA-deoxyribonucleoside adducts formed by enzymatic digestion of calf thymus DNA that had been treated for 2 h in the presence of Aroclor-induced mouse liver microsomes with (a) 2 or (b) 353 nmol [^{3}H]-DMBA per mg microsomal protein. The single-headed arrow is as defined in Figure 2. The double arrow denotes the position of elution of added DMBA K-region epoxide-deoxyribonucleoside uv-absorbing markers.

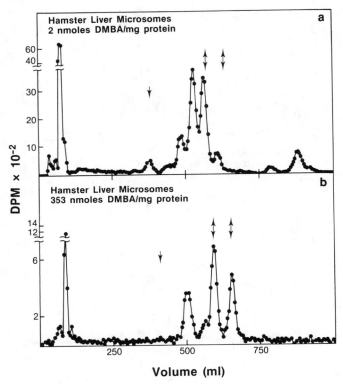

Figure 6. Comparison of Sephadex LH-20 column chromatography of DMBA-deoxyribonucleoside adducts formed by enzymatic digestion of calf thymus DNA that had been treated for 2 h in the presence of Aroclor-induced hamster liver microsomes with (a) 2 or (b) 353 nmol [^{3}H]-DMBA per mg microsomal protein. The arrows are as defined in Figures 2 and 5.

equate dosages in the two systems. However, the levels of binding to DNA in the mouse embryo cell and mouse skin studies ranged from 2 to 80 μmol/mol DNA-P and 2 to 99 μmol/mol DNA-P, respectively. These are both lower and higher than those generated in the homogenate systems (8 to 25 μmol/molDNA-P) over which the dramatic qualitative changes in adducts were observed.

We examined other intact cellular systems, [hamster embryo cells (16), rat liver cells (13) and human skin cells (13)], and found activation identical to that occurring in mouse skin and mouse embryo cells. These results suggest that cellular integrity is an important factor in reproduction of target tissue activation. To test this hypothesis, we examined the activation provided by a subcellular epidermal homogenate derived from target tissue, mouse skin. The activation generated by the skin homogenate was dramatically different from that occurring in intact skin. Fig. 7 shows the Sephadex LH-20 column chromatographic profiles for DMBA-DNA adducts generated by skin homogenates over an 800-fold DMBA concentration range. At both high and low concentrations, adducts eluting in coincidence with markers for K-region epoxide-DMBA-DNA adducts were present. They predominated at the low concentration and were accompanied by other unidentified adducts at the high concentration. There did not appear to be any adducts generated through the bay region dihydrodiol epoxide pathway, even at the low dose, though very small amounts cannot be ruled out. We lowered the concentration 10-fold but still did not see any evidence of activation through the normal target tissue activation pathway.

Table I. Summary of Results of DMBA-DNA Binding Studies in Various Cellular and Subcellular Systems

Systems Used	Adducts Formed
Subcellular	
Rat Liver microsomes (14,15) Rat liver S-9 (18) Mouse liver microsomes (16)[a] Hamster liver microsomes (16)[a] Mouse skin homogenate[a]	K-region epoxide adducts at higher doses Dihydrodiol epoxide adducts at lower doses in most cases, but always accompanied by other adducts
Cellular	
Mouse skin (9,14,15) Mouse embryo cells (11,12,23) Hamster embryo cells (16) Rat liver cells (13) Human skin cells (13)	Dihydrodiol epoxide adducts only

[a] Data presented in this paper.

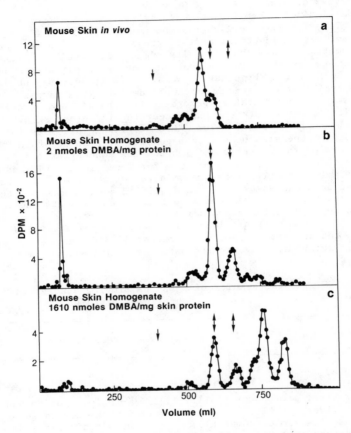

Figure 7. Comparison of Sephadex LH-20 column chromatography of DMBA-deoxyribonucleoside adducts formed by enzymatic digestion of (a) DNA from female NIH Swiss mouse skin treated <u>in vivo</u> with [³H]-DMBA (270 nmoles/mouse) for 24 h and (b,c) calf thymus DNA incubated with DMBA-induced mouse skin epidermal homogenate and (b) 2 or (c) 1610 nmoles DMBA per mg homogenate. The arrows are as defined in Figures 2 and 5.

The results of these studies, summarized in Table I, illustrate the dramatic effect of cell disruption in altering activation pathways. They also indicate that intact cells can faithfully reproduce target tissue activation and, therefore, might make good in vitro activation systems for short-term tests.

Characterization of Individual DMBA-deoxyribonucleoside Adducts Formed In Vivo in Mouse Skin. Sephadex LH-20 column chromatography is adequate to demonstrate qualitative differences in DMBA-DNA adducts formed in different systems. However, it lacks the resolution to definitively demonstrate that the adducts formed in two systems are the same (32). We had previously shown that single peaks eluted from Sephadex LH-20 columns could be separated by high pressure liquid chromatography (HPLC) into two or more components (18). Recent work on refinement of the HPLC separation of mouse embryo cell DMBA-DNA adducts provided a system with superior resolution (Figure 8) (9,33). This system demonstrated that none of the Sephadex LH-20 column peaks represented a single component. However, the major HPLC adducts A, C and D (Figure 8) were shown to be single components by subsequent chromatography on Sephadex LH-20 columns (33) and on Servacel DHB columns (20).

The chromatographic behavior of adducts A, C and D on the Servacel DHB column (20) and the fluorescence spectral properties of these adducts (33) were consistent with their formation through the reaction of two stereoisomers of the DMBA bay region dihydrodiol epoxide with DNA. Figure 1 shows the structure of these two stereoisomers, designated syn and anti, depending on whether or not the benzylic hydroxyl group is cis or trans, respectively, to the epoxide oxygen. Upon reaction with DNA, the anti, but not the syn, stereoisomer gains cis hydroxyl groups (Figure 1) which in part give rise to the different chromatographic and fluorescence spectral properties of the adducts.

In addition, double-label experiments with [^{3}H]-DMBA and [^{14}C]-adenine or [^{14}C]-guanine allowed identification of the deoxyribonucleosides associated with HPLC peaks A, C and D of DMBA-DNA adducts isolated from mouse embryo cells (34). Thus, the three major adducts formed in mouse embryo cells appear to be an anti-bay region dihydrodiol epoxide-deoxyguanosine adduct (Figure 8, peak A), a syn-bay region dihydrodiol epoxide-deoxyadenosine adduct (Figure 8, peak C) and an anti-bay region dihydrodiol epoxide-deoxyadenosine adduct (Figure 8, peak D).

With this characterization of mouse embryo cell adducts and the high resolution HPLC separation, we were able to investigate the adducts formed in mouse skin with the expectation of now being able to detect subtle differences in activation in the target tissue, if such occurred. HPLC cochromatography of adducts isolated from [^{3}H]-DMBA treated mouse skin DNA and from [^{14}C]-DMBA treated mouse embryo cells demonstrated that the adducts formed in the two systems are qualitatively identical (Figure 8) (9). Thus, as was the case with the mouse embryo cell adducts, the major adducts formed in mouse skin appear to be bay region anti-dihydrodiol epoxide-deoxyguanosine and -deoxyadenosine adducts and a bay region syn-dihydrodiol epoxide-deoxyadenosine adduct. Additional studies showed that there are no qualitative differences in the

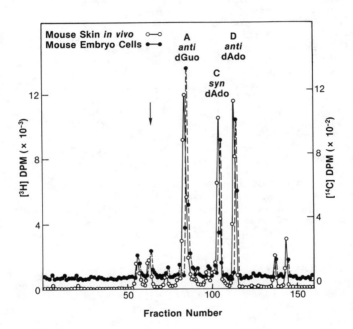

Figure 8. HPLC elution profiles for DMBA-deoxyribonucleoside
adducts from female NIH Swiss mouse skin treated with 14 nmoles
[^{3}H]-DMBA 24 h (O-O) and from mouse embryo cells exposed to [^{14}C]-
DMBA (0.14 μg/ml) 24 h (●-●). The arrow shows the position of
elution of an added uv-absorbing marker, toluene.

adducts formed in male or female mouse skin or with DMBA exposure
time (6 h to 55 h) (9).

The relative amounts of syn and anti adducts produced in mouse
embryo cells did not vary substantially with DMBA concentration
(20). However, we found a dramatic difference in the relative
amounts of these adducts when the dose of DMBA applied to mouse
skin was varied (9). Figure 9 shows the HPLC elution profiles for
adducts formed at a low dose of 14 nmol [^{3}H]-DMBA. Peaks A,C and
D are present in approximately equal amounts, i.e. 29, 21 and 22%
of total radioactivity, respectively. However, at a 100-fold
higher dose of 1400 nmol, peak C has increased to 39% while A and
D have decreased to 13% and 9%. These results indicate that the
formation of syn-bay region dihydrodiol epoxide adducts is favored
at high doses. Due to this, the total binding to deoxyadenosine
(peaks C and D) also increases with dose and ranges from 27% to
48% of the total DNA binding.

These analyses show major differences in the DNA reaction
products formed by DMBA and by BP, a weaker but much more extensively studied polycyclic aromatic hydrocarbon carcinogen (35).
Syn-dihydrodiol epoxide adducts formed in mouse skin treated with
benzo[a]pyrene constitute only about 12% of the total binding (36)
and dihydrodiol epoxide–deoxyadenosine adducts account for even
less (2 to 3%) of the total (37,38). DMBA is approximately 20
times more potent a carcinogen than BP and this difference cannot
be explained by the 2- to 4-fold difference in overall binding to
DNA by these two carcinogens in mouse skin (35). Thus, these more
subtle differences in DNA reaction products, i.e. the difference
in reaction of syn-stereoisomer with DNA or in the modification of
deoxyadenosine residues, might account for the greater tumor-initiating potential of DMBA.

Studies of the Effect of Modifiers of Carcinogenesis on DMBA–DNA
Binding In Vivo in Target Tissue. The results of our studies on
the formation of specific adducts in mouse skin prompted us to
examine adduct formation under conditions inhibiting tumor initiation to determine whether there is any correlation between the
formation of individual adducts and tumor initiation.

NIH Swiss mice are much more susceptible to initiation by
DMBA than C57BL mice (Table II) (39). Differences in the overall
binding of DMBA to skin DNA in these strains did not correlate
with their sensitivity to DMBA initiation (40) but analyses of
individual adducts had not been reported. Therefore, we treated
mice of the two strains with 0.1 μmol [^{3}H]-DMBA per mouse (the
dose used in initiation-promotion tests), isolated skin DNA at
various times and analyzed the DMBA-deoxyribonucleoside adducts by
HPLC (10). Table II shows the results of this experiment. We
confirmed the earlier finding (40) that there is no difference in
overall binding of DMBA to skin DNA of the two strains. Table II
also shows that there was no significant difference in the amounts
of individual anti-deoxyguanosine- and deoxyadenosine- and syn-
deoxyadenosine adducts formed in the two strains. Both strains
responded to increases in dose in the same way i.e. the syn-dihydrodiol epoxide adducts increased with increasing dose more than

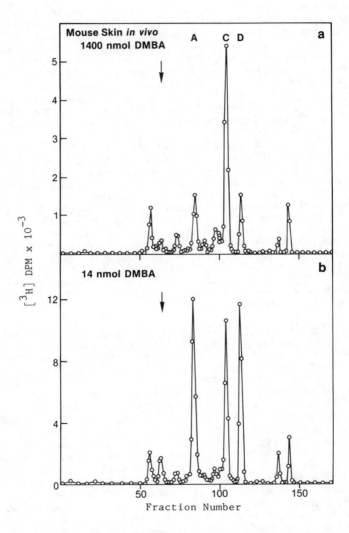

Figure 9. HPLC elution profiles for DMBA–deoxyribonucleoside
adducts from female NIH Swiss mouse skin treated with (a) 1400 or
(b) 14 nmol DMBA for 24 h. The arrow is as defined in Figure 8.

the anti-dihydrodiol epoxide adducts. Thus, differences in relative
amounts of binding of syn- and anti-dihydrodiol epoxides of DMBA to
skin DNA do not explain the difference in susceptibility to DMBA-
initiated tumorigenesis exhibited by these two strains.

Table II. DMBA-DNA Binding at Various Times in Male NIH Swiss
and C57BL mice

Mouse Strain	Tumors/ Mouse (39)	Time (h)	Adducts in μmol/mol DNA-P			
			Total	anti dGuo	syn dAdo	anti dAdo
NIH Swiss	7.32	6	2.7	0.54	0.89	0.39
		24	4.6	1.06	1.42	0.80
		48	4.2	1.03	1.26	0.73
C57BL	1.17	6	2.7	0.44	1.02	0.31
		24	5.5	1.09	1.81	0.80
		48	4.7	1.07	1.45	0.69

A number of chemicals, such as 5,6-benzoflavone, 7,8-benzo-
flavone, butylated hydroxytoluene, butylated hydroxyanisole, vitamin C and vitamin E, have been shown to partially inhibit DMBA-
initiated papilloma formation in mouse skin (39,41,42). We examined
the effect of pretreatment of mouse skin with these compounds,
using the conditions of tumor inhibition studies, on the binding
of DMBA to skin DNA and on formation of individual adducts. The
results (10) of HPLC analyses of adducts in all cases showed no
significant differences in relative amounts of individual adducts
following pretreatment with any of the six inhibitors tested. This
was surprising because in vitro studies on DMBA-DNA binding in
mouse embryo cells in culture showed that the syn-dihydrodiol
epoxide was selectively inhibited in this system following treatment with butylated hydroxyanisole (43), while the syn-dihydrodiol
epoxide was selectively enhanced following treatment with another
DMBA initiation inhibitor, benz[a]anthracene (manuscript in preparation). Thus, though cultured rodent embryo cells may be a good
model for qualitative activation in target tissue, they may not
reflect the more subtle quantitative interactions of DMBA with DNA
with respect to relative amounts of syn- and anti-dihydrodiol
epoxide stereoisomers of DMBA bound to DNA.
In contrast, with respect to the overall binding of DMBA to
DNA in mouse skin, treatment with certain inhibitors coincided with
partial inhibition of DMBA-DNA binding. Table III gives the
figures for total binding at various times following treatment
with 5,6- or 7,8-benzoflavone. Our findings, in agreement with
previous studies (39,40,44), show an inhibition of total DMBA-DNA
binding following 7,8-benzoflavone treatment. This inhibition
correlates well with inhibition of tumorigenesis (39,41) by this
compound (Table III). In the case of 5,6-benzoflavone, DMBA-DNA
binding is inhibited at 6 and 24 h by about 30% and this figure
also correlates well with the inhibition of tumors. However

by 48 h, inhibition of binding drops and, though there seems to be some effect on binding, the correlation of binding inhibition with tumor inhibition is not as clear-cut as that for 7,8-benzoflavone.

Table III. Effect of Benzoflavones on the Binding of DMBA to DNA in the Skin of Female NIH Swiss Mice

Benzo-flavone	% Inhibition (Papillomas) (39,41)	Time (h)	DMBA-DNA Binding (µmol/mol DNA-P)	%Inhibition (Binding)
None		6	1.9	0
		24	1.8	0
		48	1.2	0
5,6- (1000 µg)	35	6	1.3	~ 30
		24	1.3	~ 30
		48	1.1	~ 10
7,8- (25 µg)	74	6	0.3	~ 80
		24	0.4	~ 80
		48	0.4	~ 70
7,8- (100 µg)	74	6	0.2	~ 90
		24	0.3	~ 80
		48	0.2	~ 80

Table IV shows the effect of pretreatment with vitamins C and E on the binding of DMBA to mouse skin DNA. Vitamin E which inhibits tumor formation by about 38% (42), also inhibited total binding to a comparable extent. In contrast vitamin C, which is a somewhat better tumor inhibitor (44%) (42), had almost no effect on binding of DMBA to DNA.

Table IV. Effect of Vitamins on the Binding of DMBA to DNA in Skin of Female NIH Swiss Mice

Pretreat-ment	% Inhibition (Papillomas) (42)	Time (h)	DMBA-DNA Binding (µmol/mol DNA-P)	% Inhibition (Binding)
None	0	6	2.0	0
		24	2.0	0
		48	2.0	0
Vitamin C (1000 µg)	44	6	1.7	~ 20
		24	1.8	~ 10
		48	2.0	0
Vitamin E (1000 µg)	38	6	1.0	~ 50
		24	1.3	~ 40
		48	1.3	~ 40

Table V shows an even more dramatic disparity between tumor inhibition and effect of inhibition on total binding of DMBA to DNA. Butylated hydroxytoluene and butylated hydroxyanisole cause inhibition of DMBA initiation of tumors by 53% and 28%, respectively. There is little inhibition of binding of DMBA to DNA by these compounds and in the case of butylated hydroxyanisole, and the 24 h sample for butylated hydroxytoluene, binding of DMBA to skin DNA is actually enhanced.

Table V. Effect of Antioxidants on the Binding of DMBA to DNA in Skin of Female NIH Swiss Mice

Pretreatment	%Inhibition (Papillomas) (42)	Time (h)	DMBA–DNA Binding (μmol/mol–DNA–P)	% Inhibition (Binding)
None	0	6	2.0	0
		24	2.0	0
		48	2.0	0
Butylated hydroxytoluene (1000 μg)	53	6	1.9	~ 10
		24	2.5	0[a]
		48	1.7	~ 20
Butylated hydroxyanisole (1000 μg)	28	6	2.3	0[a]
		24	2.3	0[a]
		48	2.4	0[a]

[a] Binding enhanced over controls.

For the past twenty years, the prevailing dogma has held that the initiating event of polycyclic aromatic hydrocarbon carcinogenesis is the covalent interaction of hydrocarbon with target tissue DNA (45). While we cannot rule out some subtle effects on adduct formation in a small population of target cells, our findings, that certain antioxidant inhibitors of tumorigenesis do not alter covalent binding of the initiator to DNA, suggest that this covalent interaction of carcinogen with DNA may not be the only step involved in initiation. Our findings would be more consistent with a two-step mechanism for initiation which involved covalent interaction of carcinogen with DNA and another step mediated by the carcinogen and inhibited by antioxidants (10). This is compatible with the suggestion by Cerutti et al. (46) that polycyclic aromatic hydrocarbons can cause membrane-mediated chromosomal damage which would not involve covalent adduct formation and could be blocked by antioxidants. The hypothesis could also explain the lower tumor-initiating activity of benzo[a]pyrene dihydrodiol epoxide compared with that of benzo[a]pyrene (47). In this case, the two-step mechanism would involve a second step mediated by another benzo[a]pyrene metabolite, which could not be generated by further metabolism of the dihydrodiol epoxide.

Conclusions

These studies illustrate the utility of carcinogen–DNA binding studies in probing metabolic activation in various systems.
They enable us to identify the DNA reactive syn- and anti-dihydrodiol epoxide metabolites of DMBA generated in a target tissue,
mouse skin. Further characterization of the adducts formed in
mouse skin showed that the predominant adducts are bay region
anti-dihydrodiol epoxide-deoxyguanosine and -deoxyadenosine, and
bay region syn-dihydrodiol epoxide-deoxyadenosine. Comparison
with the adducts formed by treating mouse skin with the weaker
carcinogen benzo[a]pyrene suggests that the greater reactivity
of DMBA through the syn stereoisomer and with deoxyadenosine residues in mouse skin may play a role in determining its greater
tumor initiating potential.

We also used DNA binding studies to show that in vitro subcellular activation systems do not qualitatively duplicate target
tissue activation and thus may not be adequate as activation systems for short-term tests for detection of chemical carcinogens.
In contrast, intact cellular in vitro systems, such as rodent
embryo cells in culture, do seem capable of qualitatively mimick-
ing target tissue activation. However, when we investigated
changes in the relative involvement of syn- and anti-dihydrodiol
epoxide stereoisomers of the DNA-reactive metabolite of DMBA in
response to altered conditions we did not always see the same
response in target tissue and cultured cells. These results suggest that at this more defined level of carcinogen–DNA interaction
even the intact cellular in vitro system is not a precise model
for target tissue activation.

In other studies, we investigated the effects of different
inhibitors of DMBA-initiated carcinogenesis in mouse skin on the
interaction of DMBA with skin DNA. Our findings that some antioxidants do not alter overall binding of DMBA to DNA or the relative involvement of the syn- and anti- dihydrodiol epoxide stereoisomers, cast some doubt on the belief that covalent binding of
carcinogen to DNA is the only initiating event in DMBA-initiated
carcinogenesis. These results are more compatible with a two-step
mechanism of initiation involving covalent interaction of DMBA
with DNA and another step which can be inhibited by antioxidants.

Acknowledgments

We thank Lisa G. Raymond, Donna M. Blake and Margaret A.
Pigott for their expert assistance with these studies.
Research sponsored by the National Cancer Institute, DHHS,
under Contract No. N01-CO-23909 with Litton Bionetics, Inc.

Literature Cited

1.   Miller, E.C.; Miller, J.A. Cancer 1981, 47, 2327-2345.
2.   Baird, W.M.; Dipple, A.; Grover, P.L.; Sims, P.; Brookes, P.
     Cancer Res. 1973, 33, 2386-2392.

3. Pullman, A.; Pullman, B. In "Advances in Cancer Research"; Greenstein, J.P.; Haddow, A., Eds.; Academic Press: London, 1955; Vol. 3, pp. 117–169.

4. Borgen, A.; Darvey, H.; Castagnoli, N.; Crocker, T.T.; Rasmussen, R.E.; Wang, I.Y. J. Med. Chem. 1973, 16, 502–506.

5. Sims, P.; Grover, P.L.; Swaisland, A.; Pal, P.; Hewer, A. Nature (London) 1974, 252, 326–328.

6. Jerina, D.M.; Daly, J.W. In "Drug Metabolism"; Parke, D.V.; Smith, R.L., Eds.; Taylor and Francis: London, 1976; pp. 13–32.

7. Dipple, A.; Moschel, R.C.; Bigger, C.A.H. In "Chemical Carcinogens"; Searle, C.E.; Ed.; American Chemical Society: Washington, D.C., 1984, in press.

8. Holder, G.M.; Yagi, H.; Jerina, D.M.; Levin, W.; Lu, A.Y.H.; Conney, A.H. Arch. Biochem Biophys. 1975, 170, 557–566.

9. Bigger, C.A.H.; Sawicki, J.T.; Blake, D.M.; Raymond, L.G.; Dipple, A. Cancer Res. 1983, 43, 5647–5651.

10. Dipple, A.; Pigott, M.A.; Bigger, C.A.H., Blake, D.M. Carcinogenesis 1984, 5, in press.

11. Moschel, R.C.; Baird, W.M.; Dipple, A. Biochem. Biophys. Res. Commun. 1977, 76, 1092–1098.

12. Baird, W.M.; Dipple, A. Int. J. Cancer 1977, 20, 427–431.

13. Bigger, C.A.H.; Tomaszewski, J.E.; Dipple, A.; Lake, R.S. Science 1980, 209, 503–505.

14. Bigger, C.A.H.; Tomaszewski, J.E.; Dipple, A. Biochem. Biophys. Res. Commun. 1978, 80, 229–235.

15. Bigger, C.A.H.; Tomaszewski, J.E.; Dipple, A. Carcinogenesis 1980, 1, 15–20.

16. Bigger, C.A.H.; Dipple, A. In "Organ and Species Specificity in Chemical Carcinogenesis"; Langenbach, R.; Nesnow, S.; Rice, J.M.; Eds.; Plenum Press: New York, 1983, pp. 587–604.

17. Bigger, C.A.H.; Moschel, R.C.; Dipple, A. In "Chemical Analysis and Biological Fate: Polynuclear Aromatic Hydrocarbons"; Cooke, M.; Dennis, A.J., Eds.; Battelle Press: Columbus, Ohio, 1981, pp. 209–219.

18. Bigger, C.A.H.; Tomaszewski, J.E.; Andrews, A.W.; Dipple, A. Cancer Res. 1980, 40, 655–661.

19. Thompson, S.; Slaga, T.J. J. Invest. Dermatol. 1976, 66, 108–111.

20. Sawicki, J.T.; Moschel, R.C.; Dipple, A. Cancer Res. 1983, 43, 3212–3218.

21. Baird, W.M.; Brookes, P. Cancer Res. 1973, 33, 2378–2385.

22. Moschel, R.C.; Hudgins, W.R.; Dipple, A. Chem.–Biol. Interac. 1979, 27, 69–79.

23. Dipple, A.; Nebzydoski, J.A. Chem.–Biol. Interact. 1978, 20, 17–26.

24. Dipple, A.; Tomaszewski, J.E.; Moschel, R.C.; Bigger, C.A.H.; Nebzydoski, J.A.; Egan, M. Cancer Res. 1979, 39, 1154–1158.

25. Vigny, P.; Duquesne, M.; Coulomb, H.; Tierney, B.; Grover, P.L.; Sims, P. FEBS Lett. 1977, 82, 278–282.

26. Cooper, C.S.; Ribeiro, O.; Hewer, A.; Walsh, C.; Grover, P.L.; Sims, P. Chem.–Biol. Interac. 1980, 29, 357–367.

27. Chouroulinkov, I.; Gentil, A.; Tierney, B.; Grover, P.L.;
     Sims, P. Int. J. Cancer 1979, 24, 455-460.
28. Slaga, T.J.; Gleason, G.L.; DiGiovanni, J.; Sukumaran, K.B.;
     Harvey, R.G. Cancer Res. 1979, 39, 1934-1936.
29. Wislocki, P.G.; Gadek, K.M.; Chou, M.W.; Yang, S.K.; Lu,
     A.Y.H. Cancer Res. 1980, 40, 3661-3664.
30. de Serres, F.J.; Shelby, M.D. Science 1979, 203, 563-565.
31. Ames, B.N.; McCann, J.; Yamasaki, E. Mutat. Res. 1975, 31,
     347-364.
32. Dipple, A.; Bigger, C.A.H. In "Cellular Systems for Toxicity
     Testing"; Williams, G.M.; Dunkel, V.; Ray, V.A.; Eds.; ANNALS
     OF THE NEW YORK ACADEMY OF SCIENCE No. 407, New York Academy
     of Science: New York, 1983; pp. 26-33.
33. Moschel, R.C.; Pigott, M.A.; Costantino, N.; Dipple, A.
     Carcinogenesis 1983, 4, 1201-1204.
34. Dipple, A.; Pigott, M.; Moschel, R.C.; Costantino, N. Cancer
     Res. 1983, 43, 4132-4135.
35. Dipple, A.; Sawicki, J.T.; Moschel, R.C.; Bigger, C.A.H. In
     "Extrahepatic Drug Metabolism and Chemical Carcinogenesis";
     Rydström, J.; Montelius, J.; Bengtsson, M., Eds.; Elsevier
     Biomedical Press: Amsterdam, 1983; pp. 439-448.
36. Koreeda, M.; Moore, P.D.; Wislocki, P.G.; Levin, W.; Conney,
     A.H.; Yagi, H.; Jerina, D.M. Science 1978, 199, 778-781.
37. Ashurst, S.W.; Cohen, G.M. Int. J. Cancer 1981, 27, 357-364.
38. Ashurst, S.W.; Cohen, G.M.; Nesnow, S.; DiGiovanni, J.; Slaga,
     T. J. Cancer Res. 1983, 43, 1024-1029.
39. Kinoshita, N.; Gelboin, H.V. Cancer Res. 1972, 32, 1329-1339.
40. Phillips, D.H.; Grover, P.L.; Sims, P. Int. J. Cancer 1978,
     22, 487-494.
41. Slaga, T.J.; Thompson, S.; Berry, D.L.: DiGiovanni, J.;
     Juchau, M.R.; Viaje, A. Chem.-Biol. Interac. 1977, 17, 297-
     312.
42. Slaga, T.J.; Bracken, W.M. Cancer Res. 1977, 37, 1631-1635.
43. Sawicki, J.T.; Dipple, A. Cancer Lett. 1983, 20, 165-171.
44. Bowden, G.T.; Slaga, T.J.; Shapas, B.G.; Boutwell, R.K.
     Cancer Res. 1974, 34, 2634-2642.
45. Brookes, P.; Lawley, P.D. Nature (London) 1964, 202, 781-784.
46. Cerutti, P.; Friedman, J.; Zimmerman, R. In "Extrahepatic
     Drug Metabolism and Chemical Carcinogenesis"; Rydström, J.;
     Montelius, J.; Bengtsson, M.; Eds.; Elsevier Biomedical Press:
     Amsterdam, 1983; pp. 499-506.
47. Slaga, T.J.; Bracken, W.J.; Gleason, G.; Levin, W.; Yagi, H.;
     Jerina, D.M.; Conney, A.H. Cancer Res. 1979, 39, 67-71.

RECEIVED August 17, 1984

Effect of Nutrition on the Metabolism and Toxicity of Mycotoxins

JOHNNIE R. HAYES

Department of Pharmacology and Toxicology, Medical College of Virginia, Virginia Commonwealth University, Richmond, VA 23290-0001

The microflora of various foods and feeds worldwide contain diverse fungi, some of which are toxigenic. Whether or not a particular food or feed will contain a particular genus, species or strain of toxigenic fungus is dependent upon a number of factors; including geographical location, specific growing conditions, associated macro and micro environments and storage conditions. The presence of a toxigenic fungus does not always mean that the particular mycotoxin(s) associated with that species will be present. Whether or not a particular species and strain will actually produce its particular mycotoxin(s) is dependent upon various factors associated with mold growth, many of which are poorly understood.

Mycotoxins are generally considered to be secondary metabolites formed by biochemical pathways which represent branches off normal cellular anabolic and catabolic pathways. Their mammalian toxicity scans the range from low to extremely high and encompasses forms of toxicity ranging from acute to genotoxicity, such as cancer. Their toxicological targets are diverse and include the heart, liver, kidney and skin among others. Mycotoxin research was sporadic before the discovery that aflatoxin B_1 (AFB_1), one of several aflatoxins produced by various strains of Aspergillus flavus and found in certain commodities destined for human food and animal feed, was both highly toxic and carcinogenic. This finding not only led to intensive studies concerning this mycotoxin but also to efforts to identify and toxicologically characterize other mycotoxins.

There are currently sufficient reports in the literature to conclude that the mycotoxins may pose significant adverse human health effects at specific times and in specific locations (1).

0097–6156/85/0277–0209$06.00/0

The adverse health effects most readily associated with mycotoxin consumption are either acute or subchronic. Chronic effects, such as carcinogenicity, have been more difficult to directly relate to mycotoxin consumption. This is in spite of the fact that various data indicate that at least 45 mycotoxins are known to be either mutagenic or carcinogenic (1). The following mycotoxins may pose an adverse human health risk in respect to carcinogenicity: aflatoxin, cyclochlorotine, griseofulvin, luteoskyrin, ochratoxin, patulin, penicillic acid, sterigmatocystin, T-2 toxin, and zearalenone.

An exception to this trend is epidemiological data indicating that AFB_1 is a human hepatocarcinogen (2). However, the relationship between AFB_1 consumption and human liver cancer may not be a simple one. For instance, it has been suggested that there is an association between hepatitis B and aflatoxin carcinogenicity; with hepatitis being permissive in respect to the hepatocarcinogenicity of AFB_1 (3). Other factors may also be associated with and permissive in respect to AFB_1 hepatocarcinogenicity including nutrition, simultaneous exposure to other hepatotoxins and other types of liver disease. Promotion of the initial damage to the genome (initiation) may also be important in the expression of the hepatocarcinogenicity of AFB_1, as discussed below. Overall, there may not be a simple relationship between the exposure to a carcinogenic mycotoxin and tumor production. It is becoming apparent that carcinogenesis is a multimechanistic, multifactorial and multistage event susceptible to a large number of modulating factors, both within the host and in the host's environment. Nutrition as a modulator of an individuals susceptibility to carcinogenic mycotoxins became a major interest within our laboratories over a decade ago. This report will review selected past and current studies in this area.

Our interest in the effect of nutrition, especially dietary protein, was originally sparked by the studies of Madhavan and Gopalan (4) who were the first to show that low-protein (5% casein) diets completely protected rats from the hepatocarcinogenicity of AFB_1, whereas diets containing 20% casein resulted in rats demonstrating the expected susceptibility. Wells et.al (4) later found that an 8% casein diet protected rats from AFB_1 induced liver tumors and the severity of liver involvement increased as dietary protein levels were increased from 22 to 30%.

Our original hypothesis was that dietary protein influenced the metabolism of AFB_1 in a manner that decreased the susceptibility of rats fed low dietary protein to AFB_1 carcinogenicity. At that time little was known about the metabolism of AFB_1, but Portman et al. (6) had recently demonstrated that hepatic microsomes could hydroxylate AFB_1 to form aflatoxin M_1. Due to the lack of knowledge concerning AFB_1 metabolism, we initiated our studies employing model drugs as substrates for the cytochrome P-450 dependent hepatic polysubstrate monooxygenase system (PSMOS). The basic experimental protocol employed male, weanling rats and diets consisting of 5% casein ab libitum, 20% casein diets fed ab libitum, and 20% casein diets pair-fed to the 5% casein group (7). Due to the decreased food consumption of the 5% casein group, the 20% casein pair-fed group represents the effects of dietary protein, whereas the comparison between the 20% casein ab libitum diet and the 5% casein ab libitum diet represents protein-calorie malnutrition (imposed by self-restricted food intake by the 5% group).

The latter group is probably more representative of the human situation. The diets are generally fed for 14-days before termination of the experiment. Various modifications have been imposed upon this basic protocol, including altering the level of protein and varying in the length of the feeding trial.

Figure 1 represents the effects dietary protein level on various parameters. The data is plotted as a percent of the 20% casein ab libitum control group to simplify the graph. The 5% casein diet depresses body weight by approximately 50% compared to both 20 and 30% casein. On the other hand, liver weight is actually increased compared to the higher protein diets. The increased liver weight is due to fatty infiltration of the liver as indicated by higher total lipid content and the increase in the size and number of hepatocellular fat vacuoles (8). Total hepatic microsomal protein is depressed by approximately 50% by the low protein diet. Cytochrome P-450, the terminal oxidase of the PSMOS, is also decreased by approximately 50% by the low protein diet (9). The only parameter altered by the 30% casein diet is an increase in microsomal cytochrome P-450 concentration (10).

Figure 2 represents the effects of dietary protein on various enzymic activities of the PSMOS system. The metabolism of two model PSMOS substrates, ethylmorphine and aniline is depressed by approximately 50% by the low protein diets, and the metabolism of ethylmorphine is significantly increased by the 30% protein diet. Reduction of cytochrome c catalyzed by the flavoprotein NADPH-cytochrome P-450 reductase is depressed approximately 20% by the low protein diet and significantly enhanced by the 30% protein diet. The ability of the flavoprotein to reduce cytochrome P-450, its natural substrate, is reduced 50% by the low protein diet and significantly increased by the 30% protein diet. Overall, this data indicates that low protein diets result in a decreased ability of the PSMOS to metabolize xenobiotics, whereas diets high in protein result in enhanced PSMOS activity. The decreased PSMOS activity is, in part, due to a lower total cytochrome P-450 concentration, depressed activity of NADPH-cytochrome P-450 reductase, and decreased ability of cytochrome P-450 to accept electrons from this flavoprotein. The latter conclusion can be drawn from the greater depression of NADPH-cytochrome P-450 reductase than that of NADPH-cytochrome c reductase. The depressions of PSMOS activity occur rapidly after instituting the low protein diets in weanling rats (11, 12, 13). From the day of initiation of the low protein diet there is a decrease in ethylmorphine metabolism, whereas aniline metabolism does not actually decrease, but fails to increase over a 45-day time course of treatment. After only one day on the low protein diet, significant decreases in ethylmorphine metabolism can be detected and by eight days these decreases have reached maximum (7). At both 8 and 15 days after initiation of the low protein diets, increasing the dietary protein level to 20% results in recovery of body weight, microsomal protein levels and enzyme activity by 45 days after initiation of the study. This indicates that nutritional intervention programs in human populations have the potential to reverse the effects of low dietary proteins. We have recently demonstrated that when adult male rats are switched from normal chow diets to either 1% casein or 20% casein semipurified diets the 1% protein group shows depressed PSMOS activity compared to the 20% group after only 14 days (14). This indicates

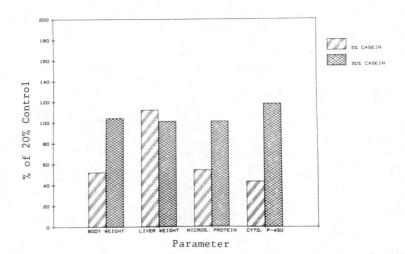

Figure 1. The effect of dietary protein levels on various parameters associated with animal growth and xenobiotic metabolism. Rats were fed semifurified diets consisting of either 5%, 20%, or 30% casein as the protein source for 14-days. Data is expressed as a percent of the 20% control diet.

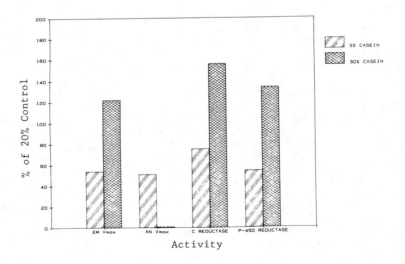

Figure 2. The effect of dietary protein levels on polysubstrate monooxygenase system activities of rat liver. Rats were fed semipurified diets consisting of either 5%, 20%, or 30% casein as the protein source for 14-days. Data is expressed as a per cent of the 20% control diet. No data is available for the Vmax of aniline (AN) at the 30% protein level.

that adults may rapidly respond to a low protein diet in a manner similar to a young animal and confirms that low protein diets depress PSMOS activity in adult rats.

Low protein diets also depress hepatic PSMOS activity by additional mechanisms. The PSMOS is a membrane bound system with the flavoprotein being an extrinsic protein bound to the membrane by a hydrophobic tail while cytochrome P-450 is an intrinsic protein. Translateral mobility of these components would be required for reduction of cytochrome P-450 (15). Since the number of cytochrome P-450 molecules far exceeds the number of reductase molecules, each reductase must be capable of reducing several cytochrome P-450 molecules. The reductase and cytochrome P-450 appear to be randomly distributed within the plane of the membrane, although they may exist in specific lipid domains different from the bulk lipid of the membrane. Alteration of either lipid-lipid or lipid-protein interactions within the membrane may modify the translateral mobility of these proteins and thereby alter the reduction of cytochrome P-450 and, consequently, rates of metabolism. By using fluoresent probes, we have demonstrated that microsomal membranes from rats fed low protein diets have decreased lipophilicity compared to 20% protein controls. Lipid content of the membranes from the low protein group is decreased even though total hepatic lipids increase. Membrane cholesterol levels appear to increase as a result of feeding the low protein diets (16). These changes may be associated with an apparent alteration of the transition temperature of the microsomal membranes obtained from rats fed the low protein diets. Figure 3 illustrates that an Arrhenius plot of the 0-deethylation of ethoxycoumarin by animals fed the 20% protein diets shows a break indicating a change in the energy of activation of the reaction. Classically the break-point is interpreted to represent the transition temperature of the membrane where it changes from a fluid mosaic to a more crystalline form. In contrast to the microsomes from the 20% protein fed rats, those from animals fed the 5% protein diets fail to elicit the break-point, although induction by phenobarbital restores the break-point (Figure 4). This indicates a fundamental change in the interactions between the components of the system probably associated with altered lipid-lipid and/or protein-lipid interactions. Studies utilizing isolated components of this enzyme system have indicated that the low protein diets also alter protein-protein interactions in this enzyme system (17). Therefore alterations in the microsomal membranes and in protein- protein interactions also have a mechanistic role in the depressed PSMOS activity observed in rats fed low protein diets.

Other enzymes associated with xenobiotic metabolism are also altered by dietary protein levels. Epoxide hydratase can hydrolyze various epoxides and appears to be important in decreasing their toxicity and carcinogenicity, although it is involved in the metabolic activation of certain carcinogens. Low dietary protein depresses epoxide hydratase activity in our dietary model (8). This may indicate both a decreased ability to detoxify epoxides and a decrease in metabolic activation of specific carcinogens, such as benzo(a)pyrene. Woodcock and Wood (19) have reported that dietary protein deficiency increases the activity of uridine diphosphate glucuronic acid (UDPG) transferase activity. This indicates that

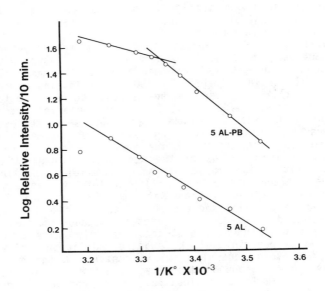

Figure 3. Arrhenius plot of the metabolism of ethoxycoumarin by hepatic microsomes isolated from rats fed a 5% casein diet for 14–days (5AL). Animals whose PSMOS was induced by phenobarbital are denoted at 5AL–PB.

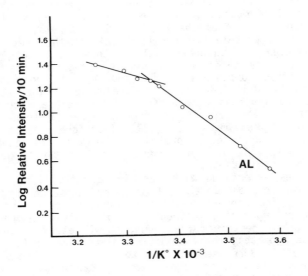

Figure 4. Arrhenius plot of the metabolism of ethoxycoumarin by hepatic microsomes isolated from rats fed a 20% casein diet for 14–days (20AL).

protein deficient animals may have greater ability to detoxify xe-nobiotics by this important pathway.

Mainigi and Campbell (20) have shown that low protein diets de-press hepatic glutathione levels. Since enzymatic conjugation and spontaneous reaction of certain xenobiotics with hepatic glutathi-one is an important detoxication step with certain compounds, this depression of glutathione levels may alter the toxicity of these compounds in animals fed low protein diets.

Figure 5 represents the in vitro metabolism of AFB_1 by rats fed diets containing either 5% or 20% casein. The production of the hydroxylated metabolites AFQ_1 and AFM_1 is depressed in animals fed the low protein diet. The depression of metabolism is similar to that seen with the N-demethylation of ethylmorphine. An exception to the depressed production of AFM_1 and AFQ_1 is the enhanced production of an unidentified aflatoxin, tentatively termed AFX_1. This metabolite is retained at the origin on TLC plates and its significance in AFB_1 toxicity and carcinogenicity is not known. The hydroxylated metabolites probably represent de-toxication products and do not have a direct role in AFB_1 carcin-ogenesis. The ultimate carcinogen of AFB_1 appears to be the 2,3 epoxide produced by the cytochrome P-450 dependent PSMOS. This me-tabolite covalently binds to DNA, predominately to the N-7 position of guanine, and initiates the biochemical lesion responsible for carcinogenesis. Although the epoxide can not be directly detected, the production of covalent adducts between it and macromolecules can be determined. Microsomes from rats fed the low protein diet have decreased ability to metabolically activate AFB_1 to the ep-oxide as measured by the in vitro covalent binding to DNA. This decrease is quantitatively similar to that found for ethylmorphine metabolism and the production of the hydroxylated metabolites of AFB_1.

Figure 6 represents the in vivo covalent binding of AFB_1 administered i.p. to male rats consuming diets containing 5%, 20% and 30% casein. Covalent binding to DNA and RNA was depressed ap-proximately 75% and binding to protein was depressed 60% in rats fed the low protein diet. On the other hand, the 30% protein diet enhanced covalent binding to DNA by approximately 30% and RNA by 10%. Covalent binding to protein was enhanced by 40% in rats fed the 30% protein diet. These data indicate that low protein diets depress the covalent binding of AFB_1 to critical tissue macro-molecules and should result in less damage to DNA than would occur at higher levels of dietary protein. The decreased DNA damage should result in a lower level of initiation which may, in part, result in decrease tumor yield and a resistance to AFB_1 carcino-genicity. This is in agreement with the studies indicating that rats fed low levels of dietary protein are resistant to AFB_1 hepatocarcinogenicity (4). Extrapolating this data to the results from rats fed the 30% protein group indicate that high protein di-ets may actually increase the susceptibility to AFB_1 hepatocar-cinogenicity.

The studies employing model drug substrates and in vitro AFB_1 metabolism suggest that the decreased covalent binding of AFB_1 to tissue macromolecules in rats fed low protein diets re-sults, in part, from the depression of the activity of the cyto-chrome P-450-dependent PSMOS. This depression would result in the

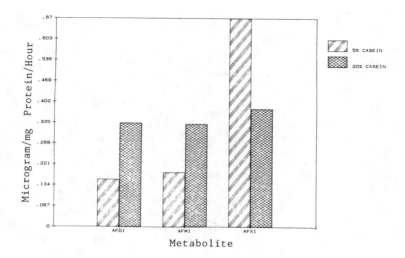

Figure 5. The effect of dietary protein levels on the metabolism of aflatoxin B_1 to hydroxylated metabolites. Rats were fed semifurified diets consisting of either 5% casein or 20% casein as the protein source.

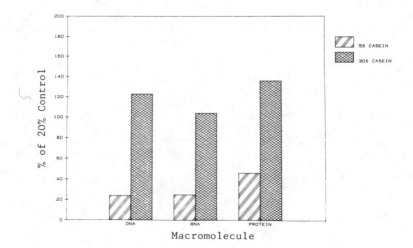

Figure 6. The effect of dietary protein levels on the covalent binding of aflatoxon B_1 to hepatic macromolecules. Rats were fed semifurified diets consisting of either 5%, 20% or 30% casein as the protein source for 14-days. Data is expressed as a percent of the 20% control diets.

production of lower levels of the 2,3 epoxide of AFB_1. However, the mechanism may be more complex. The total level of covalent adducts produced will be dependent upon the complex interplay between metabolic activation and factors which alter the level of the ultimate carcinogen. For instance, if epoxide hydratase plays a role in detoxication of the 2,3 epoxide, then the reduction in the activity of this enzyme by the low protein diets may decrease destruction of the epoxide. It is possible that the reduced activity of this enzyme does not play a role because this reduced activity may not be rate limiting in respect to covalent adduct formation. The enhanced activity of the UDPG-transferases seen in rats fed low protein diets may actually shift the equilibrium of AFB_1 metabolism toward glucuronide formation and away from epoxide production. An understanding of the effect of protein nutrition on the complex kinetic interplay between these various pathways requires further research before the various mechanisms associated with the protective effect of low protein in respect to the initiation of AFB_1 hepatocarcinogenicity can be understood. Low protein diets actually increase the acute toxicity of AFB_1 (21). The mechanism associated with this increased toxicity is not understood, in major part because the mechanism of the acute toxicity is not understood. It is not known if the acute toxicity of AFB_1 is associated with either the parent compound or a metabolite. The depressed metabolism of AFB_1 in protein deficient rats suggest that the acute toxicity may be associated with the parent compound, as opposed to a metabolite, since depressed biotransformation would result in higher levels of AFB_1 and decreased levels of metabolites.

As previously mentioned, carcinogenesis is a complex process and it would be naive to believe that dietary protein alters only the initiation phase. A series of eloquent studies by Appleton and Campbell (22, 23, 24) have indicated that the effects exerted by dietary protein during the promotional phase of AFB_1 hepatocarcinogenesis are as important, if not more so, than the effects seen during the initiation phase.

Appleton and Campbell (22) employed an initiation-promotion protocol employing varing levels of dietary protein and the assessment of gama-glutamyl transferase (GGT) positive preneoplastic foci as an early indicator of neoplastic lesions. Initiation was performed by the oral administration of 10 doses of AFB_1 over a two week period while the rats were fed a 20% casein diet. This allowed the animals to start with the same level of initiation. Following a one-week holding period after initiation, the diets of the rats were changed and then maintained constant during the 12 week promotion phase. Different groups of rats received either 5%, 20% or 40% dietary protein during the promotion phase of the study. Animals fed the 20% casein diets showed a 4-fold increase in GGT positive foci and those fed the 40% casein showed a 3-fold increase when compared to the rats fed the 5% casein diet. This indicates that even when rats are identically initiated, the level of dietary protein during the promotion phase exerts a profound influence upon lesion production. Therefore low protein diets not only decrease the level of covalent adducts between AFB_1 and DNA during the initiation phase; they also are less promoting during the promotional stage. In a second study, Appleton and Campbell

(23) employed a protocol similar to the one described above but divided the promotional phase into two six week phases. During the second six week phase of the 12 week promotion period, rats from the 20% and 5% casein groups were switched to 5% and 20% casein respectively for the duration of the study. The production of GGT positive foci in rats maintained on the 5 and 20% casein diets throughout the study followed the trends described for the previous study. However, switching rats fed 20% casein to 5% casein at the midpoint of the promotion phase produced GGT positive foci intermediate between those continued on either the 20% or 5% diets throughout the studies. Switching rats fed 5% protein to 20% protein produced a similar result. This indicates that foci production, and probably tumor production, is sensitive to changes in dietary protein during the promotion period. Therefore nutritional intervention after initiation and during promotion may inhibit carcinogenesis. This idea has important ramifications in respect to human cancer risk. To further investigate the role of dietary protein in initiation and promotion, Appleton and Campbell (24) performed experiments in which rats were initiated with AFB_1 while on either 5 or 20% casein diets. They then continued these diets in one set of animals and reversed the dietary protein levels of the other during the promotion phase. These studies indicated that even though the animals fed 5% casein diets during initiation had fewer covalent adducts, feeding the 20% casein diet increased GGT positive foci by five-fold. On the other hand, changing the 20% casein diets employed during the initiation period to 5% casein diets during the promotional period decreased foci production by six-fold. It therefore appears that modulation of dietary protein during the promotion phase is more important than modulation during the initiation phase.

In summary, it has been shown that dietary protein levels can influence the metabolism of the mycotoxin AFB_1. Altered metabolism is, in part, responsible for the protective role of low protein diets with respect to carcinogenicity and possibly with its increased toxicity in protein deficient rats. Dietary protein levels can also influence the promotional phase of carcinogenesis. Further research is required to determine the mechanisms associated with the influence of dietary protein on both the initiation and promotional phases of carcinogenesis.

Literature Cited

1. Stoloff, L. Carcinogens and Mutagens in the Environment, Vol. I, Food Products, H. F. Stich (ed.). 1982, CRC Press, Boca Raton, Fla., pp. 97-126.

2. Linsell, C.A. and Peers, F.G. Trans. Roy. Soc. Trop. Med. Hyg. 1977, 71. 471-473.

3. Munoz, N. and Linsell, A. Epidemiology of Cancer of the Digestive Organs, P. Correa and W. Haenszel (ed.). 1982, Martinus Nijhoff Publishers, The Hague. pp. 161-195.

4. Madhavan, T.V. and Gopalan, C. Arch. Pathol 1968, 85, 133.

5. Wells, P., Aftergood, L. and Alfin-Slater, R.B. J. Am. Oil Chem. Soc. 1976, 53, 559.

6. Portman, R.S., Plowman, K.M., and Campbell, T.C. Biochem. Biophys. Res. Comm. 1968, 33, 711.

7. Hayes, J.R., Mgbodile, M.U.K. and Campbell, T.C. Biochem. Pharmacol. 1973, 22, 1005.

8. Mgbodile, M.U.K. and Campbell, T.C. Personal Communication

9. Hayes, J.R. and Campbell, T.C. Biochem. Pharmacol. 1974, 23, 1721.

10. Hayes, J.R. Developments In Industrial Microbiology 1982, 23, 257.

11. Hayes, J.R., Mgbodile, M.U.K., Merrill, A.H., Nerurkar, L.S. and Campbell, T.C. J. Nutr. 1978, 108, 1788.

12. Hayes, J.R. and Campbell, T.C. Carcinogenesis, Vol. 5: Modifiers of Chemical Carcinogenesis, T. J. Slaga (ed.), 1980, Raven Press, NY, pp. 207-241.

13. Campbell, T.C., Hayes, J.R., Merrill, A.H., Maso, M. and Geotchius, M. Drug Metab. Rev. 1979, 9, 173-184.

14. Hayes, J.R., Spivey, R., Thompson, A. Unpublished observations, 1984.

15. Yang, C.S. Life Sciences 1977, 21, 1047.

16. Hayes, J.R. Unpublished observations, 1984.

17. Nerurkar, L.S., Hayes, J.R., Campbell, T.C. J. Nutr. 1978, 108, 678.

18. Adekunle, A.A., Hayes, J.R. and Campbell, T.C. Life Sci. 1977, 21, 1785.

19. Woodcock, B.G. and Wood, G.C. Biochem. Pharmacol. 1971, 20, 2703.

20. Mainigi, K.D. and Campbell, T.C. Toxicol. Appl. Pharmacol. 1981, 59, 196.

21. Madhavan, T.V. and Gopalan C. Arch. Pathol. 1965, 80, 123.

22. Appleton., B.S. and Campbell, T.C. Nutr. and Canc. 1982, 3, 200.

23. Appleton. B.S. and Campbell, T.C. J. Natl. Canc. Inst. 1983, 70, 547.

24. Appleton, B.S. and Campbell, T.C. Canc. Res. 1983, 43, 2150.

RECEIVED January 23, 1985

Food and Drug Interactions

C. JELLEFF CARR

Carr Associates, 6546 Belleview Drive, Columbia, MD 21046

Nutritional status determines effects of therapeutic drugs and recognition of these factors should lead to improved drug therapy. Pharmacokinetics are changed by a person's diet but metabolic tissue and cellular effects are not well understood. Biochemical transformations and enzyme inductions that decrease or increase toxicity of drugs are discussed and numerous examples given.

The old adage, we are what we eat, needs a new and more attractive label. We are just beginning to recognize that the composition of our diet can have a remarkable influence on a wide variety of metabolic changes. This subject requires more interest on the part of the scientific and medical community (1).

The nutritional status of a person will determine in large measure the degree of undesirable effects of therapeutic drugs and the growing literature on the impact of nutritional and environmental substances on the disposition and therapeutic efficacy of drugs reflects a complex of biochemical and pharmacologic interactions. Recognition and understanding of these reactions should lead to improved drug therapy. However, in recent years it has become clear that the impact of nutritional and environmental substances on the disposition of drugs is difficult to predict. Biochemical and pharmacologic interactions between food components, additives, chemicals and therapeutic drugs are now under study not only for their toxicologic significance, but because understanding these reactions should lead to improved drug therapy.

Absorption and utilization of drugs given orally is influenced significantly in some instances by different foods. Pharmacokinetic studies indicate plasma levels changed by the diet may be crucial for those drugs where the blood concentration must be kept within a narrow range. These are relatively elementary facts related to efficient drug therapy and wisely observed by the careful physician. On the other hand, metabolic changes and tissue interactions at the cellular level of drug actions are more arcane and frequently not recognized, indeed, are often not known.

Biochemical transformations at the target cell sites, the

0097–6156/85/0277–0221$06.00/0
© 1985 American Chemical Society

pharmacokinetic changes, metabolic significance and the detoxification and excretion of drugs as modified by nutritional influences are coming under study. We recognize that therapeutic efficacy and drug toxicity may be directly influenced by food-drug interactions, however, relatively few investigators pursue studies to develop the necessary knowledge required to understand these relationships.

A relatively new note on this subject has been added by the developing knowledge of non-nutrient food additives. These substances also may change the pharmacokinetics of therapeutic drugs. With increasing concern about carcinogens in the food supply and with more sensitive analytical methodology, these chemical biotransformations in man are being studied in terms of dietary factors that influence the action of drugs. The most recent concern, for example, has been traces of the soil fumigant ethylene dibromide (EDB) in foods arising from agricultural applications.

Dietary modifications are brought about by use of weight-reducing diets, vegetarian diets, hospitalization, or post-operative regimens. These diets are often continued for long periods of time and it is likely they result in changes in the metabolism by the body of subsequently administered drugs. We know that drug metabolism rates in the elderly average one-half to two-thirds the rate observed in younger people. However, individual variations are great and an old person may have metabolic rates well within the value normal for younger persons. Thus, generalizations cannot be drawn because the elderly, who as a group consume the greatest number of drugs, are far from a homogeneous population. It is of interest that drug regulatory guidelines do not address these issues. Generally speaking, the physician or the nutritional biochemist is confronted with a complicated clinical picture of multiple disease entities, multiple drug therapy, and a poor dietary regimen in the elderly.

Effect of Foods on Biochemical Transformation of Drugs

Living cells have a remarkable capacity to chemically modify drug molecules. The biochemical transformation frequently achieved by the non-specific enzymes present in the microsomes of cells is one of the chief oxidative pathways drug molecules undergo. These are usually hydroxylation reactions leading to detoxification of the drug. More polar metabolites are formed and hence are less capable of penetrating the lipid target cell barrier. The result is subsequent excretion of the less toxic metabolites.

The mechanism in hepatic cellular metabolism involves an electron transport system that functions for many drugs and chemical substances. These reactions include O-demethylation, N-demethylation, hydroxylation, nitro reduction and other classical biotransformations. The electron transport system contains the heme protein, cytochrome P-450 that is reduced by NADPH via a flavoprotein, cytochrome P-450 reductase. For oxidative metabolic reactions, cytochrome P-450, in its reduced state (Fe^{+2}), incorporates one atom of oxygen into the drug substrate and another into water. Many metabolic reductive reactions also utilize this system. In addition, there is a lipid component, phosphatidylcholine, which is associated with the electron transport and is an obligatory requirement for drug metabolism. It is obvious that in such a complex series of events the food, drug, or chemical elements could participate in a variety of ways.

It must be pointed out that not all enzymic reactions of drugs in liver cells produce less toxic metabolites---some are more toxic. Hepatic drug metabolizing enzymes activate some chemically stable drugs to potent alkylating, arylating or acylating agents. These bind covalently to liver cell macromolecules and may cause necrosis (1a,2). Foods yield protective substances such as glutathione, that are capable of conjugating with a toxic metabolite. However, when body stores of these substances are exhausted the toxicity of chemical substances can be increased. Thus, nutrition can greatly influence the activity of these important metabolic systems (3).

The rates of toxication or detoxication of drugs and xenobiotics in animals and man are known to be influenced by age, sex, species, strain, disease and diet. One research report lists 10 factors (3a). It appears that for man, diet is most varied and therefore most complex as a variable in ascertaining its role in either enhancing toxicity or reducing untoward effects of therapeutic drugs or environmental chemicals.

Following the prolonged administration of some drugs, hepatic microsomal enzymes may be stimulated and the process of "induction" takes place (4,5). The implications of microsomal enzyme induction are just beginning to be appreciated by clinicians. Indeed, this phenomenon explains why in some cases repeated drug dosage may lead to decreased therapeutic effectiveness. For example, the detoxification mechanisms of the liver become more efficient in metabolizing the drug and larger doses are required to elicit the desired clinical pharmacologic effects. Microsomal enzymes can also be induced by diet in such tissues as the intestine, lung, adrenals and kidney although less is known about these extra-hepatic systems (6-9).

Toxicological Significance of Enzyme Induction

A long series of experiments has demonstrated that many plant foods serve as inducers of both liver and gastrointestinal hydroxylases (10,11). Enhanced activity of some microsomal enzymes or induction of increased aryl hydrocarbon hydroxylase activity by food additives or naturally-occurring flavones, has been shown to inhibit the action of chemical carcinogens in animals. These inhibitors include both natural food ingredients, drugs, or synthetic compounds introduced into the environment (11). Phenobarbital, diphenylhydantoin, phenylbutazone, and pregnenolone-16-carbonitrile are examples of drugs that induce hepatic microsomal enzymes (12).

The significance of these findings lies in the apparent protective effects of these and related substances in inducing increased microsomal monooxygenase activity. The wide range of compounds capable of inducing this protective effect against known potent carcinogens is noteworthy. Many of these substances are present in plants consumed by man as food. These include the flavones of natural origin, e.g. 5,6-benzoflavone, and rutin from the buckwheat family. Natural indoles in the edible vegetables Brussels sprouts, cabbage, cauliflower and broccoli, are inhibitory to

benzo(a)pyrene-induced neoplasia in the forestomach of rodents and
addition of certain of these indoles to their diets inhibited pulmonary adenoma, and mammary tumor formation (13). The mechanism(s)
of action of these indoles is not known at present.

In addition, pesticide residues such as DDT and the fungicide
EDB present in low levels in man's foods, while below the level that
causes enzyme induction in rats, may also contribute to total metabolic drug effects. The influences of diet and socially used drugs
on drug oxidation has been studied in vegetarians and non-vegetarians. Major differences in diet, cigarette smoking, and use of the
steroid oral contraceptives were shown to have significant effects
on antipyrine oxidation (14,15). If one can generalize from antipyrine to other drugs, these environmental factors could play important roles in drug therapy and prevention of toxicity. Obviously,
it is difficult to control for so many different variables in any
population group, but the findings emphasize points that require
study for food and drug interactions.

Toxic substances, food ingredients and therapeutic drugs have
an altered tissue distribution depending on the diet. For example,
splanchnic blood flow is modified by oral glucose or protein feeding and hence the tissue site of action of these various substances
can be modified (15a). Tissue changes then can be induced by altering blood flow and the resulting pharmacologic effects, tissue injury or repair will be changed.

From animal studies and from human experience we know that high
fat diets promote the rapid absorption of substances from the gastrointestinal tract. This will include drugs, test substances in animal diets, and food ingredients (15b). Lipid diets with their
saturation, polyunsaturation, and essential fatty acid composition
modify nutrition of the person and added anti-oxidants in these oils
are recognized to influence metabolism. The extensive literature
in this field has been reviewed and compiled by The Nutrition Foundation. One of the noteworthy findings was the demonstration by
many investigators that tumor promotion is enhanced in experimental
animals by high fat diets (15b).

In addition, we know that changing a customary diet to one high
in protein and low in carbohydrate in some people, increases the
rates of metabolism of drugs such as antipyrine and theophylline,
and shifting to an isocaloric diet of low protein-high carbohydrate
slows the rates of metabolism of these drugs. However, numerous
studies emphasize the considerable individual variability to changes
in human diets; some people exhibit dramatic effects others exhibit
little or no response.

Metabolite Induction Enhancing Toxicity

Liver drug toxicity may be increased by enzyme inducers and a number
of examples are known. Thus, carbon tetrachloride (16), trichlor-
ethylene (17), toluene (18), hycanthone (19), acetaminophen and
isoniazid (20), and metotrexate (21), among other drugs and chemicals, have been studied in this respect.

The significance of polycyclic aromatic hydrocarbons (PCH)
formed in charcoal-broiled beef has been publicized with respect to
the ability of these substances to alter the fate of drugs in the

body. The bioavailability of phenacetin in human subjects apparently
is reduced (22) and the plasma clearance of caffeine in the rat is
altered (23). Benzanthracene, dibenzanthracene, chrysene, and pyrene, potent inducers of the cytochrome P-448 system in liver microsomes, caused a marked increase in the plasma clearance of caffeine
(23). These findings suggest that the metabolism of many drugs may
be altered in man exposed to these environmental substances or foods
containing PCH.

Long-term anticonvulsive therapy with diphenylhydantoin or
phenobarbital is known to cause osteomalacia by influencing calcium
metabolism (24,25). Alteration in the metabolism of vitamin D,
presumably secondary to induction of hepatic microsomal enzymes,
leads to the calcium and bone abnormalities (26). Patients on anticonvulsive therapy with phenytoin exhibit a decrease in serum 25-
hydroxyvitamin D (27). Adequate dietary amounts of vitamin precursors or microsomal enzyme stimulators might prevent these effects
of long-term therapy.

The ingestion of foods containing tyramine, such as cheese, and
the hypertensive crisis produced in patients taking the antidepres-
sive drug tranylcypromine is a classic example of food and drug
toxicity. Tyramine-containing foods apparently stimulate the release of norepinephrine, which results in a sharp elevation in blood
pressure. The norephinephrine release is also accelerated by the
drug itself, a monoamine oxidase inhibitor (28). Patients receiving
the monoamine oxidase inhibitors are now cautioned to avoid the foods
that are known to contain high amounts of tyramine, as result of
this well-publicized interaction. The list of foods that contain
tyramine or related amines capable of causing these reactions is
long and it is difficult for patients on drug therapy with monoamine
oxidase inhibitors to follow these dietary restrictions. This un-
fortunate food and drug toxicity reaction has limited the therapeutic usefulness of these drugs.

Enzyme Inactivation of Clinical Significance

A large number of drugs, chemical substances, and some ingredients
of foods, are known to inactivate cytochrome enzymes. The results
are significant during therapy with multiple drugs if one or more
of them is a suicide inactivator of cytochrome P-450. This subject
has been studied intensely, however, the influence of dietary ingredients on drug activity in this regard has not received very much
attention. This impaired metabolic disposition of a therapeutic
drug or food versus drug interaction is an area for future research
investigation that has important clinical ramifications. These issues have been reviewed in detail (29).

High Fiber Diets

The recent enthusiasm for high fiber foods may carry a special chal-
lenge in considering food/drug toxicities. Vegetable fiber diets
have been shown to reduce the toxicity of some drugs for animals
(30). Presumably, phytates hold inorganic ions in a clathrate matrix
that prevents absorption of the metal from the gut, other substances,
e.g. bile acids, may also be bound (31). The bioavailability of
iron as influenced by phytates in cereal foods via the formation of

insoluble iron phytates is an example of a well known but little
understood problem in gastrointestinal physiology and nutrition (32).
Magnesium, zinc and tin are covalently bound by fiber and it is possible to produce zinc deficiency in animals by feeding high soybean-
protein diets.

On the other hand, potentially toxic substances in foods such
as aflatoxins may become less toxic in the presence of fiber in the
gut. In experimental animals there is evidence that vegetable fiber
is protective against estrogen-induced ovarian and uterine tumors
(30). Natural ingredient diets protect rats against carcinogenic-
induced mammary tumors (33,34). There is an obvious need to evaluate these potentially useful or harmful effects in man as we come to
a better understanding of the effects of changing diets, on drug
toxicity and therapeutic usefulness.

Summary

Changes in man's diet produce marked and often unpredictable effects
on drug metabolism. Methods are needed to measure inter-individual
and inter-group differences in metabolism of foreign compounds in
order to accurately assess dietary influences on drug metabolism and
vice versa. Epidemiologic studies of rigorously selected human populations, coupled with the newer sensitive chemical analytical methods
will provide the necessary data base for these investigations.

Literature Cited

1. Carr, C.J. Food and drug interactions. Ann Rev Pharmacol
    Toxicol, 1983; 2219-29 (982)

1.a Mitchel, J.R. & Jollows, D.J. Metabolic activation of drugs
    to toxic substances. Gasteroenterology, 1975; 68:392-410

2. Sherlock, S. Progress report: Hepatic reactions to drugs.
    Gut, 1979; 20:634-48

3. Anderson, K.E., Conney, A.H. & Kappas, A. Nutrtional in-
    fluences on chemical biotransformations in humans. Nutr Rev,
    1983; 40:161-171

3.a Jusko, W.J., et al. Factors affecting theophylline clearances:
    Age, tobacco, marijuana, cirrhosis, congestive heart failure,
    obesity, oral contraceptives, benzodiazepines, barbiturates
    and ethanol. J Pharm Sci, 1979; 68:1358-1366

4. Conney, A.H. Pharmacological implications of microsomal enzyme
    induction. Pharmacology Reviews, 1967; 19:317-366

5. Wattenberg, L.W. Effect of dietary constituents on the metabo-
    lism of chemical carcinogens. Cancer Research, 1975; 35:3326-
    3331

6. Chhabra, R.S. & Fouts, J.R. Biochemical properties of some
    microsomal xenobiotic-metabolizing enzymes in rabbit small
    intestines. Drug Metab Dispos, 1976; 4:208-214

7. Tredger, J.M., et al. Postnatal development of mixed-function oxidation as measured in microsomes from the small intestine and liver of rabbits. Drug Metab Dispos, 1976; 4:17-23

8. James, M.O., et al. Hepatic and extrahepatic metabolism in vitro of an epoxide (8-^{14}C-styrene oxide) in the rabbit. Biochem Pharmacol, 1976; 25:187-193

9. Minchin, R.F. & Boyd, M.R. Localization of metabolic activation and deactivation systems in the lung. Ann Rev Pharmacol Toxicol, 1983; 23:217-238

10. Wattenberg, L.W. Dietary modification of intestinal and pulmonary aryl hydrocarbon activity. Toxicol Appl Pharmacol, 1972; 23:741-748

11. Wattenberg, L.W. Inhibitors of chemical carcinogens. J Environ Pathol and Toxicol, 1980; 3:35-52

12. Poland, A. & Kende, A. The genetic expression of aryl hydrocarbon hydroxylase activity: Evidence for a receptor mutation in nonresponsive mice. In Origins of Human Cancer. Cold Spring Harbor Symposium, New York, 1977; 847-967

13. Wattenberg, L.W. & Loub, W.D. Inhibition of polycyclic hydrocarbon-induced neoplasia by naturally-occurring indoles. Cancer Res, 1978; 38:1410-1413

14. Vesell, E.S., et al. Studies on the disposition of antipyrine, aminopyrine and phenacetin using plasma, saliva, and urine. Clin Pharmacol Therap, 1975; 18:259-272

15. Shively, C.A., et al. Dietary patterns and diurnal variations in aminopyrine disposition. Clin Pharmacol Therap, 1981; 29:65-73

15.a Brandt, J.L., et al. The effect of oral protein and glucose feeding on splanchnic blood flow and oxygen utilization in normal and cirrhotic subjects. J Clin Invest, 1955; 34:1017

15.b Ad Hoc Working Group Report on Oil/Gavage in Toxicology. July 14, 15, 1983. The Nutrition Foundation, Washington, DC

16. McLean, A.E.M. & McLean, E.K. Diet and Toxicity. British Med Bull, 1969; 25:278-281

17. Baerg, R.D. & Kimberg, D.V. Centrilobular hepatic necrosis and acute renal failure in "solvent sniffers." Ann Int Med, 1970; 73:713-720

18. O'Brien, E.T., et al. Hepatorenal damage from toluene in a "glue sniffer." British Med J, 1971; 2:29-30

19. Cohen, C. Liver pathology in hycanthone hepatitis. Gasteroenterology, 1978; 75:103-106

20. Mitchell, J.R., et al. Metabolic activation - Biochemical basis for many drug-induced liver injuries. Prog Liver Dis, 1976; 5:259-279

21. Almeyda, J., et al. Structural and functional abnormalities of the liver in psoriasis before and during methotrexate therapy. Br J Dermatol, 1972; 87-623-631

22. Pantuck, E.J., et al. Effect of charcoal-broiled beef on phenacetin metabolism in man. Clin Pharmacol Therap, 1979; 25:88-95

23. Welch, R.M., et al. Effect of aroclor 1254, phenobarbital, and polycyclic aromatic hydrocarbons on the plasma clearance of caffeine in the rat. Clin Pharmacol & Therap, 1977; 22:Part 2, 791-798

24. Sotaniemi, E.A., et al. Radiologic bone changes and hypocalcemia with anticonvulsant therapy in epilepsy. Ann Intern Med, 1972; 77:389-394

25. Tolman, K.G., et al. Osteomalacia associated with anticonvulsive drug therapy in mentally retarded children. Pediatrics, 1975; 56:45-51

26. Hahn, T.J. & Avioli, L.V. Anticonvulsive osteomalacia. Arch Intern Med, 1975; 135:997-1000

27. Bell, R.D., et al. Effect of phenytoin on bone and vitamin D metabolism. Ann Neurol, 1979; 5:374-378

28. Marley, E. & Blackwell, B. Interactions of monoamine oxidate inhibitors, amines, and food stuffs. Adv Pharmacol and Chemo-Therap, 1970; 8:185-239

29. Ortiz de Montellano, P.R. & Correia, M.A. Suicidal destruction of cytochrome P-450 during oxidative drug metabolism. Ann Rev Pharmacol Toxicol, 1983; 23:481-503

30. Ershoff, B.H. Antitoxic effects of plant fiber. Am J Clin Nutri, 1974; 27:1395-1398

31. Kritchevsky, D. & Story, J.A. Binding of bile salts in vitro by non-nutritive fiber. J Nutr, 1974; 104:458-461

32. Gortner, W.A. Nutrition in the United States 1900 to 1974. Cancer Res, 1975; 35:3246-3253

33. Carroll, K.K. Experimental evidence of dietary factors and hormone-dependent cancers. Cancer Res, 1975; 35:3374-3383

34. Engel, R.W. & Copeland, D.H. Protective action of stock diets against the cancer-inducing action of 2-acetylaminofluorene in rats. Cancer Res, 1952; 12:211-215

RECEIVED August 28, 1984

Dietary Vitamin E and Cigarette Smoking

CHING K. CHOW

Department of Nutrition and Food Science, University of Kentucky, Lexington, KY 40506

The effect of dietary vitamin E on cellular
susceptibility to cigarette smoke was studied in rats.
Weanling male rats maintained on a basal vitamin E
deficient diet with or without vitamin E
supplementation for 4-8 weeks were exposed to either
sham or cigarette smoke for up to 7 days. Relative to
the respective sham groups, a greater alteration of
biochemical parameters, such as levels of glutathione
and related enzymes, was found in the lungs of smoked
rats fed the deficient diet than in those of the
supplemented groups. Animals' lungs exhibited a
greater biochemical response to whole smoke than to
the gaseous phase of smoke. The results suggest that
the nutritional status of vitamin E alters cellular
susceptibility of rats to cigarette smoke.

Cigarette smoking has been implicated as a contributing factor to
the causation and exacerbation of various respiratory diseases,
cardiovascular disease and other disorders in man. The lung appears
to be the primary organ at risk to the effects of cigarette smoking.
In addition to the morphological lesions induced (1-2), cigarette
smoking has been shown to alter a number of biochemical parameters
in animal lungs (3-4).
        Cigarette smoke consists of a large variety of compounds
including oxidants and free radicals (5). The formation of reactive
oxygen species such as superoxide radical anion, hydroxy radical,
hydrogen peroxide, hypochlorous acid and singlet oxygen may be
augmented by the action of polymorphonuclear leukocytes and
macrophages following cigarette smoking (6-7). The aqueous phase of
cigarette smoke extract has been shown to be capable of initiating
autooxidation of unsaturated lipids of alveolar macrophages in vitro
(8). The reduction of elastase inhibiting capability of α_1 -
antitrypsin in the lung lavage fluid of cigarette-smoked rats has

been shown to be preventable by a reducing agent (9). These findings are suggestive that an oxidative damage mechanism may be involved in the adverse effects of cigarette smoking.

Increasing evidence indicates that diet/nutrition plays an important role in modulating the action and/or metabolism of a number of chemicals, drugs and environmental pollutants. Nutrients are essential for all fundamental cellular processes. The nutritional status of the affected subject may, therefore, influence cellular susceptibility to the effect of xenobiotics, including those from cigarette smoke. While the precise role of vitamin E in cellular metabolism is not yet clear, the vitamin may protect essential cellular components from the adverse effects of xenobiotics either via a free radical scavenging mechanism or as a component of the cell membrane (10-11). Administration of vitamin E has been shown to lessen the toxicity of a variety of compounds (12-16).

The studies reported herein deal primarily with the influence of dietary vitamin E on cellular susceptibility of rats to cigarette smoke.

Methods

Male Sprague-Dawley rats were employed as experimental animals. Weanling rats received from the supplier (Harlan Industries, Inc., Indianapolis, Indiana) were initially maintained on Purina rat chow for 5-10 days. They were then randomly divided into groups and fed a basal vitamin E-deficient diet (17) supplemented with either nothing, 100 or 200 ppm vitamin E (as d, l-α-tocopheryl acetate) for 4-8 weeks prior to smoking exposure. As determined spectrophotofluorometrically (18), the selenium content of the basal diet averaged 0.02 to 0.03 ppm. The nutritional status of vitamin E was monitored by measuring the degree of erythrocyte hemolysis (19) and activity of plasma pyruvate kinase (20).

Animals were exposed to either sham smoke, the gaseous phase of the smoke, or whole smoke at 10-120 puffs/day/exposure for up to 7 days using either a single-port reverse phase smoking machine or a peristaltic pump smoking machine (21-22). Additional animals were also maintained to serve as room controls. The single-port reverse phase smoking machine generates a rectilinear puff of two-second duration and 35 ml volume once a minute. The puff is then diluted to 10% with fresh air in the inhalation chamber and is held there for 15 seconds. The smoke-air mixture is then removed from the chamber, and fresh air is introduced for the remaining 45 seconds. The non-filtered low nicotine University of Kentucky reference cigarette, 1A1, was used for this study. Sham animals were exposed to fresh room air in the same manner as the smoked group.

The peristaltic pump smoking machine with a recycle dilution system delivered a 12.5% to 50% smoke to the animals for the first 2 seconds, and 6.25% to 25% smoke for the next 2 seconds. The smoke concentration was further reduced by half each 2 seconds until the next puff was taken (21). The gaseous phase of smoke was generated by passing whole smoke through a Cambridge filter to remove particulate matter. The University of Kentucky reference cigarette, 2R1,was employed for this study. Immediately following each exposure, blood samples were taken from tail veins for the estimation of carboxyhemoglobin levels using a microprocedure (23).

Sixteen to eighteen hours following each exposure period, animals from each group were anesthetized ethereally, blood was withdrawn, and then they were killed. Tissues (lung, kidney, heart, liver, spleen and testes) were examined for abnormal changes and were removed, blotted and weighed. Lungs, and in some cases kidneys were homogenized with isotonic phosphate buffer, pH 7.4. The tissue homogenates and 9,000 x g supernatant fraction, as well as blood plasma/serum were aliquoted for various biochemical measurements. The significance of difference between two sample means was determined using the Student's "t" test as a 95% confidence interval.

Results

Particulate Matter Intake and Carboxyhemoglobin Level. Apparent total particulate matter intake averaged about 1.5 mg/rat/smoking session (or about 6 mg/kg rat) for rats exposed to whole smoke at 50% initial concentration for 10 puffs per session using a peristaltic pump smoking machine. This is comparable to the estimated dose for humans smoking one pack per day of the same type of cigarette, taking in 6.8 mg total particulate matter per kg body weight (24). The average blood carboxyhemoglobin level after smoking exposure was 8.5% under the above mentioned smoking conditions. The carboxyhemoglobin level was, in general, proportionate to the concentration of smoke inhaled. However, it was not significantly different for rats receiving whole smoke exposure or the gaseous phase of the smoke, and was not significantly affected by the status of dietary vitamin E.

The body weight, tissue weight and protein contents in the lungs and kidneys were not significantly altered by whole smoke or the gaseous phase of the smoke in either dietary group of animals.

Blood Cell Concentrations and serum Enzymes. The lungs with their airways and alveolar surfaces exposed directly to the external environment are conceivably a primary target to injury from a variety of agents, including cigarette smoke. The blood cells may become exposed to cigarette smoke at the lung parenchyma gas exchange surface or following the infusion of the smoke components. Increased carboxyhemoglobin levels in blood with secondary tissue hypoxia have been suggested to be associated with increased hematocrit values in smokers (25). In patients who stopped smoking, hemotacrit values were found to decrease from a mean of 56% down to 4% (26). Smoking has also been linked to an increase in the white blood cell count and red cell mean corpuscular volume (27). In our studies, smoke-exposed animals were found to have higher red blood cell counts, mean cell volumes, and higher hematrocit and hemoglobin levels, while white blood cell counts were either unchanged or lower. The magnitude of the alterations was less profound in the blood of animals fed the vitamin E-supplemented diet than in the deficient group.

Alteration of serum enzyme activity has been shown to be a
sensitive parameter of tissue injury (20). While the activities of
such enzymes as pyruvate kinase, lactate dehydrogenase, glutamate
oxaloacetate transaminase, alkaline phosphatase, and creatine
phosphokinase in rat serum were significantly altered by the
deprivation of dietary vitamin E, the activities of these enzymes
were not influenced by smoking exposure under the experimental
conditions (Table I).

Table I. Effect of Dietary Vitamin E and Cigarette Smoking on
Plasma Enzymes[1]

Enzyme Activity (nmoles/min/ml)	Dietary Vitamin E (ppm)			
	0		100	
	Sham	Smoke	Sham	Smoke
Pyruvate kinase	3009+282[2](6)	2955+306(8)	209+21(4)	234+30(8)
Lactate dehydrogenase	544+95	528+113	423+84	453+92
Glutamate oxaloacetate transaminase	242+63	257+44	92+16	79+11

[1] One-month-old male rats maintained on the respective diets for 8
weeks were exposed to sham or cigarette smoke for 7 days.
[2] Mean+standard deviation; number in the parentheses represents
number of animals in each group.

Vitamin C. Studies have shown lower blood vitamin C levels and
decreased urinary excretion of vitamin C among human smokers (28).
Although the mechanism of this lowering effect is not yet clear, the
presence of such substances as nicotine, carbon monoxide, carbon
particles, acetaldehyde and nitrogen dioxide in cigarette smoke has
been attributed to a reduced bioavailability of vitamin C. In
corroboration with the results of human studies, the plasma level of
vitamin C (L-ascorbic acid) in rats was found to decrease
significantly following cigarette smoking (Table II). The degree of
the decline was relatively greater in animals fed the vitamin E-
deficient diet than in the supplemented group. On the other hand,
the levels of vitamin C in the lungs of vitamin E-deficient rats,
but not the supplemented animals, were found to increase
significantly following smoking exposure. It appears that an
increased amount of ascorbic acid may be synthesized in the tissues
of cigarette-smoked rats maintained on the vitamin E-deficient diet
to meet their increased need. A marked stimulation of hepatic
ascorbic acid biosynthesis in rats and mice has been reported upon
exposure to various noxious compounds (29-30). The levels of
vitamin C in the kidneys were not found to be altered by cigarette
smoking.

Table II. Dietary Vitamin E and Levels of Ascorbic Acid in the Plasma, Lung and Kidney of Cigarette-Smoked Rats[1]

Dietary Vitamin E (ppm)	Treatment	Plasma (mg/100 ml)	Lung (mg/g)	Kidney (mg/ml)
0	Smoke	1.29 ± 0.12[2] (8)	147.0 ± 9.3	82.3 ± 5.3
	Sham	1.53 ± 0.14 (6)	115.8 ± 9.3	80.5 ± 7.8
	p[3]	< 0.01	< 0.001	NS[4]
100	Smoke	1.37 ± 0.11 (8)	119.5 ± 8.5	74.3 ± 6.8
	Sham	1.56 ± 0.10 (4)	130.3 ± 11.0	72.5 ± 4.5
	p	< 0.02	NS	NS

[1] One-month-old male rats maintained on the respective diets for 8 weeks were exposed to either sham or cigarette smoke for 7 days (31).
[2] Mean±standard deviation; number in the parentheses represents number of animals in each group.
[3] Student's "t" test.
[4] Not significant ($p < 0.05$).

The functional interrelationship between vitamin C and vitamin E has been known for a number of years (11). While dietary vitamin E appears to play a role in determining the levels of vitamin C in the plasma and lungs of cigarette smoked rats, the levels of vitamin E in plasma were not significantly altered by the smoke exposure (31).

Lipid Peroxidation Products and the Glutathione Peroxidase System.
Cigarette smoke contains a large variety of compounds including oxidants and free radicals (5). Nitrogen dioxide, for example, has been found in cigarette smoke at the level of up to 250 ppm. Animal experiments indicate nitrogen dioxide can cause pulmonary effects at a concentration as low as 1 ppm (32). A number of reports also suggest that an oxidative damage mechanism may be involved in the adverse effects of cigarette smoking (7-9).

In our attempts to determine the possible role of free radical lipid peroxidation in smoke induced injury, the levels of lipid peroxidation products – thiobarbituric acid reactants, mainly malondialdehyde – were measured in lung homogenates with or without prior incubation at 37°C for one hour. contrary to our expectation, the levels of thiobarbituric acid reactants were found to be decreased, rather than increased, in the lungs of cigarette-smoke-exposed rats (Table III). Such a depression effect, however, was observed only when animals were exposed to whole smoke, and not to the gaseous phase of smoke.

Table III. Dietary Vitamin E and Thiobarbituric Acid Reactants in the Lungs of Cigarette-Smoked Rats [1]

Dietary vitamin E (ppm)	Sham smoke	Gaseous phase	Whole smoke
0	59 ± 9 [2,3,a]	53 ± 6 [a]	45 ± 6 [b]
100	21 ± 6 [c]	24 ± 5 [c]	17 ± 2 [d]

[1] One-month-old male rats maintained on the respective diets for 4 weeks were exposed to 10 puffs/exposure/day for 4 days (42).
[2] Mean+standard deviation; eight animals in each group. The means do not share the same superscript letter, indicating a significant difference ($p < 0.05$).
[3] The data are expressed as umoles/lung. The homogenate was incubated at 37°C for 1 hour.

Similar to the report of York et al. (5), the levels of reduced glutathione (GSH) and activities of the potentially protective enzyme, glutathione peroxidase, and its metabolically related enzymes, glutathione reductase and glucose-6-phosphate (G-6-P) dehydrogenase (11) were variably increased in the lungs following cigarette smoking exposure (Tables IV and V). However, the magnitude of the alterations was, in general, dose dependent, and was greater in the lungs of animals fed the vitamin E-deficient diet than in those of the supplemented group. Similar results were also observed for such pulmonary enzymes as pyruvate kinase and lactate dehydrogenase.

Table IV. Dietary Vitamin E and GSH Peroxidase System in the Lungs of Cigarette-Smoked Rats[1]

Biochemical parameter	Dietary vitamin E (ppm)			
	0		100	
	Smoke	Sham	Smoke	Sham
GSH (umoles/lung)	1.28 ± 0.08 [a]	1.10 ± 0.05 [b]	1.07 ± 0.08 [a]	0.96 ± 0.10 [a]
GSH peroxidase (umoles/min/lung)	2.42 ± 0.30 [a]	2.25 ± 0.25 [a]	2.27 ± 0.27 [a]	2.16 ± 0.23 [a]
GSH reductase (umoles/min/lung)	1.83 ± 0.30 [a]	1.38 ± 0.23 [b]	1.41 ± 0.18 [a]	1.29 ± 0.20 [a]
G-6-P dehydrogenase (umoles/min/lung)	2.54 ± 0.22 [a]	1.96 ± 0.14 [b]	1.68 ± 0.22 [a]	1.76 ± 0.24 [a]

[1] One-month-old male rats maintained on the respective diets for 5 weeks were exposed to 120 puffs of cigarette smoke or sham per day for the first day and 50 puffs/day for 2 more days. (42). Mean+standard deviation. The means do not share the same superscript letter, indicating a significant difference (p<0.05).

Table V.   Dietary Vitamin E and GSH Peroxidase System in the Lungs
of Cigarette-Smoked Rats[1]

Dietary Vitamin E (ppm)	Biochemical parameter	Sham smoke	Gaseous phase	Whole smoke
0	GSH (umoles/lung)	0.99 ± 0.08[2],a	1.29 ± 0.24[b]	1.40 ± 0.33[b]
	GSH peroxidase (umoles/min/lung)	1.44 ± 0.20[a]	1.54 ± 0.28[a]	1.56 ± 0.20[b]
	GSH reductase (umoles/min/lung)	1.53 ± 0.23[a]	1.45 ± 0.12[a]	1.53 ± 0.19[a]
	G-6-P dehydrogenase (umoles/min/lung)	1.64 ± 0.14[a]	1.74 ± 0.18[a]	2.00 ± 0.19[b]
100	GSH (umoles/lung)	1.09 ± 0.16[a]	1.10 ± 0.12[a]	1.29 ± 0.14[b]
	GSH peroxidase (umoles/min/lung)	1.46 ± 0.32[a]	1.62 ± 0.24[a]	1.50 ± 0.16[a]
	GSH reductase (umoles/min/lung)	1.53 ± 0.20[a]	1.58 ± 0.20[a]	1.58 ± 0.15[a]
	G-6-P dehydrogenase (umoles/min/lung)	1.83 ± 0.21[a]	1.79 ± 0.19[a]	1.95 ± 0.23[a]

[1] One-month-old male rats maintained on the respective diets for 4
weeks were exposed to 10 puffs/exposure/day for 4 days (31).
[2] Mean±standard deviation; eight animals in each group. The means
do not share the same superscript letter, indicating a significant
difference ($p < 0.05$).

Aryl Hydrocarbon hydroxylase and Glutathione-S-Transferase.   Aryl
hydrocrabon hydroxylase is the most thoroughly studied microsomal
monooxygenase, and is considered to be a good indicator of
cytochrome P-450 mediated metabolism.   Induction of this mixed-
function oxidase has been shown to be a biochemical change that
occurs in the lungs and other tissues as a direct response to
cigarette smoking in both animals and humans (33,34).   As expected,
the activity of aryl hydrocarbon hydroxylase was found to be
significantly increased in the lungs of cigarette-smoke-exposed rats
fed either the vitamin E-deficient or -supplemented diet.   The
activity of this enzyme was also found to be significantly increased
in the kidneys of smoke-exposed rats maintained on the vitamin E-
deficient diet, but not those on the supplemented diet.

Glutathione-S-transferases are a group of important enzymes
that catalyze the metabolism of diverse foreign compounds (35).
They are known to bind certain drugs non-enzymatically both
reversibly and covalently and thereby decrease the drugs' potential
activity (36).   The activity of glutathione-S-transferase was found
to increase significantly in the lungs of cigarette-smoke-exposed
rats maintained on the vitamin E-deficient diet, but not in the
supplemented group (Table VI).   The activity of this enzyme in the
kidney was not significantly altered by cigarette smoking in either
dietary group of animals.

Table VI.   Effect of Dietary Vitamin E and Cigarette Smoking on
            GSH S-Transferase Activity[1]

Tissue	Dietary Vitamin E (ppm)	Enzyme Activity (nmoles/min/g tissue)		p[3]
		Sham	Smoke	
Lung	0	729 ± 116[2] (6)	1016 ± 91 (8)	<0.001
	100	724 ± 50 (4)	795 ± 116 (8)	NS[4]
Kidney	0	1489 ± 60 (6)	1444 ± 121 (8)	NS
	100	1796 ± 111 (4)	1675 ± 1.1 (8)	NS

[1] One-month-old male rats maintained on the respective diets for 8 weeks were exposed to sham or cigarette smoke for 7 days (31).
[2] Mean $\pm$ standard deviation; number in the parentheses represents number of animals in each group.
[3] Student's "t" test.
[4] Not significant ($p < 0.05$).

Discussion

As nutrients are essential for all fundamental cellular processes, the action and metabolism of a given xenobiotic may be modified by the nutritional status of the affected subject. A number of reports, for example, have suggested that higher vitamin A intake may serve to protect the lungs from the deleterious effects of cigarette smoking (37–38). While no epidemiological evidence linking vitamin E intake with protection from lung disease has been demonstrated, patients with primary lung carcinoma have been shown to have significantly lower serum vitamin E levels compared to the hospitalized controls or free living subjects (39). Our preliminary human study, however, indicates that the plasma levels of vitamin E were not significantly different between smokers and non-smokers (unpublished results). This agrees well with the results obtained from our animal studies.

Cigarette smoke is a composite of numerous constituents which can be inhaled in rather high concentrations, especially carbon monoxide and nicotine. Inhaled nicotine may increase the demand of the heart for oxygen, while carbon monoxide may decrease the ability of blood to furnish needed oxygen. Both nicotine and carbon monoxide have been linked to the development of cardiovascular disease (40–41). As expected, a marked increase in carboxyhemoglobin levels in animal blood was detected following exposure to either whole smoke or the gaseous phase of the smoke. Dietary vitamin E was not found to have an influence on the blood levels of carboxyhemoglobin.

Previous studies have shown that rats maintained on a vitamin E-deficient diet had higher mortality rate than those of the - supplemented group when subjected to an acute dose of smoking exposure (42). Relatively greater increases in the levels of ascorbic acid, glutathione and related enzymes, glutathione-S-transferase and pyruvate kinase were also observed in the lungs of vitamin E-deficient rats than in those of the supplemented group following smoking exposure. The observations suggest that deprivation of dietary vitamin E renders animals more susceptible to the effects of cigarette smoking. Although the mechanism of this effect is not yet clear, it is possible that vitamin E deprivation may alter membrane stability and permeability of pulmonary cells and thus alter the cellular sensitivity to the effects of cigarette smoking. The nutritional status of vitamin E has been shown to alter the cellular responses to both oxidants and nonoxidants (12–16).

As cigarette smoke contains a large variety of compounds, it is not surprising that many of them are oxidants or prooxidants capable of initiating or promoting free radical lipid peroxidation damage. While the information available (7–9) suggests that an oxidative damage mechanism may be involved in the toxicity of cigarette smoking, the results obtained show that the levels of lipid peroxidation products were decreased, rather than increased, in the lung homogenates of rats exposed to whole smoke. This finding is in agreement with the report that cigarette smoke consists largely of reducing rather than oxidizing agents (43). Since the depressant effect on lipid peroxidation products was observed only when animals were exposed to whole smoke but not the gaseous phase of the smoke, it is indicative that the reducing compounds present in the particulate matter fraction of the smoke may be mainly responsible for the decreased lipid peroxidation products observed.

In addition to lipid peroxidation products, the biochemical changes resulting from smoking exposure were found to be more profound in the lungs of rats exposed to whole smoke than those exposed to the gaseous phase of the smoke. These results suggest that the Cambridge filter used was effective in removing at least portions of the reactive or harmful substances from the whole smoke, and that the particulate matter of the smoke may be mainly responsible for the pulmonary effect of cigarette smoking.

The mechanism of the pulmonary biochemical changes resulting from cigarette smoking is yet to be elucidated. Since no significant alterations in lung weight and protein levels were observed following cigarette smoking, it is possible that the increased enzymatic activities in the lungs of cigarette-smoked rats may be due to an increased rate of biosynthesis of enzymes and/or a decrease in the rate of their turnover. Increased activities of such enzymes as aryl hydrocarbon hydroxylase, glutathione-S-transferase and glutathione peroxidase may enable the pulmonary tissue to defend better against the adverse effects of cigarette smoke. On the other hand, the biochemical changes may also simply be a result of nonspecific injury-response processes of pulmonary cells as in the case of insults caused by a variety of irritants (44–46). Further studies are needed to provide a better understanding towards the significance and role of type 2 or other types of pulmonary cells in the biochemical responses to cigarette smoking. Nevertheless, the results obtained suggest that deprivation of dietary vitamin E renders rats more susceptible to the effects of cigarette smoking, and that smoke particulate matter appears to be mainly responsible for the pulmonary effects of cigarette smoking.

Acknowledgments

Supported by the University of Kentucky Agricultural Experiment Station and Tobacco and Health Research Institute, and by Hoffmann-La Roche, Inc., Nutley, New Jersey. I thank Dr. R.B. Griffith, Dr. L.H. Chen, Dr. G.C. Gairola, and Mr. R.R. Thacker for their collaboration and assistance.

Literature Cited

1. Frasca, J.M.; Auerbach, O.; Parks, V.R.; Jamieson, J.D. Exp. Mol. Pathol. 1974, 21, 300–312.
2. Costa, M.G.; Hale, K.A.; Niewoehner, D.E. Amer. Rev. Resp. Dis. 1980, 122, 265–271.
3. Akin, F.J.; Benner, J.F. Toxicol. Appl. Pharmacol. 1976, 36, 311–337.
4. Arnold, W.P.; Aldred, W.; Murad, F. Science 1977, 198, 934–936.
5. York, G.K.; Peirce, T.H.; Schwarz, L.W.; Cross, C.E. Arch. Environ. Health 1976, 31, 286–290.
6. Fantone, J.C.; Ward, P.A. Amer. Assoc. Pathol. 1982, 107, 397–418.
7. Babior, B.M. New Engl. J. Med. 1978, 298, 659–668.
8. Lentz, P.E.; Di Luzio, N.R. Arch. Environ. Health 1974, 28, 279–282.
9. Janoff, A.; Carp, H.; Lee, D.K. Science 1979, 206, 1313–1314.
10. Lucy, J.A. Ann. New York Acad. Sci. 1972, 203, 4–11.
11. Chow, C.K. Amer. J. Clin. Nutr. 1979, 32, 1066–1081.
12. Goldstein, B.D.; Buckley, R.D.; Cardenas, R.; Balchum, O.J. Science 1970, 169, 605–606.
13. Mino, M. J. Nutr. Sci. Vitaminol. 1973, 19, 95–104.
14. Block, E.R. Lung 1979, 156, 195–203.
15. Doroshow, J.H.; Locker, G.Y.; Myers, C.E. Cancer Treat. Rep. 1979, 63, 855–860.
16. Dashman, T.; Kamm, J.J. Biochem. Pharmacol. 1979, 28, 1485–1490.
17. Schwarz, K.; Fredga, A. J. Biol. Chem. 1969, 244, 2103–2110.
18. Spallholz, J.E.; Collins, G.F.; Schwarz, K. Bioinorg. Chem. 1978, 9, 453–459.
19. Draper, H.H.; Csallany, A.S. J. Nutr. 1969, 98, 390–394.
20. Chow, C.K. J. Nutr. 1975, 105, 1221–1224.
21. Griffith, R.B. Proc. 34th Tobacco Chemist's Res. Conf. 1980, paper no. 21.
22. Griffith, R.B.; Benner, J.F.; Owens, S.S.; Hancock, R.L. Proc. 3rd Univ. Kentucky Tobacco Health Res. Inst. Conf. 1972, pp. 71–84.
23. Lubway, W.C.; Perrier, D.G. Environ. Res. 1980, 21, 438–445.
24. Binns, R. Toxicology 1977, 7, 189–195.
25. Smith, J.R.; Landaw, S.A. New Engl. J. Med. 1978, 298, 6–10.

26. McAloon, E.J.; Streiff, R.R.; Kitchens, C.S. <u>South. Med. J.</u> 1980, 73, 137-139.
27. Helman, N.; Rubenstein, L.S. <u>Amer. J. Clin. Pathol.</u> 1975, 63, 35-44.
28. Pelletier, O. <u>Amer. J. Clin. Nutr.</u> 1970, 23, 520-528.
29. Boyland, E.; Grove, P.L. <u>Biochem.</u> J. 1961, 81, 163-168.
30. Conney, A.H.; Burns, J.J. <u>Nature</u> 1959, 184, 363-364.
31. Chow, C.K. <u>Ann. New York Acad. Sci.</u> 1982, 393, 426-436.
32. Parkinson, D.R.; Stephens, R.J. <u>Environ. Res.</u> 1973, 6, 37-51.
33. Akin, F.J.; Benner, J.F. <u>Toxicol. Appl. Pharmacol.</u> 1976, 36, 331-337.
34. Contrell, E.T.; Warr, G.A.; Busbee, D.L.; Martin, R.R. <u>J. Clin. Invest.</u> 1973, 52, 1881-1884.
35. Smith, G.J.; Ohl, V.S.; Litwack, G. <u>Cancer Res.</u> 1977, 37, 8-14.
36. Chasseaul, L. In "Glutathione: Metabolism and Function"; Arias, I.M.; Jacob, B.B. eds., Raven Press, New York, 1976, pp. 77-114.
37. Gram, S.; Mettlin, C.; Marshall, J.; Priore, R.; Rzepks, T.; Shedds, D. <u>Amer. J. Epidemiol.</u> 1981, 113, 675-680.
38. Bjelke, E. <u>Int. J. Cancer</u> 1975, 15, 561-565.
39. Lopez, S.A.; Legardeur, B.Y. <u>Amer. J. Clin. Nutr.</u> 1982, 35, 851A.
40. Doyle, J.T.; Dawler, T.R.; Kannel, W.B.; Kinch, S.H., Khan, H.A. <u>J. Amer. Med. Assoc.</u> 1964, 190, 886-890.
41. Seltzer, C.C. <u>Arch. Environ. Health</u> 1978, 20, 418-423.
42. Chow, C.K.; Chen, L.H.; Thacker, R.T.; Griffith, R.B. <u>Environ. Res.</u> 1984, 34, 8-17.
43. Horrman, D.; Hecht, S.S.; Schmeltz, I.; Brunnemann, K.D.; Wynder, E.L. <u>Rec. Advan. Tob. Sci.</u> 1975, 1, 97-122.
44. Bus, J.A.; Vinegar, A.; Brooks, S.M. <u>Amer. Rev. Resp. Dis.</u> 1978, 118, 573-580.
45. Witschi, H.; Saheb, W. <u>Proc. Soc. Exp. Biol. Med.</u> 1974, 147, 690-693.

RECEIVED November 30, 1984

Effect of the Antioxidant Butylated Hydroxyanisole on In Vivo Formation of Benzo[a]pyrene Metabolite–DNA Adducts

Correlation with Inhibition of Benzo[a]pyrene-Induced Neoplasia by Butylated Hydroxyanisole

MARSHALL W. ANDERSON, PETER I. ADRIAENSSENS, CATHERINE M. WHITE, Y. M. IOANNOU, and ALAN G. E. WILSON

Laboratory of Biochemical Risk Analysis, The National Institute of Environmental Health Sciences, National Institutes of Health, Research Triangle Park, NC 27709

Phenolic antioxidants such as BHA[1] and ethoxyquin can inhibit the induction of tumors in rodents by a variety of carcinogens, including several PAH (1, 2). For example, BP-induced neoplasia of the forestomach and lung in mice is inhibited by BHA in the diet (1-3). The initiation of papilloma formation in the skin of mice is inhibited by prior administration of BHA (4).

There is compelling evidence that a large number of mutagens and carcinogens are able to react with cellular DNA either directly or following metabolic activation to reactive metabolites. If DNA replication proceeds on such a modified template before altered bases or nucleotides are removed by enzymic repair processes, DNA damage may be genetically fixed. Thus, the extent of carcinogen-induced promutagenic DNA damage and the capacity of cells to repair such damage represent critical events in the initiation of carcinogenesis. Implicit in all of the suggested mechanisms of anticarcinogenic action of BHA is that they result in a decreased level of carcinogen metabolite-DNA adduct formation. In this report we describe our results of the effects of BHA on the in vivo formation of BP metabolite-DNA adduct formation and the relationship of these effects to the anticarcinogenic property of BHA.

Abbreviations
The abbreviations used are: BHA, butylated hydroxyanisole; BP, benzo(a)pyrene; BPDEI, (+)-7ß,8a-dihydroxy-9a,10a-epoxy-7,8,9,10-tetrahydrobenzo(a)pyrene; BPDEII, (+)-7ß,8a-dihydroxy-9ß,10ß-epoxy-7,8,9,10-tetrahydrobenzo(a)pyrene; BPDE, BPDEI plus BPDEII; DMBA, 7,12-dimethylbenz(a,h)anthracene; PAH, polycyclic aromatic hydrocarbons; TCDD, 2,3,7,8-tetrachlorodibenzo-p-dioxin.

Effects of BHA Treatment on in Vivo Formation of Benzo(a)pyrene-
DNA Accucts in Target Tissues for Benzo(a)Pyrene-Induced Neoplasia

We have investigated BP metabolite-DNA adduct formation in lung
and forestomach of female A/HeJ and ICR/Ha mice under conditions
known to result in inhibition of BP-induced neoplasia by BHA. In
an earlier study (5), the experimental protocol followed was that
used by Wattenberg (6) which resulted in 53% inhibition of
BP-induced pulmonary adenoma formation in female A/HeJ mice by
BHA feeding, 0.5% of diet for twenty-one days. BP was
administered orally (6 mg/mouse) on the fourth and eighteenth
days of the diet. This BHA treatment regimen resulted in a 53%
reduction of BP-induced pulmonary adenomas. In our study (5),
^{3}H-BP (6 mg/mouse) was administered to one group (A) of
animals, both BHA-treated and control, on the fourth day of the
diet. To another group (B) of mice, BHA-treated and control,
unlabelled-BP (6 mg/mouse) was given on the fourth day of the
diet and ^{3}H-BP (6 mg/mouse) was administered on the eighteenth
day of the diet. Animals were returned to control diets after
administration of ^{3}H-BP and sacrificed forty-eight hours
later. DNA isolated from lung, as well as liver, was
enzymatically digested and the deoxyribonucleosides were
chromatographed on HPLC. The major adduct in lung, as well as
liver, was the BPDEI-deoxyguanosine adduct (Peak II, Figure 1).
The BPDEII-deoxyguanosine adduct (Peak III, Figure 1) was 10 to
15% of the BPDEI adduct in both lung and liver and the
unidentified Peak I was 10 to 20% of BPDEI adduct. A detailed
discussion of the identification of these adducts is given in
Anderson et al. (5). As seen in Figure 1, BHA significantly
inhibited the formation of the BP-DNA adducts in the lungs of
Group B animals. Table I gives the percentage decrease in
BPDE-DNA adducts ((BPDEI plus BPDEII) formed in the lung of
BHA-treated mice for Group A and Group B animals and in the
inhibition of pulmonary adenoma formation. The decrease in the
amount of the BPDE-DNA adducts in the lung, 53-62%, appears to
correlate with the inhibition of pulmonary adenoma formation
(53%). BHA treatment also inhibited the formation of the
BPDE-DNA adducts in the liver by approximately 75% in both Group
A and Group B animals (5).
        The effect of BHA on the in vivo formation of BP metabolite-
DNA adducts in the forestomach of female A/HeJ mice was also
examined (7). In this study, mice were fed BHA, 0.5% of diet,
for eighteen days. ^{3}H-BP (6 mg/mouse) was adminitered and the
animals were sacrificed 48 hours later. As in lung and liver,
the BPDEI-deoxyguanosine adduct was the predominant adduct formed
in the forestomach. BHA treatment inhibited the formation of
BPDE-DNA adducts in the forestomach by 50%. Wattenberg (8) has
shown that BHA treatment inhibits BP-induced forestomach tumors
approximately 90%. Although our protocol for administration of
BP was not identical to that used in the tumorigenicity studies,
we can still see a definite trend between BHA inhibition of
BPDE-DNA adduct formation in the forestomach of A/HeJ mice and
reduction in tumor formation.
        Ioannou et al. (9) examined the effect of dietary BHA on the
in vivo formation of BP metabolite-DNA adducts in the lung,
forestomach, and liver of ICR/Ha mice. As with the A/HeJ strain
of mice, the major adduct formed in lung, liver and forestomach

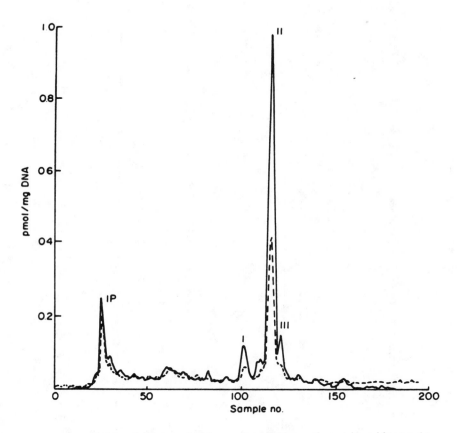

Figure 1.   HPLC of BP metabolites–deoxyribonucleoside adducts in
lung of untreated (–) and BHA-treated (– – –) mice.   Untreated or
BHA-treated mice (Group B) were killed 48 hours after an oral dose
of ^{3}H–BP (6mg/mouse).   DNA isolated from lung was enzymatically
digested and the deoxyribonucleosides were chromatographed on
HPLC.   The observed peaks are discussed in the text.   Abscissas
fraction number, and each fraction represents 0.5 minutes:
ordinate, specific activity (pmole/mg DNA).

Table I. Comparison between inhibitory effects of BHA treatment on benzo(a)pyrene-induced neoplasia and on BPDE-DNA adduct formation.

Treatment[a]	Tissue (Mice Strain)	% Decrease in BPDE-DNA Adducts Formation in Mice	% Decrease in Benzo(a)Pyrene induced neoplasia
4 Day Dietary BHA (Group A)	Lung (A/HeJ)	53[b]	53[c]
18 Day Dietary BHA (Group B)	Lung (A/HeJ)	55 to 62[b]	53[c]
18 Day Dietary BHA	Forestomach (A/HeJ)	50[d]	90[e]
16 Day Dietary BHA	Forestomach (ICR/Ha)	60[f]	50 to 90[g]
16 Day Dietary BHA	Lung (IRC/Ha)	14 to 50[h]	0 to 50[i]
BHA, p.o.	Lung (A/HeJ)	44[b]	64[j]

a Treatment for adduct studies corresponds in some cases to tumor studies.

b-j Data from references 5(b); 6 (c); 7 (d); 8 (e); 9 (f); 10-12 (g); 9 and unpublished
    data (h); 3 and unpublished data (i); and 32 (j).

was the BPDEI-deoxyguanosine adduct and, in general, the adduct
profiles were similar to those in the A/HeJ strain. In the
forestomach BPDE-DNA adduct formation was inhibited by 60% while
in tumorigenicity studies, dietary BHA reduced tumors in the
forestomach by 50 to 90% (10-12) (Table I). Thus, although our
protocol for BP administration was not identical to those used in
the tumorigenicity studies, we can see a correlation between BHA
inhibition of BPDE-DNA adduct formation in the forestomach of
ICR/Ha mice and reduction in tumor formation. The results of BHA
treatment on adduct formation and BP-induced neoplasia in the
lung of ICR/Ha mice is more variable, although the variability is
in the same range. BPDE-DNA adduct formation was inhibited by
60% in liver of ICR/Ha mice as compared to 75% in liver of A/HeJ
mice (5, 9).

These results suggest that BHA treatment inhibits BP-induced
neoplasia in the lung and forestomach of mice by inhibiting the
amount of the BPDE-DNA adducts formed in the target tissue. BHA
treatment also inhibited BP-induced DNA damage in liver, a non-
target tissue for BP-induced neoplasia. A recent study has shown
that BP metabolite-DNA adducts are formed in numerous tissues
after exposure of animals to this environmental pollutant (13).
Since BPDE-DNA adducts are very persistent (14), toxic responses
other than neoplasia could result from exposure to BP and other
PAHs. Thus, the ability of BHA to inhibit BPDE-DNA adduct
formation in tissues would serve as a protective mechanism for
various toxic responses resulting from BP-induced DNA damage.

BHA inhibition of in vivo BPDE-DNA adduct formation as a function
of benzo(a)pyrene dose

Most investigations on the effects of dietary BHA on BP-induced
neoplasia and on in vivo formation of BP metabolite-DNA adducts
have been done at doses of BP that are much higher than the usual
environmental exposure levels. The tumor studies were performed
at high BP doses for various practical reasons; however, adduct
studies can be done over a wide dose range. In a recent study
(15), the formation of benzo(a)pyrene (BP) metabolite-DNA adducts
in lung, liver, and forestomach of control and BHA-treated
(5 mg/g diet) female A/HeJ mice was examined as a function of BP
dose (p.o), ranging from 2 to 1351 umol/kg. The results from
this study demonstrate that dietary BHA inhibits the formation of
BPDE-DNA adducts in mouse lung, liver and forestomach over a wide
BP dose range (Figure 2). In forestomach, the dose-response
curve for BPDEI-DNA adducts in BHA-treated mice, 0.5% of diet for
2 weeks, was parallel to the curve for control animals and thus,
the inhibition (45%) of adduct formation is independent of BP
dose. In contrast, BHA treatment diminished the curvilinear
nature of the dose-response curves for BPDE adducts in lung and
liver. The inhibition of BPDEI-DNA adduct formation by BHA in
lung and liver was dose dependent. The inhibition of lung (68%)
and liver (82%) adduct formation was highest at a BP dose of 270
umol/kg. As the BP dose approached zero, the inhibition of
BPDEI-DNA adduct formation by BHA decreased with BP dose and
approached values of approximately 40% (lung) and 55% (liver).

The results from the study by Adriaenssens et al. (15), in
conjunction with previous findings, suggest that dietary BHA will

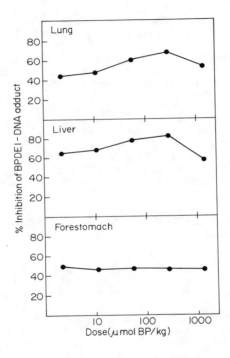

Figure 2.   Dose dependency for inhibition of BPDEI–DNA adduct
formation by BHA treatment. The percentage of inhibition of BPDEI–
DNA adduct formation by BHA treatment is plotted versus BP dose
for lung, liver, and forestomach of mice. (Reprinted from
Adriaenssens et al., Cancer Research, Vol. 43, pp. 3712–3719, 1983.)

also inhibit the neoplastic effects of BP at low doses. However, the BHA dose of approximately 1 g/kg/day, which was used in all of the reported studies, is very high, reative to the estimated consumption of several mg of BHA per day in the human diet (2,16). Examination of the anticarcinogenic effect of BHA at lower doses is required in order to assess the practical use of BHA. Since tumor studies themselves are usually not practical at low doses of a carcinogen, the examination of the dose dependency of pertinent biochemical parameters, i.e. adduct formation, is one way to attempt to extrapolate carcinogenic effects to low doses.

Possible Mechanisms by Which BHA Treatment Inhibits Benzo(a)pyrene Metabolite–DNA Adduct Formation

There are several known effects of BHA treatment which have been proposed to reduce the levels of reactive metabolites of BP which bind to DNA. It has been demonstrated that BHA feeding alters the microsomal mixed-function oxidase system in mice and rats (7,17–19). Several studies suggest that BHA treatment does not decrease the amounts of BP-7, 8-diol formed (7,20,21) whereas there is some indirect evidence that BHA treatment alters the metabolism of BP-7,8-diol (3,20). An induction by BHA of an isozyme(s) of cytochrome P-450, which has kinetics of metabolism of BP-7,8-diol different than that of the constitutive isozyme(s), could account for the BHA-induced shifts in the dose-response curve for BPDEI-DNA adduct levels (15).

The enhancement of glutathione transferase(s) activity by BHA has been postulated to play a role in the anticarcinogenis action of BHA (22,23). Benson et al. (23) showed that the levels of constitutive isozymes of glutathione transferase were elevated, but did not observe the induction of any new isozyme. In this case, the capacity of the enzyme system is increased (maximum volocity) but the inherent affinity for substrate is not altered. This would predict a parallel shift in the dose response curve for BPDEI adduct levels, and thus is not consistent with the observed BHA-induced shifts in lung and liver (15). Recent results by Dock et al. (20) also suggest that elevation of glutathion transferase may not be invoilded in the inhibition of binding of PB metabolites to DNA in lever since BHA treatment did not increase the levels of glutathione conjucates of BP metabolites formed from metabolism of BP by hepatocytes.

It has also been shown that the direct addition of BHA to microsomal incubations and/or tissue cultures can inhibit metabolism, DNA binding, and mutagenicity of BP (19,24–27). For a constant dose of BHA and varying doses of BP, these direct actions of BHA would predict a parallel shift in the dose response curve for BPDEI-DNA adduct levels, as was observed in forestomach (15). It is very possible that different mechanisms may be responsible for the inhibition of adduct formation in lung and liver than those in forestomach. It is obvious that further work is required to clarify the exact mechanism(s) by which dietary BHA Inhibits BPDEI-DNA adduct formation in the various tissues. A better understanding of the mechanism of action of BHA might allow the design of more potent "BHA-like" anticarcinogenic agents.

Anticarcinogenic Agents Other Than Phenolic Antioxidants

There are numerous compounds other than antioxidants which will also inhibit chemical-induced neoplasia in rodents (2). For example, ß-naphthoflavone treatment inhibits DMBA-and BP-induced neoplasia in lung and forestomach of mice (28,29). TCDD inhibits BP- and DMBA-induced initiation of papilloma formation in mouse skin (30). ß-naphthoflavone and TCDD, both aryl hydrocarbon hydroxylase inducers, are very potent anticarcinogenic agents. a-angelicalactone, a naturally occurring lactone, inhibits BP-induced neoplasia in forestomach of mice (31). The effect that these anticarcinogenic agents have on BP metabolite-DNA adduct formation has been examined in some cases. As seen in Table II these agents, like BHA, inhibit BP-induced neoplasia to the same degree that BPDE-DNA adduct formation is inhibited in the target tissue. The mechanism(s) of inhibition of BPDE-DNA adduct formation is probably different among the various classes of anticarcinogenic agents.

No consideration has been given to possible synergistic effects with the various anticarcinogenic agents. It is possible that combinations of relatively small nontoxic doses of the anticarcinogenic compounds would protect against chemical-induced neoplasia for a variety of carcinogens.

Table II. Comparison of the inhibitory effects of aryl hydrocarbon hydroxylase inducers and a-angelicalactone on benzo(a)pyrene-induced neoplasia and on BPDE-DNA adduct formation.

Treatment	Tissue (Mice Strain)	%Decrease in BPDE Adduct Formation	% Decrease in Benzo(a)pyrene induced neoplasia
ß-Naphthoflavone	Lung (A/HeJ)	85 to 92[a]	94[b]
TCDD	Forestomach (ICR/Ha)	100[c-f]	92[c]
a-Angelicalactone	Skin (Sencar)	56[d]	80[e]

[a-e] Data from references 33(a); 29(b); 30 (c); 9(d); and 31 (e).
[f] BPDE-DNA adducts were not detectable in treated animals.

Literature Cited

1. Wattenberg, L.W. Inhibition of carcinogenic and Toxic Effects of Polycyclic Hydrocarbons by Phenolic Antioxidants and Ethoxyquin. J. Natl. Cancer Inst., 48: 1425–1430, 1972.
2. Wattengerg, L.S. Inhibitors of Carcinogenesis. In: A.C. Griffin and C.R. Shaw (eds.), Carcinogens: Identification and Mechanisms
3. Wattenberg, L.W., Jerina, D.M., Lam, L.K.T., and Yagi, H. Neoplastic Effects of Oral Administration of (+)-trans-7,8-dihydroxy–7,8-dihydroxy=7,8-dihydrobenzo(a)pyrene and their inhibition by butylated hydroxyanisole. J. Natl. Cancer Inst., 62: 1103–1106, 1979.
4. Slaga, T.J., and Bracken, W.M. The Effect of Antioxidants on Skin Tumor Initiation and Aryl Hydrocarbon Hydroxylase. Cancer Res., 37: 1631–1635, 1977.
5. Anderson, M.W., Boroujerdi, M., and Wilson, A.G.E. Inhibition in Vivo of the Formation of Adducts Between Metabolites of Benzo(a)pyrene and DNA by Buylated Hydroxyanisole. Cancer Res., 41: 4309–4315, 1981.
6. Wattenberg, L.W. Inhibition of chemical–carcinogen–induced pulmonary neoplasia by butylated hydroxyanisole. J. Natl. Cancer Inst., 50: 1541–1544, 1973.
7. Ionnou, Y.M., Wilson, A.G.E., and Anderson, M.W. Effect of Butylated Hydroxyanisole and the in Vivo and in Vitro metabolism and DNA binding of benzo(a)pyrene in the A/HeJ mouse. Carinogenesis (Lond.), 3:739–745, 1982.
8. Wattenberg, L.W. Inhibition of carcinogenic and Toxic Effects of Polycyclic Hydrocarbons by Phenolic Antioxidants and Ethoxyquin. J. Natl. Cancer Inst., 48: 1425–1430, 1972.
9. Ioannou, Y.M., Wilson, A.G.E., and Anderson, M.W. Effect of Butylated Hydroxyanisole, a-angelicalactone and ß-naphtho-flavone on Benzo(a)pyrene–DNA Adduct Formation in Vivo in the Forestomach, Lung and Liver of Mice. Cancer Res., 42: 1199–1205, 1982.
10. Lam, L.K.T., Pai, R.P., and Wattenberg, L.W. Synthesis and Chemical Carcinogen Inhibitory Activity of 2-tert-butyl-4-hydroxyanisole. J. Med. Chem., 22: 569–571, 1979.
11. Wattenberg, L.W., Jerina, D.M., Lam, L.K.T., and Yagi, H. Neoplastic Effects of Oral Administration of (+)-trans-7,8-dihydroxy–7,8-dihydrobenzo(a)pyrene and their inhibition by Butylated Hydroxyanisole. J. Natl. Cancer Inst., 62: 1103–1106, 1979.
12. Wattenberg, L.W. Inhibition of Carcinogenic and Toxic Effects of Polycyclic Hydrocarbons by Phenolic Antioxidants and Ethoxyquin. J. Natl. Cancer Inst. 48: 1425–4130, 1972.
13. Stowers, S.J., and Anderson, M.W. Ubiquitous binding of benzo(a)pyrene metabolites to DNA and protein in tissues of the mouse and rabbit. Chem. Biol. Interact. 51: 151–166, 1984.
14. Kulkarni, M.S., and Anderson, M.W. Persistence of Benzo(a)pyrene metabolite: DNA Adducts in Lung and Liver of Mice. Cancer Res. 44: 97–101, 1984.

15. Adriaenssens, P.I., White, C.M., and Anderson, M.W.
    Dose-response Relationships for the Binding of Benzo(a)pyrene
    Metabolites to DNA and Protein in Lung, Liver and Forestomach
    of Control and Butylated Hydroxyanisole-treated Mice. Cancer
    Res. 43: 3712–3719, 1983.
16. Branen, A.L. Toxicology and Biochemistry of Butylated
    Hydroxyanisole and Butylated Hydroxytoluene. J. Am. Oil
    Chem. Soc., 52: 59–63, 1975.
17. Lam, L.K., and Wattenberg, L.W. Effects of Butylated
    Hydroxyanisole on the Metabolism of Benzo(a)pyrene by Mouse
    Liver Microsomes. J. Natl. Cancer Inst., 58: 413–417, 1977.
18. Speier, J.L., and Wattenberg, L.W. Alterations in Microsomal
    Metabolism of Benzo(a)pyrene in Mice Fed Butylated Hydroxyan-
    isole. J. Natl. Cancer Inst., 55: 469–472, 1975.
19. Wiebel, F.J., and Waters, H.L. Effect of Butylated
    Hydroxytoluene and Hydroxyanisole on Benzo(a)pyrene
    Metabolism and Binding. In: J.R. Fouts and I. Gut (eds.).
    Industrial and Environmental Xenobiotics, pp. 258–260.
    Amsterdam: Excerpta Medica, 1978.
20. Dock, L., Cha, Y-N., Jernstrom, B., and Moldeus, P. Effect
    of 2(3)-tert-butyl-4-hydroxyanisole on benzo(a)pyrene
    Metabolism and NDA-binding of Benzo(a)pyrene Metabolites in
    Isolated Mouse Hepatocytes. Chem. Biol. Interact., 41:
    25–38, 1982.
21. Dock, L., Cha, Y-N., Jernstrom, B., and Moldeus, P.
    Differential Effects of Dietary BHA on Hepatic Enzyme
    Activities and Benzo(a)pyrene metabolism in male and female
    NMRI mice. Carcinogenesis (Lond.), 3: 15–19, 1982.
22. Batzinger, R.P., Ou, Suh-Yun L., and Bueding, E.
    Antimutagenic Effects of 2(3)-tert-butyl-4-hydroxyanisole and
    of antimicrobial agents. Cancer Res. 38: 4478–4485, 1978.
23. Benson, A.M., Batzinger, R.P., Ou, S-y. L., Bueding, E., Cha,
    Y.-N., and Talalay, P. Elevation of Hepatic Glutathione
    S-transferase Activities and Protection Against Mutagenic
    Metabolites of Benzo(a)pyrene By Dietary Antioxidants.
    Cancer Res., 38: 4486–4495, 1978.
24. Calle, L.M., Sullivan, P.D., Nettleman, M.D., Ocasio, I.J.,
    Balzyk, J., and Jollick, J. Antioxidants and the
    Mutagenicity of Benzo(a)pyrene and Some Derivatives.
    Biochem. Biophys. Res. Commun., 85: 351–356, 1978.
25. Harris, C.C., Frank, A.L., Haaften, C.V., Kaufman, D.G.,
    Connor, R., Jackson, F., Barrett, L.A., McDowell, E.M., and
    Trump, B.F. Binding of [^{3}H]benzo(a)pyrene to DNA in
    Culture Human Bronchus. Cancer REs., 36: 1011–1018, 1976.
26. Rahimtula, A.D.. Zachariah, P.K., and O'Brien, P.J. The
    effects of antioxidants on the Metabolism and Mutagenicity of
    Benzo(a)pyrene in Vitro. Biochem,. J., 164: 473–475, 1977.
27. Rahimtula, A.D., Zachariah, P.K., and O'Brien, P.J.
    Differential Effects of Antioxidants, Steroids, and Other
    Compounds on Benzo(2)pyrene-3-hydroxylase Activity in Various
    Tissues of Rat. Br. J. Cancer, 40: 105–112, 1979
28. Wattenberg, L.W., and Leong, J.L. Inhibition of the
    Carcinogenic action of 7,12-dimethylbenzo(a)anthracene by
    Beta-napthoflavone. Proc. Soc. Exp. Biol. Med., 128:
    940–943, 1968.

29. Wattenberg, L.W., and Leong, J.L.   Inhibition of Carcinogenic Action of Benzo(a)pyrene by Flavones.   Cancer Res. 30: 1922–1925, 1970.
30. Cohen, G.M., Bracken, W.M., Iyer, R.P., Berry, D.L., Selkirk, J.K., and Slaga, T.J.   Anticarcinogenic Effects of 2,3,7,8-tetrachlorodibenzo–p–dioxin on Benzo(a)pyrene and 7,12–di-emthylbenz(a)anthracene Tumor Initiation and its Relationship to DNA Binding.   Cancer Res., 39: 4027–4033, 1979.
31. Wattenberg, L.W., Lam, L.K.T., and Fladmoe, A.R.   Inhibition of Chemical Carcinogen–induced Neoplasia by Coumarins and a–angelicalactone.   Cancer Res., 39: 1651–1654, 1979.
32. Speier, J.L., Lam, L.K., and Wattenberg, L.W.   Effects of Administration to Mice of Butylated Hydroxyanisole by Oral Intubation on Benzo(a)pyrene–induced Pulmonary Adenoma Formation and Metabolism of Benzo(a)pyrene.   J. Natl. Cancer Inst., 60: 605–609, 1978.
33. Wilson, A.G.E., Kung, H.–C., Boroujerdi, M., and Anderson, M.W.   Inhibition in Vivo of the Formation of Adducts Between Metabolites of Benzo(a)pyrene and DNA by Aryl Hydrocarbon Hydroxylase Inducers.   Cancer Res., 41: 3453–3460, 1981.

RECEIVED March 15, 1985

Inadequate Vitamin E and Selenium Nutrition
Effect on Enzymes Associated with Hydroperoxide Metabolism

C. CHANNA REDDY, CRAIG E. THOMAS, and RICHARD W. SCHOLZ

Department of Veterinary Science and Center for Air Environment Studies, The Pennsylvania State University, University Park, PA 16802

Hydroperoxides are the immediate oxygenase products of various polyenoic fatty acids formed via the cyclooxygenase pathway and the lipoxygenase(s) pathway. Not only are these semistable intermediates further metabolized to prostaglandins and leukotrienes, but they have been shown to influence various enzyme activities including cyclooxygenase, 5-lipoxygenase, etc. In addition they can be readily decomposed by transition metals to produce extremely reactive free radicals which in turn, might cause peroxidative damage to biological membranes. By sequestering free radicals and reducing hydroperoxides, dietary vitamin E and selenium (Se) have been implicated respectively in the protection of membranes from oxidative damage. In these studies, we have investigated the effects of altered vitamin E and/or Se nutrition on cytochrome P-450 peroxidase, prostaglandin H synthase and glutathione peroxidases (GSH-Pxs). In general, vitamin E deficiency had no effect on GSH-Px activities whereas opposite effects were observed on heme peroxidase (significantly decreased) and PGH synthase (two fold increase). Se deficiency resulted in a marked decrease of Se-GSH-Px activity but caused significant elevation of non-GSH-Px and heme peroxidase activities. These differential effects have been interpreted as a compensatory mechanism to one another to protect cell from peroxidative damage.

Recent investigations in many laboratories indicate that lipid peroxidation may be a fundamental mechanism of oxidant toxicity which can be initiated by atmospheric oxidants such as O_3 and NO_2 or by enzymatically produced reactive oxygen intermediates like hydroxyl radical, singlet oxygen, etc. ([1-6]). These short-lived oxygen intermediates can be generated by several enzymatic and non-enzymatic processes (Figure 1). It is evident from the figure that the cellular production of H_2O_2 seems to be a physiological

0097–6156/85/0277–0253$06.00/0

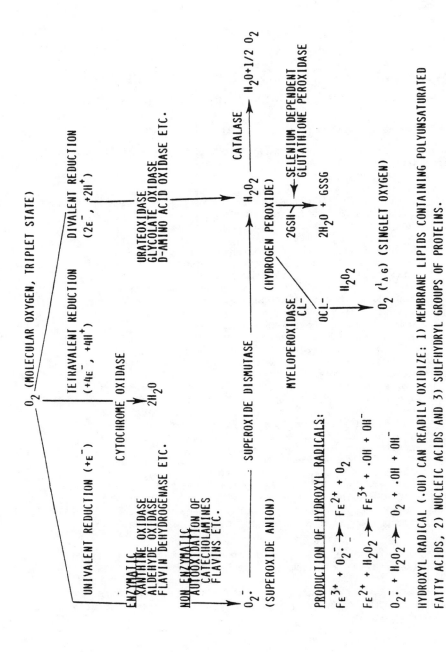

Figure 1. Cellular production of reactive oxygen intermediates.

event and the generation of extremely reactive oxygen intermediates such as hydroxyl radical is potentially a dangerous
factor in living cells. It is well known that methylene-inter-
rupted polyunsaturated fatty acids (PUFA) exhibit marked
vulnerability to peroxidative attack induced by free radical
processes (7-8). Most biological membranes are rich in PUFA,
thus, rendering them particularly susceptible to oxidative damage.
     Peroxidation of membrane lipids involves the production of
labile fatty acid hydroperoxides from free radical intermediates,
which can readily decompose in the presence of transition metals
to give rise to extremely reactive free radicals such as alkyl
peroxy (ROO·), alkoxyl (RO·) and hydroxyl (·OH) radicals (2).
These short-lived species, in turn, promote the propagation of
chain peroxidation of membrane lipids, thus disrupting the
cellular integrity, or they may oxidize also various xenobiotics
that are in the vicinity. Indeed, the hydroperoxide dependent
oxidation process has been implicated as one of the mechanisms of
conversion of procarcinogens to carcinogens (6,9).
     Dietary vitamin E and selenium (Se) have been implicated in
the protection of membrane lipids from oxidative damage (10-12).
But the precise mechanism(s) by which vitamin E and Se function
together as antioxidants to prevent cellular damage mediated by
reactive oxygen intermediates remains enigmatic and a challenging
issue to the scientists of various disciplines. Nevertheless,
vitamin E, as an integral part of membranes, is visualized as a
biological antioxidant which by sequestering free radicals
functions to terminate the propagation of autooxidation processes
such as lipid peroxidation. On the other hand Se, as an essential
component of Se-glutathione peroxidase (Se-GSH-Px) (EC.1.11.1.9),
has been proposed to function in the reduction of fatty acid
hydroperoxides to less reactive alcohols (10,13,14). Each
nutrient, therefore, acts to control lipid peroxidation by
interrelated but independent mechanisms. Thus, increased lipid
peroxidation, as a consequence of inadequate vitamin E and Se
nutrition, can exert marked deleterious effects both on the
structural integrity and biochemical properties of subcellular
organells.
     Often times, lipid peroxidation has been associated with the
deleterious proceses such as cancer, atherosclerosis, thrombosis,
aging etc., however, more recent studies suggest that it is involved also in the normal function of cell (15-16). For example,
enzymatically regulated lipid peroxidation is associated with
arachidonic acid (AA) metabolism via the lipoxygenase(s) and
cyclooxygenase pathways and with phagocytosis. Fatty acid
hydroperides are the immediate oxidation products of AA metabolism
via the former process. The hydroperoxides formed in the AA
cascade include 5-hydroperoxy eicosatetraenoic acid (5-HPETE),
12-HPETE, 15-HPETE, etc., products of lipoxygenases, and PGG_2 and
PGH_2, cyclooxygenase products. Not only are these hydroperoxides
and cyclic endoperoxides the precursors of biologically active
compounds like leukotrienes (LTs), prostaglandins (PGs),
thromboxanes (Txs) and prostacyclins (PGIs) but they have been
implicated in the modulation of catalytic activities of various
enzymes including PGH_2 synthase, 5-Lipoxygenase and PGI_2 synthase
of AA cascade (Figure 2) (15-17). Therefore, an enzyme or enzyme

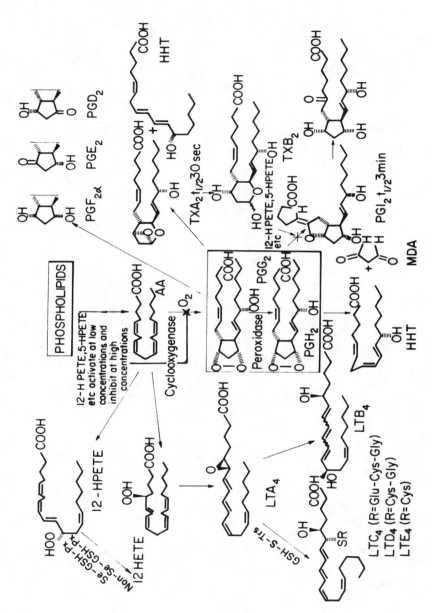

Figure 2. Biosynthesis of prostaglandins, thromboxanes, prostacyclins, and leukotrienes.

system that can reduce these hydroperoxides effectively to less reactive alcohols has the potential to modulate enzyme activities themselves and the profile of AA products. Important to this discussion is the fact that Se-GSH-Px together with non-Se-GSH-Px associated with glutathione S-transferases (GSH-S-Trs) (EC.2.5.1.18) have been shown to reduce fatty acid hydroperoxides effectively and, thus, may plan an important regulatory role in AA cascade (Figure 2) (10,13,15,18,19). Recently, the presence of an additional enzyme associated with cytochrome P-450 mixed function oxidase system (Cyt P-450 MFO) has been reported in many tissues which is capable of reducing various organic hydroperoxides including HPETEs (20). However, the latter class of enzymes are known to produce extremely reaactive oxidizing radicals during hydroperoxide metabolism. These free radicals have been implicated in the conversion of pre-carcinogens to proximate carcinogens (9,21,22). In contrast, free radicals are not generated during GSH-Pxs catalyzed reduction of hydroperoxides (C. C. Reddy and R. A. Floyd, unpublished results). Also, it is well known that extremely reactive radicals are generated during the formation and decomposition of HPETEs in AA cascade which have been implicated in the inactivation of enzymes as well as co-oxidation of xenobiotics (9,21,22). Therefore antioxidants like vitamin E have the potential to affect the activity of enzymes as well as the profile of products formed. Thus, vitamin E and Se-GSH-Px have the potential to modulate the activities of enzymes involved in the turnover of AA and the profile of intermediates/ products of AA cascade.

In these studies, employing the Long-Evans Hooded rat as a model mammalian system, we have investigated the effects of inadequate vitamin E and/or Se nutrition, on the catalytic activities of enzymes involved in the detoxification of hydro-peroxides in order to help define the role of these enzymes in AA metabolism.

Experimental Methods

Animals and Diets. Post-weanling male Long-Evans Hooded rats (Charles Rivers Laboratory, Wilmington, MA) weighing approximately 50g were fed on chemically defined, purified diets for a minimum of 5 weeks. The torula yeast-based diets were formulated to provide adequate amounts of all known nutrients except vitamin E and Se. The composition of diet was: 300.0g torula yeast; 3.0g D,L-Methionine; 40.0g cellulose; 10.0g vitamin mixture (minus tocopherol) as formulated by Harper (23); 2.1g choline chloride (70%); 40g mineral mixture (USPXVII Salt Mixture); 100.0g tocopherol-stripped corn oil; 60.0g tocopherol-stripped lard; 444.9g sucrose per kg diet. Four following experimental groups diets were established based on supplementation or deficiency of vitamin E and/or Se: +E, +Se; -E, +Se; +E, -Se; -E, -Se. Vitamin E was supplied as a d-α-tocopherol acetate, 150 I.U/kg diet and Se as sodium selenite, 0.5mg/kg diet. The diets with Se-deficiency were found to contain less than 0.01 mg Se/kg diet as measured by the method of Whetter and Ullrey (24). The diets with inadequate vitamin E had undetectable tocopherol levels as determined by the procedure of Taylor, et al. (25). Fat supplied 36% of the total

calories in these diets, reflecting the average dietary calories
obtained from fat in human diets. The diets were prepared approximately every 2 weeks and stored under refrigeration (0-4°C). All
animals were housed individually in stainless steel cages with
raised wire floors and had free access to deionized water.
Temperature and relative humidity were controlled at 22°C ± 0.2°
and 50% ± 0.5%, respectively. A 12-hour photoperiod was employed.

Preparation of Microsomal and Cytosolic Fractions. At the end of
the 5 week period on experimental diets, all animals were killed
via sodium pentobarbital anesthesia (120mg/kg body weight). The
tissues were perfused in situ with ice-cold normal saline via the
right ventricle of the heart, excised, trimmed free of connective
tissue, minced, and washed thoroughly with ice-cold deionized
water. The subcellular fractions of liver, lungs, kidneys, etc.,
were prepared as previously described (26).

Determination of Vitamin E and Se Levels in Tissues. Vitamin E
levels (at total tocopherol) were determined by the spectro-
fluorometric method of Taylor, et al. (25). Selenium levels were
determined spectrofluorometrically as described by Whetter and
Ullrey (24).

Preparation of Fatty Acid Hydroperoxides. Linoleic acid hydroperoxide and 15-HPETE were prepared enzymatically employing
soybean lipoxygenase (Sigma Chemical Co., St. Louis, MO). The
total reaction mixture (100ml) contained: 50mM Tris-Hcl, pH 8.5
(prior to the addition of other components, the buffer was
saturated with oxygen); 1.0mM Linoleic acid or Arachidonic acid
and 5 million units soybean lipoxygenase. The reaction was
started by the addition of enzyme and incubated at 30°C for 5 min.
under oxygen atmosphere. The reaction was arrested by the addition of 5ml HCl (6.0N) and the hydroperoxides were extracted twice
with pre-cooled (-20°C) hexane:ether (1:1) solvent. The extracts
were pooled, dried with anhydrous sodium sulfate and evaporated to
dryness under vacuum. The residue was dissolved in hexane:iso-
propanol:acetic acid (987:12:1) solvent and purified by HPLC on a
preparative porasil column using the same solvent system. The
eluates were monitored at 235nm and the major hydroperoxide peak
was collected. Hydroperoxides were quantitated by employing a
molar extinction coefficient of $2.8 \times 10^4 cm^{-1}$ and stored in
Hexane:acetic acid (99:1) at -20°C. Hydroperoxides, thus, stored
were found to be stable for several months.

Enzyme Assays. Cytochrome P-450 peroxidase activity was determined by the method of O'Brien and Rahimthula (27) as modified by
Reddy, et al, with cumene hydroperoxide (CHP), linoleic acid
hydroperoxide (LHP) and 15-HPETE as substrates and tetramethyl-
P-phenylene diamine (TMPD) as electron donor. Prostaglandin H
synthase activity was measured as previously described (19).
    Glutathione-peroxidase activity was measured spectrophoto-
metrically at 340nm by an enzyme coupled assay procedure of Paglia
and Valentine (28) as modified by Reddy, et al. (26). A molar
extinction coefficient of $6.2 \times 10^3 cm^{-1}$ was used in calculations.

Protein Determination. Protein concentration was determined by the method of Lowry, et al., (29) with bovine serum albumin as standard.

Statistics. Where appropriate, the data in each experiment were subjected to analysis of variance. Means were tested for signifi-cant differences ($P < 0.05$) by the sequential methods of Newman and Keuls multiple range test.

Results and Discussion

Table I summarizes the status of vitamin E and Se in various tissues obtained from rats subjected to altered vitamin E and/or Se nutrition. It is evident from the Table that the animals fed on vitamini E and/or Se-deficient diets showed marked decrease in tissue levels of vitamin E and/or Se respectively. This indicates that the diets employed in these experiments induced desirable deficiency states of vitamin and/or Se. In general, vitamin E levels were affected more in microsomes than in cytosols under vitamin E-deficiency states.

Table I.   Vitamin E and Selenium Status of Rats Fed Diets
            Deficient in Vitamin E and/or Se for 5 weeks

Organ or Tissue	Diet			
	+E,+Se	−E,+Se	+E,−Se	−E,−Se
Tocopherol				
Serum (mg/dl)	1.18±0.08	0.11±0.02	1.33±0.15	0.15±0.01
Liver (µg/g protein)				
Microsome-rich	221±18	35±2	217±23	33±7
Cytosol	52±4	11±2	42±2	9±1
Lung (µg/g protein)				
Microsome-rich	343±59	81±23	422±35	64±2
Cytosol	90±12	40±6	92±11	42±4
Brain (µg/g protein)				
Microsome-rich	318±39	96±18	300±18	168±21
Cytosol	75±3	51±15	74±18	54±9
Blood Selenium (µg/ml)	0.49±0.02	0.50±0.01	0.02±0.005	0.03±0.006

Values are means ± SE for 6 animals.

It is true that almost every mammalian tissue has the ability to form various hydroperoxides, especially the fatty acid hydro-peroxides, and it is also true that cyt P-450 MFO system is ubiquitously distributed in almost all tissues. Therefore, it is conceivable that the heme peroxidase activity associated with cyt P-450 MFO system in which P-450 moiety is extremely susceptible to free radical attack, may be severely compromised under reduced antioxidant defense potential, thus, imparing the hydroperoxide metabolism within the cell. Accordingly, we measured the effects of vitamin E and/or Se deficiency on the catalytic activity of

heme peroxidase associated with cyt P-450 MFO system which are
shown in Table II. Generally, liver microsomes exhibited much
higher specific activity than lung microsomes toward CHP, LHP and
15-HPETE in that decreasing order.

Table II. Microsomal Heme Peroxidase Activity in Rats Fed Diets
with Altered Vitamin E and/or Selenium Nutrition for 5 Weeks

	Diet			
Tissue	+E,+Se	-E,+Se	+E,-Se	-E,-Se
Liver:				
CHP	120.0±11.5[1]	26.2±3.0	290.6±18.6	89.4±13.0
LHP	43.4± 9.8	12.4±2.9	98.2±14.3	27.3± 4.8
15-HPETE	79.6± 9.0	19.8±5.0	185.3±17.0	69.2± 6.0
Lung:				
CHP	26.3± 4.3	3.8±0.6	43.7± 9.7	14.5± 3.2
LHP	10.6± 1.3	1.2±0.1	18.3± 6.2	7.3± 1.1
15-HPETE	24.4± 2.1	0.9±0.2	36.4± 4.1	15.3± 3.3

Enzyme activity is expressed as nmoles TMPD oxidized per min. per
mg protein.
[1]Values are means ± SE for 6 animals.

   It is interesting to note that vitamin E- and Se-deficiency
states appear to have opposing effects on microsomal heme peroxidase activity, more so in liver than in lung. In vitamin E
deficiency, the hydroperoxidase activity of liver microsomes was
decreased by approximately 80% (+E, +Se vs. -E, +Se groups), even
higher reduction was observed in lung. However, in the Se-deficient states, hydroperoxidase activity of both liver and lung was
increased nearly two fold (compare the +E, +Se and +E, -Se groups).
In the combined deficiency state, hydroperoxidase activity was
reduced only marginally, less than 30% (+E, +Se vs. -E, -Se).
This may be, in part, due to a combination of the reducing effect
of vitamin E deficiency and elevating effect of Se deficiency
exerted simultaneously.
   Prostaglandin H synthase, also referred to as cyclooxygenase,
is a microsomal enzyme with a molecular weight of 72,000. The
same polypeptide has been shown to catalyze two distinct reactions: the bisdioxygenation of linoleic acid, arachidonic acid,
etc., to form PGG_1, PGG_2, etc., respectively (cyclooxygenase
activity) and the reduction of hydroperoxide function of endoperoxides like PGG_1 and PGG_2 (peroxidase activity) (30). Heme is
an essential cofactor for both activities. Thus, it is reasonable
to assume that PGH synthase might be influenced by the altered
antioxidant defense mechanisms. As shown in Table III, PGH
synthase activity was elevated significantly ($P < 0.05$) in liver
and lung microsomes from vitamin E-deficient animals. However, Se
deficiency had no effect on PGH synthase activity in all the
tissues measured.

Table III. Effects of Vitamin E and/or Selenium Deficiency on
Prostaglandin Synthetase Activity

	+E,+Se	−E,+Se	+E,−Se	−E,−Se
Liver Microsomes	94.8±12.0[1]	138.6±19	99.0±18	139.8±19
Lung Microsomes	201±24.6	334±32	141±13.8	297.6±35
Kidney Microsomes	49.8±12.6	53.4±6.6	42.0±9.0	59.0±1.0

Enzyme activity is expressed as nmoles of O_2 consumed per minute
per mg of protein.
[1]Values expressed as means ± Se for 6 animals.

These observations suggest that vitamin E may play a regulatory
role in PG biosynthesis by controlling the formation of key
intermediates such as hydroperoxides and cyclic endoperoxides. In
these experiments, peroxidase activity associated with the PGH
synthase could not be measured because of the contamination of
other peroxidases like cyt P-450 hydroperoxidase in crude microsomal preparations. Our attempts to measure the differences in
catalytic rates employing indomethacin were not successful. Nevertheless, it is not too unreasonable to assume that probably both
activities of PGH synthase are equally affected by vitamin E
deficiency, since both require heme as cofactor.
    The capacity of superoxide anion (O_2^-) to reduce H_2O_2 with
the resulting formation hydroxyl radicals in an iron-catalyzed
Haber-Weiss reaction renders O_2^- a potentially dangerous factor in
living cells which are also producing H_2O_2. Under normal circumstances, the catalytic activity of superoxide dismutases is
effective in maintaining O_2^- at low levels whereas catalase and
Se-GSH-Px control the H_2O_2 level of the cell. Catalase is
localized mainly in peroxisomes and has a high Km for H_2O_2 (the
enzyme is not easily saturatable with substrate) whereas Se-GSH-Px
is present in the cytosol as well as mitochondria and has very low
Km for H_2O_2 (1.0 μM) (14). The metabolism of H_2O_2 is equally as
important as the metabolism of organic hydroperoxides. As shown
in figure 1, H_2O_2 is produced in tissues by different enzymatic as
well as non-enzymatic mechanisms. In addition to catalase and
Se-GSH-Px, cyt P-450 peroxidase has been implicated in the
metabolism of H_2O_2 (20). Also, glutathione S-transferases
exhibiting peroxidase activity may play an important role in
reducing membrane bound lipid hydroperoxides, since hydrophobic
nature of the substrates is an absolute requirement for these
enzymes. Selenium-GSH-Px is not particularly effective with
membrane bound hydroperoxides (31). Obviously, a balance among
the activities of the hydroperoxide metabolizing enzymes together
with free radical scavengers like vitamin E is essential not only
to protect the cell from peroxidative damage, but also to regulate
various metabolic pathways in AA cascade.
    In these studies, we have assessed the effects of altered
vitamin E and/or Se nutrition on Se-GSH-Px and Non-Se-GSH-Px
activities of rat tissues. It is known that Se-GSH-Px acts both
on H_2O_2 and organic hydroperoxides and non-Se-GSH-Px acts only on
organic hydroperoxides. Therefore, GSH-Px activity was measured
in crude cytosols with two substrates; H_2O_2, which measures only
Se-GSH-Px, and CHP, which measures both Se-GSH-Px and Non-Se-GSH-Px.

XENOBIOTIC METABOLISM: NUTRITIONAL EFFECTS

262

Values with H_2O_2 were subtracted from those of CHP to obtain Non-Se-GSH-Px activities as previously described ([18]). However, from our previous experience, the estimation of non-Se-GSH-Px activity with fatty acid hydroperoxides could not be done in a similar way. Because, catalytic rates of purified Se-GSH-Px toward LHP and 15-HPETE are not identical with those for H_2O_2 whereas CHP and H_2O_2 exhibit identical rates ([13,32]). This is further complicated by the presence of different Non-Se-GSH-Px isozymes exhibiting different catalytic rates toward fatty acid hydroperoxides ([33]). Therefore, the values for LHP and 15-HPETE are presented as total GSH-Px activity rather than individually.

Table IV summarizes cytosolic Se-GSH-Px activity in various tissues. It is evident from the Table that Se-GSH-Px activity of all tissues measured was markedly reduced in Se-deficient states, especially in liver where it was reduced to about 1% that of the Se-supplemented groups and the activity in other tissues was reduced to about 10%. Vitamin E deficiency had no influence on

Table IV. Cytosolic Se-GSH-Px Activity in Tissues of Rats Fed Diets Deficient in Vitamin E and/or Se for 5 Weeks

Tissue	Diet			
	+E,+Se	-E,+Se	+E,-Se	-E,-Se
Blood	97.8± 8.5[1]	89.6± 9.8	14.5±2.4	18.1±3.0
Liver	347.4±18.9	348.0±13.5	3.2±0.3	3.5±0.3
Lung	103.4± 6.6	101.1± 6.2	7.7±0.9	8.3±0.7
Kidney	39.0± 1.9	39.8± 1.6	4.5±0.6	6.9±0.7
Heart	257.0±14.4	247.4±12.1	10±3.4	11.6±1.5
Brain	66.8± 5.6	64.9± 3.9	7.2±0.7	6.6±0.6

With hydrogen peroxide as substrate.
Enzyme units are expressed as munits/mg protein.
[1]Values are means ± Se for 6 animals.

the enzyme. Thus, Se deficiency resulting in lowered Se-GSH-Px activity might be expected to result in tissue damage due to reduced ability of the cell to eliminate H_2O_2 generated by various metabolic pathways. Again, it should be emphasized that catalase is not an effective scavenger of H_2O_2 at low levels and these low levels produced in cytosol are probably more dangerous than the high peroxisomal H_2O_2 levels where they are readily decomposed by catalase.

Non-Se GSH-Px activity is associated with one or more forms of the glutathioine S-transferases. In these experiments, we have measured the total GSH-Px activity associated with these multifunctional enzymes employing CHP as substrate. As shown in Table V, Non-Se GSH-Px activity of liver, kidney, and lung were significantly ($p < 0.05$) increased under Se-deficient states.

Table V.   Effects of Vitamin E and/or Selenium Deficiency on
            Non-Se-Glutathione Peroxidase Activity

	+E,+Se[1]	−E,+Se	+E,−Se	−E,−Se
Liver	113.5±11.8	101.7±7.5	189.6±9.5	173.2±7.5
Lung	18.6± 1.4	16.6±2.0	23.3±1.7	21.4±1.7
Kidney	12.6± 1.8	5.9±0.9	58.3±4.3	44.0±4.4
Stomach	7.4± 2.8	7.9±0.9	4.2±2.2	6.2±0.6

With cumene hydroperoxide as substrate.
Enzyme units are expressed as munits/mg protein.
[1]Values are means ± Se for 6 animals.

Once again vitamin E deficiency had no effect on this enzyme.
There were no differences in the enzyme activity of stomach among
different dietary groups. Heart showed little non-Se GSH-Px
activity (data not shown). These results suggest that, at least
in some tissues, non-Se GSH-Px may partially compensate for the
decreased Se-GSH-Px activity observed in Se deficiency.
   Table VI summarizes total GSH-Px activity toward LHP and
15-HPETE in tissues from rats fed on vitamin E and/or Se deficient
diets. GSH-Px activity toward fatty acid hydroperoxides was
reduced markedly in liver and lung under Se-deficient states
whereas kidney enzyme levels were only marginally affected. It
should be noted that these total enzyme activities were contributed by both Se-GSH-Px and non-Se GSH-Px in crude cytosols of Se
supplemented animals. However, in Se-deficient

Table VI.   Effects of Vitamin E and/or Se Deficiency on Cytosolic
             GSH-Px Activity with Fatty Acid Hydroperoxides

Tissue	Diet			
	+E,+Se	−E,+Se	+E,−Se	−E,−Se
Liver:				
LHP	476.0±23.9[1]	479.0±21.0	164.0±30.1	158.0±14.2
15-HPETE	516.0±27.6	503.0±19.8	189.0±16.4	174.0±13.9
Lung:				
LHP	134.2±11.7	138.0±12.2	21.00± 4.6	39.10± 4.7
15-HPETE	140.0±12.4	152.4±14.1	29.80± 5.3	47.80± 5.4
Kidney:				
LHP	46.10± 4.9	41.30± 3.5	32.40± 4.2	36.90± 8.5
15-HPETE	56.50± 6.6	50.90± 5.4	41.80± 7.3	44.80± 7.1

Enzyme activity is expressed as nmoles product formed per min.
per mg protein.
[1]Values expressed as Means ± SE for 6 animals.

states, greater than 95% of the GSH-Px activity toward LHP and
15-HPETE is due to non-GSH-Px, since Se-GSH-Px is completely
abolished in Se-deficiency. Thus, Se deficiency appears to have
an affect on the total capacity of hydroperoxide metabolism in
liver and lung. Interestingly, kidney appears to be compensating
with Non-Se GSH-Px for the decreased Se-GSH-Px activity observed
in Se deficiency. In general, vitamin E had no effect on GSH-Px
activity.

In summary, Se-GSH-Px and Non-GSH-Px along with cyt P-450 peroxidase appear to play an important role in the metabolism of hydroperoxides and, thus, in the control of the hydroperoxide tone of the cell. Based on recent reports, hydroperoxide tone of the cell plays a crucial role in the regulation of enzymes involved in the biosynthesis of PGs, PGIs, TXs and LTs (15,16). Conceivably, under adequate nutritional status, a balance in the level of the various peroxidases is maintained. However, when one enzyme is affected, for example Se-GSH-Px in Se deficiency, other enzymes may be elevated to compensate for the deficiency. This is supported by our results presented here on non-Se GSH-Px and cyt P-450 peroxidase activities which indicate that, at least in some tissues, the back-up systems may partially compensate for one another. Nevertheless, the total capacity of the cell to metabolize hydroperoxides appears to be markedly reduced under Se deficiency. Since Non-GSH Px acts only on organic hydroperoxides, and catalase, which is localized primarily in peroxisomes, has low affinity for H_2O_2, drastic reduction in Se-GSH-Px activity observed in these studies, could severely impair H_2O_2 metabolism. Accumulated H_2O_2 can lead to the formation of highly reactive free radicals which may affect vital cellular processes including AA cascade deleteriously. Experiments are currently in progress in our laboratory to assess the effects of altered vitamin E and/or Se nutrition on the intermediates/product profile of AA cascade.

Acknowledgments

C. Channa Reddy is a recipient of the Research Career Development Award, (K04HL01240) from NHLBI. This research was supported by research grants from NIH (R01HL31245), U.S. Environmental Protection Agency (R807746) and American Heart Association, National Chapter (84-898). We thank Mrs. Linda Cook and John R. Burgess for their valuable technical assistance.

Literature Cited

1. Pryor, W. A. In "Molecular Basis of Environmental Toxicology", Bhatnager, R. S. ed,; Ann Arbor: Science Publishers, Inc., 1980; pp. 3-36.
2. Schaiach, K. M. CRC Critical Reviews in Food Science and Nutrition, 1980, 13, 189-244.
3. Menzel, D. B. In "Vitamin E", Machlin, L. J., ed.; New York: Marcel Dekker, Inc., 1980; pp. 474-494.
4. Walton, J. R.; Packer, L. IBID, pp. 495-517.
5. Bus, J. S.; Gibson, J. E. Rev. Biochem. Toxicol., 1979, 1, 125-149.
6. Mason, R. P. Free Radicals in Biology, 1982, 5, 161-217.
7. Pryor, W. A. Free Radicals in Biology, 1976, 1, 1-49.
8. Mead, J. IBID, 51-68.
9. Marnett, L. J. Free Radicals in Biology, 1984, 6, 63-94.
10. Tappel, A. L. Ann. N.Y. Acad. Sci., 1980, 355, 18-31.
11. McCay, P. B.; King, M. M. In "Vitamin E', Machlin, L. J., ed.; New York: Marcel Dekker, Inc., 1980; pp. 289-317.

12. Reddy, C. C.; Scholz, R. W.; Thomas, C. E.; Massaro, E. J. Life Sci., 1982, 31, 571-576.

13. Rao, M. K.; Kumar, M.S.; Scholz, R.W.; Reddy, C.C. In "Prostaglandins and Leukotrienes '84", Intl. Symp. on Prostaglandins and Leukotrienes; Baily, J. M., Ed.; #170, 1984.

14. Flohe, L. Free Radicals in Biology, 1982, 5, 223-254.

15. Lands, W. E. M.; Kulmacz, R. J.; Marshall, P. J. Free Radicals in Biology, 1984, 6, 39-61.

16. Cornwell, D. G.; Morisaki, N. IBID, 95-148.

17. Pace-Asciak, C. R.; Smith, W. L. The Enzymes, 1983, 16, 543-603.

18. Reddy, C. C.; Tu, C.-P. D.; Burgess, J. R.; Ho, C.-Y.; Scholz, R. W.; Massaro, E. J. Biochem. Biophys. Res. Commun, 1981, 101, 970-978.

19. Reddy, C. C.; Grasso, T. L.; Scholz, R. W.; Labosh, T. J.; Thomas, C. E.; Massaro, E. J. Prostaglandins and Cancer, Powells, T. J.; Ramwell, P. W.; Honn, K. V.; Bockman, R. S., Eds.; Alan R. Liss: New York, 1982, Vol. 2, pp. 149-154.

20. O'Brien, P. J. In "Autooxidation in Food and Biological Systems", Simic, M. G.; Karel, M., Eds.; Plenum Press: New York, 1980, pp. 563-587.

21. Gale, P. H.; Egan, R. W. Free Radicals in Biology, 1984, 6, 1-38.

22. Kalyanaraman, B.; Sivarajah, K. IBID, 149-198.

23. Harper, A. E. J. Nutr., 1959, 68, 405-418.

24. Whetter, P. A.; Ullrey, D. E. J. Assoc. Official Anal. Chemists, 1978, 61, 927-930.

25. Taylor, S. C.; Lamden, M. P.; Tappel, A. L. Lipids, 1976, 11, 530-538.

26. Reddy, C. C.; Thomas, C. E.; Scholz, R. W.; Labosh, T. J.; Massaro, E. J. Adv. Modern Environ. Toxicol., 1983, 5, 395-410.

27. O'Brien, P. J.; Rahimthula, A. D. Methods Enzymol., 22, 407-412.

28. Paglia, D. E.; Valentine, W. N. J. Lab. Clin. Med., 1967, 70, 158-159.

29. Lowry, O. H.; Rosebrough, N. J.; Farr, A. L.; Randall, R. J. J. Biol. Chem., 1951, 193, 265-275.

30. Ohki, S.; Ogino, N.; Yamamoto, S.; Hayaishi, O. J. Biol. Chem., 1979, 254, 829-834.

31. McCay, P. B.; King, M. M. In "Vitamin E"; Machlin, L. J., Ed.; Marcel Dekker: New York, pp. 289-317.

32. Reddy, C. C.; Rao, M. K.; Mastro, A. M.; Egan, R. W. Biochem. Intl., 1984, 9, 755-761.

33. Reddy, C. C.; Burgess, J. R.; Gong, Z. Z.; Massaro, E. J.; Tu, C.-P. D. Arch. Biochem. Biophy, 1983, 224, 87-101.

RECEIVED January 23, 1985

Selenium and Carcinogenesis

JOHN A. MILNER

Department of Food Science, University of Illinois, Urbana, IL 61801

Selenium has been shown to be effective in inhibiting
the incidence of chemically and virally induced tumors.
Continuous selenium intake by the host appears to be
needed to achieve maximal inhibition of both of these
models of carcinogenesis. Present information suggests
that selenium inhibits both the initiation and promotion
phases of chemical carcinogenesis. The anticarcinogenic
property of selenium does not appear to be mediated
through its association with glutathione peroxidase
activity. Selenium is also effective in inhibiting the
proliferation of neoplastic cells. Selenium has been
shown to inhibit the growth of various neoplastic
cells in vitro and in vivo. However, differences in the
sensitivity of various tumor cell lines to selenium are
evident. The efficacy of selenium as an antitumorigenic
agent depends on the form and mode of administration of
this trace element. Total tumor mass also appears to
effect the efficacy of selenium. Evidence now suggests
that selenodiglutathione or some other intermediate in
selenium metabolism is responsible for the antitumorigenic
properties of this trace element.

In the early 1950s the only known biological action of selenium was
associated with its toxicity. However, by the late 50's and 60's
increasing evidence indicated this trace element had a role in
intermediary metabolism since a dietary source prevented a variety
of disorders including exudative diathesis in chicks, hepatosis
dietetica in swine, unthriftness in cattle and white muscle disease
in young ruminants. A metabolic function of selenium was proposed
(1) but not completely appreciated until the early 70's (2) when it
was shown to be an integral component of glutathione peroxidase, an
enzyme involved in the destruction of hydroperoxides (3) . To date
this enzymatic function remains the only known biological function
of selenium in mammals.
   Selenium is now believed by many to be an essential dietary

0097–6156/85/0277–0267$06.00/0

trace element for all mammals. Tissues of man and other mammals
have been shown to have a selenium-dependent glutathione peroxidase
activity (4) . Prolonged total parenteral nutrition (TPN) therapy
with solutions practically devoid of selenium have been reported to
produce severe muscular pain and tenderness (5, 6) . These symptoms
were correctable by daily selenium supplementation. Selenium has
also been shown to be effective in preventing the cardiac myopathy
associated with Keshan disease. Additional support for the
essentiality of this element comes from its ability to maximize
growth of mammalian cells in culture (7-9) . Generally, the
concentration of selenium need to stimulate cellular growth is 5 X
10^{-8} M.

Epidemiological Cancer Data
Shamberger and Frost (10) were among the first to report an inverse
relationship between cancer mortality and selenium content of forage
plants. Additional studies suggested that enhanced cancer mortality
occurred in geographic regions where selenium content of soils was
deficient (11-14) . Schrauzer et al., (15) examined the
age-correlated mortalities from cancer and their relationship to
apparent selenium intakes. Mortality rates in 27 countries from
cancer at 17 major body sites in individuals residing in various
countries correlated inversely with apparent dietary selenium
intakes. A significant inverse correlation of the mortality
resulting from cancer of the large intestine, rectum, prostate,
breast, ovary, lung and leukemia was observed with selenium intakes.
Similar inverse correlations were observed between the mortalities
of patients with the above cancer sites and the blood selenium
concentrations of apparently healthy subjects located in the same
geographical region. It is of interest to note, a "Cancer Test"
described in 1947 by Savignac (16), which consisted of measuring
methylene blue reduction time was shown to respond to the selenium
content of human plasma (17, 18) . Thus, considerable
epidemiological data indicate that selenium serves as a naturally
occurring anticarcinogenic agent.

Chemical Carcinogenesis
Numerous scientists have also demonstrated that dietary selenium
supplementation can inhibit chemical carcinogen induced
tumorigenesis in skin, liver, colon and mammary tissue (19-45)
(Table I). Most studies have used inorganic or organic selenium
addition to the drinking water or the diet at concentrations ranging
from 0.5 to 6.0 ug/g. These quantities are considerably higher than
the NRC recommendations of 0.1 ug/g (46) . However, this
anticarcinogenic property is generally observed without any
detectable detrimental effect on the host. Selenium supplementation
reduces the incidence and/or total tumor number in animals treated
with various carcinogens including 3'-methyl-4-dimethyl-
aminoazobenzene, 7,12-dimethylbenz(a)anthracene (DMBA),
benzo(a)pyrene, 2-acetylaminofluorene, 1,2-dimethylhydrazine (DMH),
methylazoxymethanol acetate (MAM), aflatoxin B1, and
methylnitrosourea (MNU). The ability of selenium to inhibit tumor
formation induced by such a wide variety of carcinogens and in such
a variety of tissues indicates a general mechanism rather than a
tissue specific reaction.
    The anticarcinogenic action of selenium does not appear to be

Table I. Influence of Selenium on Chemically Induced Cancer

Quantity Selenium[1]	Tumor Site	Carcinogen[2]	Species	Tumor Reduction (% Controls)	Reference
1 ppm	Breast	DMBA	Rat	38	27
1.5 ppm	Breast	DMBA	Rat	28	25
2.0 ppm	Breast	DMBA	Mice	57	42
4 ppm	Breast	DMBA	Mice	48	42
6 ppm	Breast	DMBA	Mice	62	36
4 ppm	Colon	DMH	Rat	54	31
1.0 ppm	Colon	BNA	Rat	45	22
2.0 ppm	Colon	AZM	Rat	15	39
2.0 ppm	Colon	AZM	Rat	7	37
1.0 ppm	Lungs	BNA	Rat	100	22
5.0 ppm	Liver	DMBA	Rat	48	19
0.5 ppm	Liver	AAF	Rat	83	24
4 ppm	Liver	AAF	Rat	48	35
1 ppm	Liver	Afl. B	Rat	80	23
1.0 ppm	Skin	DMBA	Mice	35	91
5 ppm	Trachea	MNU	Hamster	−23	40

Calculated as a percent reduction of tumors in animals receiving supplemental selenium plus the carcinogen compared to animals receiving the carcinogen only.

[1] Selenium and the carcinogen were applied in solution to the skin.

[2] MC=3-methylcholanthrene; DMAB = 3-methyl-4-dimethylamino-azobenzene; AAF = 2-acetylaminofluorene; MNU = 1 methyl-1-nitrosourea; DMBA = 7,12 dimethylbenz(a)anthracene; DMH = 1,2 dimethylhydrazine; BMA = bis(2-oxopropyl) nitrosamine; Afl B = aflatoxin B and AZM = azoxymethane.

mediated by its antioxidant function as a component of glutathione peroxidase (47) . Vitamin E is a much more potent antioxidant than selenium. Ip (47) examined vitamin E and selenium or a combination on the carcinogenicity of DMBA, and reported that suppression of lipid peroxidation by vitamin E alone is not sufficient to inhibit tumor formation. However, vitamin E may provide a favorable environment against oxidant stress to facilitate selenium in exerting its anticarcinogenic action.

Selenium may alter the initiation phase of carcinogenesis by modifying the activation of procarcinogens. Rasco et al., (38) provided evidence that selenium impedes activation and accelerates detoxification of chemical carcinogens, thereby reducing cancer susceptibility. Daoud and Griffin (20) indicated that selenium may enhance the detoxification of the carcinogen AAF by altering the enzymes that are involved in its metabolic activation. Studies by Harbach and Swenberg (48) reported that addition of selenium to the drinking water of rats decreased hepatic DMH metabolism, as measured by decreased expiration of azoxymethane, and suggested depressed metabolic activation accounted for the decrease in colon cancer incidence in rats treated with this carcinogen. Studies in our laboratory indicate that dietary selenium can modify the metabolism of DMBA (49) . These studies indicate that selenium reduces those intermediates considered the most carcinogenic and mutagenic. Recent studies also show that selenium can specifically inhibit the binding of DMBA and shift the types of adducts that bind in mouse embyro cells in culture (Milner and Dipple, unpublished). Selenium may also inhibit the initiation phase of carcinogenesis by protecting DNA from single-strand break induced by carcinogens or by facilitating DNA repair (34, 50) . Additional support for an alteration in the initiation phase comes from studies indicating that selenium is less effective in inhibiting the total cancer incidence of animals treated with carcinogens that do not require metabolic activation (31, 41) .

Inhibition of the initiation phase of carcinogenesis does not appear to totally explain the anticarcinogenicity of selenium. Banner et al., (21) found that selenium did not influence the acute alterations induced by 2-acetylaminofluorene or methylazoxymethanol and suggested that the anticarcinogenic properties of selenium were due to a mechanism other than an interference with carcinogen activation and interaction with cellular macromolecules. Furthermore, while the effect of selenium on the action of direct acting carcinogens is less than observed with compounds requiring metabolic activation, a reduction in total tumor number is often observed. Therefore, selenium probably inhibits both the initiation and promotion phases of carcinogenesis.

Viral Induced Tumors and Selenium

Another model often used in cancer research is the spontaneous or virally induced tumor. Mouse mammary tumorigenesis is characterized by the presence of preneoplastic hyperplastic alveolar nodules that arise from normal mammary gland cells to develop mammary adenocarcinomas (51) . Female inbred C_3H/St mice infected with the" Bittner Milk Factor", a B-type ribonucleic tumor virus (52) or Murine Mammary Tumor Virus-S (MuMTV-S) develop mammary adenocarcinoma. Addition of 2 ug/ml of selenite in the drinking

water of female virgin C_3H/St mice for 15 months lowered the
incidence of spontaneous mammary tumors to 10% relative to a 82%
incidence in unsupplemented controls (53) . Tumors in selenium
treated mice grew more slowly and appeared less malignant since
death occurred after five to six months as compared to four months
in the control group.

Selenium supplementation also significantly inhibits mammary
tumorigenesis in BALB/cfC$_3$H mice containing the highly oncogenic
exogenic MuMTV-S (53) . BALB/cfC$_3$H (MuMTV-S positive) given 2
and 6 ppm selenium in the drinking water and maintained as breeding
mice, had a significantly lower incidence of mammary tumors (50 and
80% respectively) than unsupplemented controls (54) .

Dietary supplementation with selenium has also been shown to
inhibit virally induced mammary tumorigenesis (55, 56) . The
incidence of adenocarcinoma was reduced to 27% if the mice are fed a
torula yeast diet supplemented with 1 ug/g of selenium as selenium
yeast (55) (Table II). Animals reaching the age of 13.8 months and
switched from this diet to a diet containing only 0.15 ug/g selenium
developed mammary tumors rapidly during their remaining life-span.
The overall tumor incidence reached 69%, not statistically different
from the 77% incidence of tumors observed in animals fed the basal
diet over their entire post-weaning life span. Conversely, mice,
13.8 months old, changed from the basal diet to one containing 1.0
ug/g selenium developed mammary tumors with a total incidence of
only 46%, significantly lower than in controls. This study
demonstrates that dietary selenium prevents and retards tumor
development only as long as it is supplied in adequate amounts
(55) .

More recent data indicate the efficacy of selenium in
inhibiting virally induced tumors can be markedly influenced by the
type of diet fed. While selenium addition to the drinking water
inhibited tumor formation in mice fed the Oregon State University
chow, it had little effect on mice fed Wayne Lab Blocs (56) .
Studies by Whanger et al., (56) has also shown that selenium
addition to the drinking water had no influence on tumor incidence
of C_3H/St mice fed a casein based diet regardless of the lipid
source used. What dietary factor(s) are accounting for these
differences in efficacy remain to be determined.

The mechanism by which selenium retards virally induced
tumorigenesis is unknown. Selenium may inhibit tumor formation by
interfering with the replication or transforming action of viruses.
Selenium may simply be reducing the proliferation of the transformed
cells such that the presence of tumors is not detectable.

Human Tumors and Selenium Intakes
Broghamer et al., (57) examined the association between blood
selenium concentrations of 110 patients with various types of
carcinomas and the biological behavior pattern of the tumor.
Although the range of serum selenium concentrations of these 110
patients was wide, the majority had levels lower than healthy
controls. Low serum selenium concentrations were associated with a
higher frequency of distant metastases, multiple primary tumors,
multiple recurrances, and a shortened survival time. Patients with
selenium concentrations approaching or exceeding the mean value of
all cancer patients had tumors that remained confined to the region

Table II. Effect of Dietary Selenium on the Incidence of
           Mammary Tumors in C_3H/St Mice

Dietary Selenium	0.15	1.0	0.15 to 1.0	1.0 to 0.15
Age tumor onset (months 0.5)	8.0	13.5	8.0	13.5
Tumors/Treatment	20/26	7/26	12/26	18/26
Percent Incidence	77[a]	27[b]	46[c]	69[a]

Adapted from Schrauzer et al., 1980 (55). Female virgin
C_3H/St mice were fed a Torula yeast diet supplemented
with selenium yeast as indicated above from weaning until
death. In some mice reaching 13.8 months of age the diet
was switched as indicated. Means not sharing a common
superscript letter differ significantly.

of origin, developed less distant metastasis, had fewer primary neoplasms and had a decreased frequency of recurrences. However, other observations (58) revealed that serum selenium concentration of patients with reticuloendothelial tumors did not correlate with the behavioral patterns of the tumor, i.e., extent of organ involvement, patient survival time and the incidence of multiple primary neoplasms. Therefore, the efficacy of selenium as a antitumorigenic agent may depend heavily on the tumor cell examined.

Almost 70 years ago selenium was proclaimed as a cancer therapeutic agent (59, 60) . In 1956, Weisburger and Surhland (61) reported that selenocystine was effective in reducing the leukocyte count and spleen size of patients suffering from acute leukemia. At a dose of 50–200 milligrams per day symptoms of nausea, vomiting and diarrhea were observed. Interestingly, these authors indicated that at this dosage hepatic and renal function were normal and the symptoms described were no worse than those occurring with normally employed therapeutic agents.

Inorganic and organic selenium have been reported to localize in several types of human tumors (62, 63) . Uptake of both Se^{73} selenate and selenite were similar (64) . Ehrlich carcinoma, Crocker sarcoma and Mecca lymphosarcoma tumors were found to accumulate the radioselenium slowly and continuously in contrast to rapid uptake and clearance of the label from most normal organs. Clinically, the affinity of tumors for selenium has been the basis for utilizing a radioactive nuclide of selenium as a tumor localizing agent (62, 64) . The reason for the localization of selenium is not readily apparent but may reflect enhanced division rates, protein and chondroitin sulfate biosynthesis, or a decrease in the detoxification of selenium. An outgrowth of these observations has been to examine the in vitro effects of selenium supplementation on cellular propagation.

Experimentally Transplanted Tumors and Selenium Inhibition

Considerable evidence has shown that selenium can inhibit the growth of experimentally transplanted tumors (65-74) . One of the principal cell lines that has been used for many of these studies has been the Ehrlich ascites tumor cell (65-68) . Abdullaev et al., (65) showed that the parenteral administration of sodium selenite at a dose of 1 ug per g body weight of the host retarded the growth of this tumor cell line. Additional studies also revealed that similar quantities of selenium inhibited the growth of Guerin carcinoma, sarcomatous M^{-1} neoplasms and L-1210 leukemic cells (65, 74) . An enhanced effect of tumor inhibition was observed when selenium was given in combination with X-ray (65) or chemotherapy (74) .

Recent studies in various laboratories (66-74) have extended the observation of the antitumorigenic property of selenium. Non-tumor bearing mice receiving up to 2 ug/g body weight are not significantly influenced by selenium administration. The only abnormal symptom observed with these high dosages of selenium is a slight increase in irritability and a reduction in intestinal tissue mass. The hyperirritability was found to subside once selenium injections were stopped.

Intraperitoneal treatment with 1 microgram of selenium per gram body weight results in a 90 to 100% reduction in tumor incidence (68) (Table III). Corresponding to this reduced incidence of

Table III.   Effect of Form of Selenium Administered on
Tumor Propagation

Treatment	Dosage u/g Body Weight	Weight Gain % Controls		Ascites Tumor Incidence
		−EATC	+EATC	
Buffer	---	100	100	15/15
Selenium Dioxide	2.0	87	63	0/10
	1.0	105	58	0/5
	0.25	94	58	0/4
Sodium Selenite	2.0	92	51	0/10
	1.0	93	48	0/5
	0.25	104	64	0/5
Sodium Selenate	2.0	76	47	0/10
	1.0	81	38	0/5
	0.25	85	43	0/5
Selenomethionine	2.0	83	69	0/10
	1.0	114	102	5/5
	0.25	96	103	5/5
Selenocystine	2.0	83	52	0/10
	1.0	113	51	0/5
	0.25	85	65	2/5
Pooled SEM		13	8	

On day zero mice weighing approximately 20 g were inoculated
with 5 X 10^5 Ehrlich ascites tumor cells (EATC).   SEM =
standard error of the mean.   All test solutions were prepared in
Krebs Ringers Phosphate buffer and administered by i.p. injection
on days 0, 1, 3, 5, 7, 9, 12, 15, and 18.

ascites tumor, was a reduction in weight gain of selenium treated
mice. The excessive weight gain occurring in controls resulted from
ascites fluid accumulation. This conclusion is easily appreciated
by gross examination of the massive abdominal distention of the
buffer treated tumor bearing mice (67) .

Delaying the time of injection of selenium to three days
post-tumor inoculation completely retarded tumor development in only
50% of the mice (68) . Initiation of selenium injections 5 days
after tumor inoculation did not significantly inhibit the percentage
of animals developing ascitic tumors but significantly reduced the
growth of the tumors as indicated by enhanced longevity of the mice.
Thus, these data and those obtained with L-1210 cells (74) suggest
that efficacy of this trace element is dependent on the total tumor
cell mass.

The observed tumor inhibition is not limited to ascitic tumors
since the growth of solid neoplasms such as those resulting from the
inoculation of SV 40-3T3, MCF-7, MBA-MD 231, and several canine
mammary tumor lines, is also significantly inhibited by treatment
with selenium (69-73) . In 1956, Weisberger and Suhrland (66)
showed that selenocystine reduced the growth of the Murphy
lymphosarcoma tumor cell inoculated into rats. Selenocystine was
administered at a dose of 1 mg per kg for 14 days. The reduced
growth was associated with a decrease in the incorporation of 35S
L-cystine into the tumor both in vivo and in vitro. Since this
quantity of selenium reduced growth of the rats, an additional study
was conducted to determine the influence of starvation on the growth
of this tumor. While starvation had little influence on the growth
of this tumor, selenocystine caused an approximate 75% reduction in
tumor size. Interestingly, the growth or this tumor appeared to be
quiescent since additional growth of the tumor was not observed 7
days after selenium treatment was discontinued. Selenium also
inhibits the growth of canine or human mammary tumor cell lines
established from a carcinoma of the solid type (70, 72) . Again,
selenium administration did not significantly alter the growth of
non-tumor bearing mice. However, body weight of tumor bearing mice
was reduced approximately 10%. Similarly, the average volume of
canine or human mammary tumors transplanted into mice in selenium
treated mice was reduced by approximately 75% by selenium
administration (72, 73) .

Studies of Medina and Oborn (75) examined the growth potential
of normal, preneoplastic and neoplastic mammary cells grown in
primary monolayer cell cultures and on three established mammary
cell lines. Selenium, present as sodium selenite in serum-free
medium inhibited all mammary cell cultures at 1×10^{-5} M.
Selenium, at 5×10^{-8} M, stimulated the growth of primary cell
cultures of normal mammary cells and C4 preneoplastic cells and the
established cell line YN-4 but not the growth of D2 preneoplastic
cells and tumors in primary cell cultures and of established cell
lines CL-S1 and Waz-2t. The differential response of cells from
preneoplastic outgrowth lines C4 and D2 and of D2 primary tumors in
vitro correlated with the sensitivity of these same cell populations
to selenium mediated inhibition of growth and tumorigenesis in vivo.
Selenium had little effect on 3 or 4 preneoplastic mammary outgrowth
lines. Recent studies by Poirier et al., (70) have shown that

selenium as sodium selenite preferentially inhibits neoplastic
tissue of canine or human origin compared to non-neoplastic cells.
However, differences in tumor susceptibility were also evident. One
tumor cell line CMT-13 was extremely sensitive to selenite, while
another line CMT-11 was virtually resistant to exposure to media
containing 1 ug selenium/ml. Therefore, selenium inhibition of
mammary tumorigenesis may act by inhibiting one or more different
cell populations. The differential responses among these cell lines
should allow further comparative studies on the cell biological
basis of selenium function.   These data indicate that tumor cells
may vary in their sensitivity to selenium.

     Ip et al., (71) reported the effect of dietary selenium
deficiency and supplementation on the growth of the transplantable
MT-W9B mammary tumor in female Wistar-Furth rats. Selenium
deficiency had no influence on the growth of this tumor.
Supplementation of the diet with 2 ppm of selenium inhibited tumor
growth and reduced the final tumor weight by approximately 50%
compared to the control rats receiving 0.1 ppm of selenium. The
inhibitory response was selective, without inducing any weight loss
in the animals. Recent studies by Poirier and Milner (69), compared
the efficacy of sodium selenite was administration by either
intraperitoneal injection or gastric gavage and a dose of 2.0 ug
selenium six times over a nine day period. Survival time was
significantly increased in Ehrlich ascites tumor bearing mice by 170
and 20% respectively, compared to controls. Dietary supplementation
with 2.5 or 5.0 ppm selenium as sodium selenite also increased the
survival time of tumor bearing mice but by about 15% (69) . The
mode of administration of selenium is an additional factor that may
influence the antitumorigenic properties of this trace element.

Forms of Selenium
     Selenium is generally reduced during cellular metabolism (76) .
Therefore, selenate would yield selenite, followed by a further
reduction to selenide (77, 79) . Greeder and Milner (67) and Milner
and Hsu (74) have reported little difference exists in the efficacy
of sodium selenite, sodium selenate and selenium dioxide to inhibit
tumor proliferation.

     The effect of selenomethionine and selenocystine on the growth
of various neoplastic cells has also been made. These studies
indicate that when selenium is administrated in large quantities
form becomes of less importance. However, when the quantity of
selenium administered is reduced the inorganic forms of selenium
appear to be from 4 to 10 times more effective in inhibiting tumor
proliferation that are the organic forms, selenomethionine or
selenocystine (Table III). Selenomethionine can either be
incorporated into general body proteins in place of methionine or
degraded through the transsulfuration pathway thereby forming
selenocystine (77, 78) . Alternatively, selenomethionine may be
transaminated and decarboxylated, with final release of methane
selenol in a manner similar to the methionine transamination pathway
described by Steele and Benevenga (80) . Selenocystine may be
degraded to release selenite in a manner similar to the degradation
of cystine, however the high reduction potential would favor the
direct release of selenide (81) . Thus, a slower metabolism of the
organic forms to selenite or other intermediates may explain these

differences in their ability to inhibit tumor propagation.

A GSH/glutathione reductase/NADPH pathway leading to a reduction of selenium has been proposed (76-79) (Figure 1). In this pathway selenide is methylated to form $(CH_3)_3$ Se (trimethyl selenonium ion) and excreted in the urine when moderate levels of selenium are ingested (82, 83). With acute selenium toxicity the volatile compound, dimethyl selenide, is formed and expired via the lung (79, 82). Hydrogen selenide appears to be a central compound in selenium metabolism (84). HSe or a close metabolite may be the form inserted posttranslationally into a pre-glutathione peroxidase polypeptide to form the active glutathione peroxidase subunits (85). As postulated by Diplock (84) selenide could also be the chemical form that binds to microsomes. While selenide is highly toxic (86), the intracellular toxicity of this species may be lessened by the non-specific binding to proteins.

Sodium selenite and selenodiglutathione have been found to be more effective in inhibiting the growth of Ehrlich ascites tumors than sodium selenide, dimethyl selenide or seleno-DL-cystine. Preincubation of tumor cells with either 1 or 3 ppm Se as GSSeSG, Na_2SeO_3 or dimethylselenide before reinoculated into mice resulted in a significant increase in survival in mice inoculated with cells pretreated with GSSeSG (69) (Table IV). Vernie et al., (87) also reported that intraperitoneal injections of selenodiglutathione or selenodicysteine inhibited tumor growth and increased the life span of mice treated with malignant lymphoblasts, strain MBVIA cells. Based on available data obtained with selenodiglutathione, some intermediate in the normal pathway for selenium detoxification is probably responsible for this trace element's antitumorigenic properties.

Conclusions

Evidence from several lines of inquiry show that selenium has a protective effect against carcinogenesis in a number of laboratory animals. A comparison of cancer death rate indicates that the mortality is lower in areas with abundant or high dietary selenium intakes than regions where intake is low. Selenium may alter cancer susceptibility or the growth of transformed cell through various mechanisms. Pharmacological levels of selenium have been reported to potentiate the immune response of the host (88, 89). Exposure to high concentration of selenium is known to inhibit DNA synthesis (90) such that cells are blocked in the S-G2 phase of the cell cycle (90). A modulation of mitochondrial function by selenium has also been suggested as one of the early effects of growth inhibition (91). Whatever the mechanism, a degree of specificity for inhibiting neoplastic tissue is evident. The mechanism(s) by which selenium leads to a depression in experimentally induced cancer is unknown but clearly deserves further investigation.

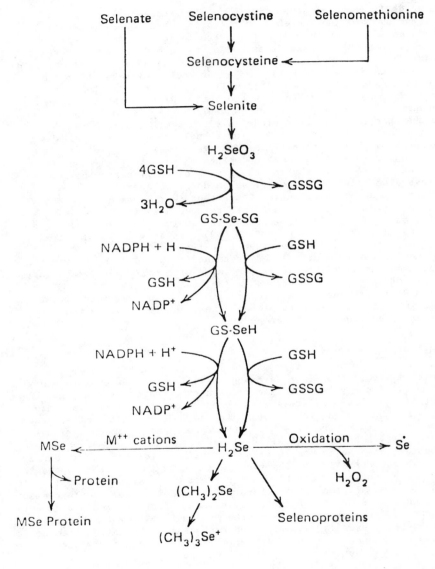

Figure 1. Proposed pathway for selenium detoxification in Mammals.

Table IV. Longevity of Mice Inoculated with Tumor Cells
Preincubated with Various Forms of Selenium

Treatment	Selenium ug/ml	Tumor Incidence	Time First Death (Hr)	Mean Longevity (Hr)
Buffer	---	10/10	480	622 ± 30
Sodium Selenite	1.0	10/10	480	626 ± 33
	3.0	10/10	480	607 ± 35
Selenodiglutathione	1.0	9/10	600	789 ± 52
	3.0	7/10	672	1069 ± 145
Dimethylselenide	1.0	10/10	528	605 ± 24
	3.0	10/10	552	607 ± 14

Adapted from Poirier and Milner (69). All tumor cells were
preincubated for 15 minutes in buffer in the presence or absence
of selenium as sodium selenite, selenodiglutathione or dimethylselenide, before inoculation into Swiss mice. Each received
5×10^5 Ehrlich ascites tumor cells. Vertical means ± SEM not
sharing a common superscript letter differ $P < 0.05$.

Literature Cited
1. Schwarz, K.; Foltz, C. M. J. Am. Chem. Soc. 1957, 79, 3292-3.
2. Rotruck, J. T.; Pope, A. L.; Ganther, H. E.; Swanson, A. B.;
Hafeman, D. G.; Hoekstra, W. G. Science 1973, 179, 588-90.
3. Little, C.; O'Brien, P. J. Biochem. Biophys. Res. Comm. 1968,
31, 145-50.
4. Ganther, H. E.; Hafeman, D. G.; Lawrence, R. A.; Serfass,
R. E.; Hoekstra, W. G. In "Trace Elements in Human Health and

Disease. Volume II. Essential and Toxic Elements"; Prasad,
A. S., Ed.; Academic Press: New York, 1976.

5.   Van Rij, A. M.; Thomson, C. D.; McKenzie, J. M.; Robinson,
     M. F. Am. J. Clin. Nutr. 1979, 32, 2076-85.
6.   Kein, C. L.; Ganther, H. E. Am. J. Clin. Nutr. 1983, 37,
     319-28.
7.   Giasuddin, A. S. M.; Diplock, A. T. Archives Biochem.
     Biophys. 1979, 196(1), 270-80.
8.   McKeehan, W. L.; Hamilton, W. G.; Ham, R. G. Proc. Natl. Acad.
     Sci. USA 1976, 73, 2023-7.
9.   Malan-Shibley, L.; Iype, P. T. In Vitro 1983, 19, 749-58.
10. Shamberger, R. J.; Frost, D. V. Canad. Med. Assoc. J. 1969,
     100, 682.
11. Shamberger, R. J. Experientia 1966, 22, 116-21.
12. Shamberger, R. J.; Willis, C. E. CRC Crit. Rev. Clin. Lab.
     Sci. 1971, 2, 211-21.
13. Shamberger, R. J.; Tytko, S. A.; Willis, C. E. Arch. Environ.
     Health 1976, 31,231-5.
14. Cowgill, U. M. Biol. Trace Elem. Res. 1983, 5, 345-61.
15. Schrauzer, G. N.; White, D. A.; Schneider, C. J. Bioinorg.
     Chem. 1977, 7, 23-34.
16. Savignac, R. J.; Jant, J. C.; Sizel, I. W. AAAS Res. Conf. on
     Cancer 1945, 245-52.
17. Schrauzer, G. N.; Rhead, W. J. Experientia 1971, 27, 1069-71.
18. Schrauzer, G. N.; Rhead, W. J.; Evans, G. A. Bioinorg. Chem.
     1973, 2, 329-40.
19. Clayton, C. C.; Baumann, C. A. Cancer Res. 1949, 9, 575-82.
20. Daoud, A. H.; Griffin, A. C. Cancer Letters 1978, 5, 231-7.
21. Banner, W. P.; Tan, Q. H.; Zedeck, M. S. Cancer Res. 1982, 42,
     2985-9.
22. Birt, D. F.; Lawson, T. A.; Julius, A. D.; Runice, C. E.;
     Salmasi, S. Cancer Res. 1982, 42, 4455-9.
23. Grant, K. E.; Conner, M. W.; Newberne, P. M. Toxicol. Appl.
     Pharm. 1977, 41, 166.
24. Harr, J. R.; Exon, J. H.; Whanger, P. D.; Weswig, P. H. Clin.
     Toxicol. 1972, 5, 187-94.
25. Ip, C. Cancer Res. 1981, 41, 2683-6.
26. Ip, C. Biol. Trace Elem. Res. 1983, 5, 317-30.
27. Ip, C.; Sinha, D. K. Cancer Res. 1981, 41, 31-4.
28. Riley, J. F. Experientia 1968, 24, 1237-8.
29. Ip, C.; Sinha, D. Carcinogenesis 1981, 2, 435-8.
30. Jacobs, M. M. Cancer Res. 1983, 43, 1646-9.
31. Jacobs, M. M.; Jansson, B.; Griffin, A. C. Cancer Letters
     1977, 2, 133-8.
32. Jacobs, M. M.; Frost, C. F.; Beams, F. A. Cancer Res. 1981,
     41, 4458-65.
33. Lalor, J. H.; Llewellyn, G. C. J. Toxicol. Environ. Health
     1981, 8, 387-400.
34. Lawson, T.; Birt, D. Proc. Am. Assoc. Cancer Res. 1981,
     22, 93-8.
35. Marshall, M. V.; Arnott, M. S.; Jacobs, M. M.; Griffin, A. C.
     Cancer Lett. 1979, 7, 331-8.
36. Medina, D.; Shepherd, F. Carcinogenesis 1981, 2, 451-5.
37. Nigro, N. D.; Bull, A. W.; Wilson, P. S.; Soullier, B. K.;
     Alousi, M. A. J. Natl. Cancer Inst. 1982, 69, 103-7.

38. Rasco, M. A.; Jacobs, M. M.; Griffin, A. C. Cancer Letters 1977, 3, 295-301.
39. Soullier, B. K.; Wilson, P. S.; Nigro, N. D. Cancer Lett. 1981, 12, 343-8.
40. Thompson, H. J.; Becci, P. J. Cancer Letters 1979, 7, 215-9.
41. Thompson, H. J.; Becci, P. J. Cancer Res. 1981, 41, 1413-6.
42. Welsch, C. W.; Goodrich-Smith, M.; Brown, C. K.; Greene, H. D.; Hamel, E. J. Carcinogenesis 1981, 2,519-22.
43. Whanger, P. D. Fundam. Appl. Toxicol. 1983, 3, 424-30.
44. Wortzman, M. S.; Besbris, H. J.; Cohen, A. M. Cancer Res. 1980, 40, 2670-6.
45. Ankerst, J.; Sjogren, H. O. Int. J. Cancer 1982, 29, 707-10.
46. "Nutrient Requirements of Laboratory Animals," National Academy of Sciences, 1983, 15th ed.
47. Ip, C. J. Ag. Food Chem. 1984, in press.
48. Harbach, P. R.; Swenberg, J. A. Carcinogenesis 1981, 2, 575-80.
49. Grunau, J. A.; Milner, J. A. Fed. Proc. 1983, 42, 928.
50. Russell, G. R.; Nader, C. J.; Patuck, E. J. Cancer Lett. 1980, 10, 75-81.
51. Medina, D. Cancer Res. 1973, 7, 3-53.
52. Lyons, M. J.; Moore, D. H. Nature (Lond.) 1962, 194, 1141-2.
53. Schrauzer, G. N.; Ishmael, D. Annals Clin. Lab. Sci. 1974, 4, 441-7.
54. Medina, D.; Shepherd, F. Cancer Letters 1980, 8, 241-5.
55. Schrauzer, G. N.; McGinness, J. E.; Kuehn, K. Carcinogenesis 1980, 1, 199-201.
56. Whanger, P. D.; Schmitz, J. A.; Exon, J. H. Nutr. Cancer 1982, 3, 240-8.
57. Broghamer, W. L., Jr.; McConnell, K. P.; Blotcky, A. L. Cancer 1976, 37, 1384-8.
58. Broghamer, W. L., Jr.; McConnell, K. P.; Grimaldi, M.; Blotcky, A. J. Cancer 1978, 41(4), 1462-6.
59. Walker, C. H.; Klein, F. Amer. Med. 1915, 628-33.
60. Dalbert, P. Bull. Assoc. Franc. Etude Cancer 1912, 121-5.
61. Weisberger, A. S.; Suhrland, L. G. Blood 1956b, 11, 19-30.
62. Cavalieri, R. R.; Scott, K. C.; Sairene, E. J. Nucl. Med. 1966, 7, 197-208.
63. Spencer, R. P.; Montana, G.; Seanlon, G. T.; Evans, O. R. J. Nuclear Med. 1967, 8, 197-208.
64. Hara, T.; Tilbury, R. S.; Freed, B. R.; Woodard, H. Q.; Laughlin, J. S. Intl. J. Appl. Rad. Isotopes 1973, 24, 377-84.
65. Abdullaev, G. B.; Gasanov, G. G.; Ragimov, R. N.; Teplyakova, G. V.; Mekhutiev, M. A.; Dzhafarov, A. I. Doklady Akademiia Nauk Azerbaidzhanskoi SSR. 1973, 29, 18-24.
66. Weisberger, A. S.; Suhrland, L. G. Blood 1956a, 11,11-6.
67. Greeder, G. A.; Milner, J. A. Science 1980, 209, 825-7.
68. Poirier, K. A.; Milner, J. A. Biol. Trace Elem. Res. 1979, 1, 25-34.
69. Poirier, K. A; Milner, J. A. J. Nutr. 1984, 113, 2147-54.
70. Poirier, K. A.; Watrach, A. M.; Milner, J. A. Submitted 1984.
71. Ip, C.; Ip, M. M.; Kim, U. Cancer Letters 1981, 14, 101-7.
72. Watrach, A. M.; Milner, J. A.; Watrach, M. A. Cancer Letters 1982, 15, 137-43.

73. Watrach, A. M.; Watrach, M. A.; Milner, J. A.; Poirier, K. A.
     Cancer Letters 1983, (accepted).
74. Milner, J. A.; Hsu, C. Y. Cancer Res. 1981, 41,1652-6.
75. Medina, D.; Oborn, C. J. Cancer Letters 1981, 13, 333-44.
76. Levander, O. A. In "Trace Elements in Human Health and
     Disease"; Prasad, A. S., Ed.; Academic Press: New York, 1976;
     Vol. II, p. 135-63.
77. Shrift, A. In "Organic Selenium Compounds: Their Chemistry and
     Biology"; Klayman, D. L.; Gunther, W. H. H., Eds.; Wiley and
     Sons, Inc.: New York, 1973; p. 763-814.
78. Sunde, R. A.; Gutzke, G. E.; Hoekstra, W. G. J. Nutr. 1981,
     111(1), 76-86.
79. Hsieh, H. S.; Ganther, H. E. Biochim. Biophys. Acta 1977, 497,
     205-17.
80. Steele, R. D.; Benevenga, N. J. J. Biol. Chem. 1979, 254,
     8885-90.
81. Esaki, N.; Nakamura, T.; Tanaka, H.; Soda, K. J. Biol. Chem.
     1982, 257(8), 4386-91.
82. Ganther, H. E.; Levander, O. A.; Baumann, C. A. J. Nutr. 1966,
     88, 55-60.
83. Palmer, I. S.; Gunsalus, R. P.; Halverson, A. W.; Olson, O. E.
     Biochim. Biophys. Acta 1970, 208, 260-6.
84. Diplock, A. T. CRC Crit. Rev. Toxicol. 1976, 4, 271-392.
85. Dudley, H. C.; Miller, J. W. J. Ind. Hyg. Toxicol. 1941, 23,
     470-7.
86. Sunde, R. A.; Hoekstra, W. G. Nutr. Rev. 1980, 38, 265-73.
87. Vernie, L. N.; Hamburg, C. J.; Bont, W. S. Cancer Letters
     1981, 14, 303-8.
88. Spallholtz, J. E.; Martin, J. L.; Gerlach, M. L.; Heinzerling,
     R. H. Proc. Soc. Exp. Biol. Med. 1973, 143, 685-9.
89. Spallholtz, J. E.; Martin, J. L.; Gerlach, M. L.; Heinzerling,
     R. H. Proc. Soc. Exp. Biol. Med. 1975, 148, 37-40.
90. Medina, D.; Lane, H. W.; Tracey, C. M. Cancer Res. 1983, 43,
     2460s-4s.
91. Shamberger, R. J. J. Natl. Cancer Inst. 1970, 44, 931-6.

RECEIVED August 17, 1984

In Vitro Effects of Soybean Protease Inhibitors

JONATHAN YAVELOW[1], KENNETH A. BECK[1], MORTIMER LEVITZ[2], and
WALTER TROLL[3]

[1]Department of Biology/Biochemistry, Rider College, Lawrenceville, NJ 08648
[2]Department of Obstetrics and Gynecology, New York University Medical Center, New York,
NY 10022
[3]Institute of Environmental Medicine, New York University Medical Center, New York, NY 10016

We have recently reported that the action of
protease inhibitors as dietary anticarcinogens
may work via two mechanisms: 1) An indirect
effect on protein absorption; and 2) A direct
effect on cell transformation (Cancer Res.,
Suppl. 43: 2454S-2459S, 1983). The direct
effect on cell transformation has been demonstrated in vitro using several protease inhibitors. The following studies have been designed
to assess the effect of protease inhibitors on
transformed cell growth and to determine which
protease inhibitory activity (antitrypsin or
antichymotrypsin) is responsible for these effects. A number of protease inhibitors have
been tested, among them the Kunitz soybean
trypsin inhibitor and the Bowman-Birk soybean
trypsin and chymotrypsin inhibitor. The cell
lines which have been examined are LoVo (human
colon cancer) and MCF-7 (human breast cancer).
In cells tested, the Bowman-Birk inhibitor is
more potent than the Kunitz inhibitor in decreasing cell growth. Thus, it appears that the
antichymotrypsin activity is modulating growth
of these cells.

The role of diet in cancer causation and prevention was originally derived from epidemiological data. More recently these
studies have been followed up with laboratory experiments
where variables can be more carefully controlled. For example, the correlation between meat consumption and elevated
colon and breast cancer incidence (1) has been confirmed in
animal studies showing high fat and/or protein dietary levels
result in an increased number of colon tumors (2). Also
mutagens have been isolated from cooked beef (3). With regard
to cancer prevention recent work has defined several classes
of dietary anti-carcinogens; for example, retinoids (4), antioxidants (5), prostaglandin antagonists (6); and protease in-

0097-6156/85/0277-0283$06.00/0

hibitors (7). Indeed, it may be that our risk for developing cancer relates to the balance of ingested carcinogens/ promoters and anticarcinogens (8).

As well as being of potential public health interest, anticarcinogens can serve as useful probes into the mechanism of carcinogenesis. For example, antioxidants, prostaglandin antagonists and protease inhibitors (classes of chemopreventive agents) strongly suggest free oxygen radicals, prostaglandins and proteases, respectively, as important chemical mediators of transformation. With respect to proteases, tumor cells elaborate the means for invasion through the connective tissue and into the vasculature. In vitro studies have also revealed that tumor cells secrete proteases (e.g. lysosomal hydrolases, collagenase, plasminogen activator). These enzymes may mediate invasion and metastasis. (See 9 for review). In addition to secreted proteases, intracellular and/or membrane-associated proteases may be important in the establishment and maintenance of the transformed cell. This could occur via activation of precursor enzymes or hormones which may not be present or present at different levels in normal cells. Protease inhibitors may therefore be effective anticarcinogens or antitumor drugs via effecting proteases at different sites.

The Bowman-Birk type protease inhibitors represent a class of low molecular weight, cysteine-rich proteins found in legume seeds (10). The major Bowman-Birk inhibitor in soybean seeds is a double-headed protein capable of blocking the activity of both trypsin and chymotrypsin. This protein represents approximately 4% of the total protein in soybean seeds (11). In contrast to the soybean trypsin inhibitor (Kunitz), the "double-headed" inhibitor (referred to as BB) is typical of protease inhibitors present in a large number of legume seeds: for example, peanuts (12); chick peas (13); kidney beans (14); adzuki beans (15); lima beans (16).

The BB protease inhibitors are heat and acid stable, thus they survive both cooking (17) and digestion (18). BB complexes with proteases in the small intestine of rodents and is excreted primarily as protease-protease inhibitor complexes in the feces. The decreased efficiency of protein utilization from foods rich in protease inhibitors may indirectly lower an individual's effective protein intake (19). This may, in part, protect animals on protease inhibitor-rich diets as shown in a lower incidence of skin, breast and liver tumors (20,21).

The Bowman-Birk inhibitor also blocks the transformation of $C_3H/10T1/2$ cells (18). This raises the speculation that BB may represent a direct acting nutritionally relevant anticarcinogen particularly in the case of colon cancer. In this regard it was recently reported that ε-aminocaproic acid (a trypsin inhibitor) inhibits dimethylhydrazine-induced colon tumors in mice (22).

Does the active form of the Bowman-Birk inhibitor reach the colon? If so, what is the effect on colon tumor cells? Is the effect of BB specific or might it effect many cell types? Studies described below localize active BB in the

colon wall and assess the inhibitory effect of BB on human
colon and breast cancer cell growth. Studies concerning its
mechanism of action suggest the antichymotrypsin activity
associated with BB is affecting growth inhibition.

Methods and Materials

<u>Isolation, iodination and metabolic studies with 125I-BB</u>: The
Bowman-Birk inhibitor was isolated as previously described
(11). For metabolic studies BB was iodinated and purified
using chymotrypsin-sepharose (18). C_3H/HEN mice were administered ^{125}I-BB by gavage and sacrificed after one hour.
Colon was excised, irrigated free of feces, homogenized and
chromatographed on chymotrypsin sepharose (18).
      <u>Cell Culture</u>: Human colon cancer cells (LoVo) were ob-
tained from Dr. M. Lipkin (Cornell University Medical Center)
and human breast cancer cells (MCF-7) were obtained from Dr.
H. Leon Bradlow (Rockefeller University). Cells were grown in
RPMI 1640 supplemented with 10% Fetal Calf Serum (Gibco) and
pen/strep/ fungizone. Experiments were performed in microtiter wells or 35mm tissue culture dishes. Cells were
enumerated using a hemocytometer.
      <u>Protease inhibitors and assays</u>: BB modified enzymatically
by sequential trypsin and carboxypeptidase B digestions was a
kind gift from Dr. Y. Birk (23). This inhibitor which contains only chymotrypsin inhibitory activity is referred to as
BBchy. Soybean trypsin inhibitor (Kunitz) (Worthington,
Freehold, NJ), BB and BBchy were assayed for trypsin and
chymotrypsin inhibitory activities using benzoyl arginine para
nitroanilide (BAPNA) and benzoyl tyrosine para nitroanilide
(BTPNA) respectively (Sigma) (24). Protease activity secreted
into serum-free medium was assayed using ^{3}H casein (17).

Results

The Bowman-Birk protease inhibitor was purified from defatted
soybean flour. Activity and purity were assessed by inhibition of trypsin and chymotrypsin, SDS and native polyacrylamide gel electrophoresis, high performance liquid chromatography and amino acid analysis (data not shown). The
^{125}I-BB derivative was administered to mice by gavage and
after 1 hour the lower intestine was dissected and irrigated
free of feces. Approximately 1% of the ingested BB is associated with colon wall. Figure 1 illustrates the chymotrypsin-sepharose elution profile of a clarified homogenate of
intestinal wall. The ^{125}I-BB peak that is not sticking to the
affinity column most likely represents a protease-protease
inhibitor complex because this elutes as a 33,000 dalton peak
on HPLC (18). Counts eluting at pH 2.6 represent free BB capable of binding protease. The molecular weight of the peak
tube eluting with acid was similar to the material administered to the animals by gavage. (Data not shown).
      Human colon cancer cell growth (LoVo) is effected by
protease inhibitors. In the presence of 62.5 μ<u>M</u> BB both the
doubling time and saturation density are considerably

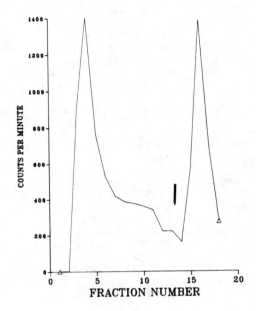

Figure 1 - Chymotrypsin-sepharose elution profile of
colon wall homogenate 1 hour after i.g.
administration of ^{125}I-BB. Arrow (↓)
denotes changing elution buffer to pH 2.6.

depressed (Figure 2). An independent series of experiments
performed in the presence of 25,50 and 62.5 μM BB demonstrated
25%, 35% and 40% inhibition, respectively in cell number after
4 days of growth. (62.5 μM bovine serum albumin inhibited day
4 cell number by 5%). Additional studies are needed to precisely define decreases in doubling time as a function of BB
concentration. Higher concentrations of BB further depress
growth, however, the protease inhibitory effects can not be
differentiated from a general protein inhibitory effect.

In order to assess the relative inhibition of BB and the
Kunitz soybean trypsin inhibitor (SBTI) plating efficiency and
cell growth experiments were performed. BB blocks growth and
plating efficiency 50 and 53%, respectively at 62.5 μM whereas
47.5 μM SBTI blocks growth and plating efficiency 14 and 20%,
respectively. (Table I) At 190 μM the SBTI blocked cell
growth 30% after 3 days. (Data not shown)

Table I. Comparison of BB and SBTI on LoVo Growth and
Plating Efficiency

	P.E.(%)	(%I)	Growth (Day 3)	(%I)
Control	44.25 ± .75		4.43×10^4 ± .475	
BB 62.50 μM	21.0 ± 4.5	(53%)	2.28×10^4 ± .98	(50%)
SBTI 47.50 μM	35.5 ± 4.5	(20%)	3.80×10^4 ± .10	(14%)

Plating efficiency experiments were performed by plating
200 viable cells into 60 mm tissue culture dishes and counting
colonies after 7-10 days. Growth experiments were performed
using microtiter wells with 1×10^4 cells/well on day 0 (N=3).

In an effort to assess the site of action of BB on LoVo cell
growth, proteases secreted from these cells into serum-free
medium were analyzed in the presence and absence of BB and the
α1 protease inhibitor. BB inhibited secreted protease
activity 80% and the α1 protease inhibitor blocked secreted
protease activity 99% (Table II).

Table II. Effect of BB and α1PI on Proteases Secreted
from LoVo Cells

	CPM	%I
Control	5685 ± 545	-
BB	1158 ± 189	80%
α1 PI	70 ± 7	99%

10^4 cells were plated in microtiter wells (o.2 ml). Serum was
removed, cells washed with PBS and incubated in serum-free
medium. 100 μl of conditioned medium was incubated with ^{3}H-
casein ± 10 μl of 1 μg/ml solutions of protease inhibitor.

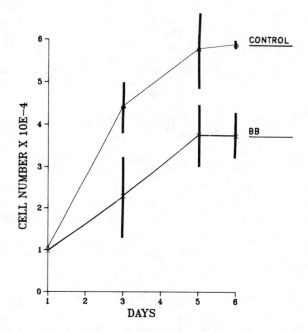

Figure 2 – LoVo cells were grown in microtiter wells in
         the presence and absence of 62.5 µM BB.
         Triplicate cultures were counted on days
         indicated. 10⁴ cells were plated on day 0.
         Data is expressed as mean ± S.D. (N=3).

The effects of BB on cells in vitro are not confined to LoVo. Several other transformed cell lines are also inhibited by BB (hamster amelanotic melanoma, AM, and its revertant, FF, methylcholanthaene transformed $C_3H/10T1/2$ cells, MCA6, (data not shown). In all cases BB is a more potent inhibitor than equimolar concentrations of the Kunitz SBTI.

The effects of BB and Kunitz SBTI on MCF-7 cell growth are summarized in Table III. The cell number after 10 days of growth in the presence of estradiol was decreased from 45 to 79% by 200 µg/ml BB, whereas Kunitz SBTI had no effect. In the absence of estradiol the effect of BB was more variable resulting in no effect in 3 experiments and approximately 50% inhibition in the other 2 experiments. Parameters effecting this variability are currently being investigated.

The Bowman-Birk inhibitor also effects MCF-7 cell growth in media containing unstripped serum. In a single experiment (with triplicate plates) we observed a decrease in MCF-7 cell number after 6 days of growth (approximately 70% of control). BB derivatized such that it was a chymotrypsin inhibitor only and native BB equally effected growth modulation. Equimolar concentrations of the Kunitz SBTI was ineffective in modulating cell growth.

Discussion

The Bowman-Birk soybean trypsin and chymotrypsin inhibitor modulates the growth of human colon and breast cancer cells. In parallel experiments the Kunitz soybean trypsin inhibitor proved ineffective in modulating cell growth. These results suggest the chymotrypsin inhibitory activity is more important in effecting growth inhibition. One must be cautious in interpreting this data because it must be confirmed with the isolation of the cellular target of BB. Unfortunately one is unable to assess the effects of BB on growth of "normal" colon and breast epithelia in vitro because they do not grow in culture. Schnebli and Berger ([25]) observed selective growth inhibition of only SV40 transformed 3T3 cells with TLCK (tosyl lysine chloromethyl ketone). This selective inhibition has been discussed by Quigley ([9]) as resulting from cytotoxic events independent of a protease specific to transformed cells.

There are three possible sites where BB may act to modulate cell growth: 1) proteases secreted from cells; 2) proteases on the plasma membrane; 3) intracellular proteases. The possibility of secreted proteases as mediating cell growth seems not to be the case because the endogenous serum α1 protease inhibitor is capable of blocking secreted proteases from LoVo cells more efficiently than BB. (Cells also grow normally in serum containing active protease inhibitor). Preliminary studies using ^{125}I-BB suggest the protease inhibitor is not being taken up by cells (Yavelow- unpublished data). The possibility remains that BB is interacting with the plasma membrane. Indeed it has been reported that ovomucoid (at similar concentrations to those used in the above studies) blocks growth of polyoma transformed 3T3 cells and ovomucoid

Table III. The effect of BB and Kunitz SBTI on modulating MCF-7 Cell Growth in the Presence and Absence of Estradiol

	Estradiol (+) (Day 10 cell number x10^{-6})			Estradiol (−) (Day 10 cell number x10^{-6})		
Expt. #	Control	+BB	+Kunitz	Control	+BB	+Kunitz
1	2.83 ± .13	2.17 ± .32 (77%)	N.D.	1.73 ± .22	1.65 ± .25 (95%)	N.D.
2	1.14 ± .04	0.90 ± .15 (79%)	1.07 ± .10 (94%)	.51 ± .12	0.59 ± .10 (115%)	0.61 ± .11 (120%)
3	1.94 ± .15	1.00 ± .02 (52%)	1.88 ± .15 (97%)	1.10 ± .10	1.31 ± .25 (119%)	1.31 ± .25 (120%)
4	1.23 ± .06	0.90 ± .13 (73%)	N. D.	1.42 ± .27	0.69 ± .40 (49%)	N.D.
5	3.08 ± .64	1.38 ± .20 (45%)	N.D.	3.37 ± .41	1.71 ± .05 (51%)	N.D.

Legend: 5 x 10^4 cells were plated in 35 mm tissue culture dishes containing RPMI 1640 + 5% Estrogen-stripped serum. For the estradiol (+) condition plates were supplemented with 10^{-8} M estradiol. The final concentration of protease inhibitors was 200 µg/ml. Data is expressed as mean ± SD, N=3. Percent of control cell number is in parenthesis.

immobilized on polyacrylamide beads affects growth inhibition at lower protease inhibitor concentrations (26). Membranes isolated from transformed chick embryo fibroblasts also possess chymotrypsin- like protease activity (27). These studies establish the possibility that the chymotrypsin inhibitory activity associated with BB may be interacting with a membrane associated protease. Clearly, more studies need to be done to directly assess the nature of the cellular target of BB. From the variety of cells affected by BB it suggests that the target protease may be common to many cell types.

The Bowman-Birk protease inhibitor is exceedingly stable, easy to immobilize to affinity supports and seems not to penentrate cells. For these reasons it is an ideal probe for the putative membrane-associated targets that may mediate cell growth. Until the cellular target is identified it is premature to assume the cellular target of BB to be a protease. Several interesting in vivo studies are suggested from this work, for example: 1) does BB bind to colon cancer cells preferentially over normal colon epithelia in vivo?; 2) does pure BB decrease colon cancer incidence in carcinogen treated animals? Completion of these studies will further assess the role of BB as a dietary anticarcinogen.

Acknowledgments

This work was supported in part by NIH Grants CA-02071 (M.L.) and CA-16060 (W.T.) The technical assistance of Monica Gidund is greatly appreciated. We thank Ms. Geraldine Holley and Mrs. Helen Hudzina for preparation of the manuscript.

Literature Cited

1. Armstrong, B. and Doll, R.   Int. J. Cancer, 1975, 15, 617.
2. Reddy, B.U., Narisawa, T. and Weisberger, J.H.   J. Nat'l Cancer Institute. 1976, 57, 567.
3. Sugimura, T. and Sato, S.   Cancer Research (Suppl.) 1983, 45, 2415S.
4. Moon, R.G., McCormick, D.L. and Mehta, R.G.   Cancer Research (Suppl.) 1983, 43, 2469S.
5. Wattenberg, L.W.   Cancer Research (Suppl.) 1984, 43, 2448S.
6. Narisawa, T., Sato, M., Tani, M., Kudo, T., Takahashi, T. and Gota, A.   Cancer Research, 1981, 41, 1954.
7. Troll, W. and Yavelow, J. In "Current Topics in Nutrition and Disease," Vol. 9. Roe, D.A., Ed., Alan R. Liss, New York, 1983, p. 167-176.
8. Ames, B.N. Science 1983, 221, 1256.
9. Quigley, J.P. In "Surfaces of Normal and Malignant Cells", John Wiley and Sons, New York, 1979, pp. 247-285.
10. Laskowski, M.J. and Kato, I.   Ann. Review of Blochem. 1980, 49, 593.
11. Hwang, D.L.R., Davis Lin, K.T., Yang, W-K. and Foard, D.E. Biochem. Biophys. Acta. 1977, 495, 369.
12. Norioka, S. and Ikenaka, T. J. Biochem. 1983, 93, 479.

13. Smirnoff, P., Khalef, S., Birk, Y., Applebaum, S.W.
     Int'l. J. Peptide Protein Res. 1979, 14, 186.
14. Pusztai, A. Eur. J. Biochem, 1968, 5, 252.
15. Toshibawa, M., Kiyohava, T., Iasaki, T., Kawata, N.,
     Ohtaki, Y. and Nakkao, C. J. Biochem. 1980, 87, 619.
16. Stevens, F.C., Wuerz, S. and Krahn, J. In Bayer
     Symposium V "Proteinase Inhibitors", Springer-Verlag,
     Berlin 1974. pp. 344-354.
17. Yavelow, J., Gidlund, M. and Troll, W. Carcinogensis,
     1982, 3, 135.
18. Yavelow, J., Finlay, T.H., Kennedy, A.R. and Troll, W.
     Cancer Research (Suppl.) 1983, 43, 2454S.
19. Navarette, D.A. and Bressani, R. Am. J. Clinical Nutr.
     1981, 34, 1893.
20. Becker, F.F. Carcinogensis, 1981, 2, 1213.
21. Troll, W., Weisner, R., Shellabarger, C.J., Holtzman, S.
     and Stone, J.P. Carcinogensis 1980, 1, 469.
22. Corasanti, J.G., Hobika, G.H. and Markus, G. Science
     1982, 216, 1020.
23. Birk, Y. In Bayer Symposium V "Proteinase Inhibitors",
     Springer Verlag, Berlin, 1974, pp. 355-361.
24. Abramovitz, A.S., Yavelow, J. Randolph, V. and Troll, W.
     J. Biol. Chem. 1983, 258, 15153.
25. Schnebli, H.P. and Burger, M.M. Proc. Nat'l Acad. Sci.
     (USA) 1972, 69, 3825.
26. Talmadge, K.W., Noonan, K.D, and Burger, M.M. In
     "Control of Proliferation in Animal Cells", Cold Spring
     Harbor, NY, 1974, pp. 313-325.
27. O'Donnell-Tormey, J. and Quigley, J.P. Proc. Nat'l Acad.
     Sci. (USA) 1983, 50, 344.

RECEIVED August 17, 1984

Dietary Protein and the Carcinogenesis, Metabolism, and Toxicity of 1,2-Dimethylhydrazine

WILLARD J. VISEK and STEVEN K. CLINTON

University of Illinois College of Medicine at Urbana-Champaign, Urbana, IL 61801

The hydrazines are a diverse class of compounds used in the manufacture of therapeutic drugs, agricultural chemicals, rocket fuels and other industrial products. They show a variety of toxic effects and some are carcinogenic in laboratory animals (1). Naturally occurring hydrazines have also been identified in tobacco, mushrooms and other plants (1). Scientists studying colon cancer have frequently used 1,2-dimethylhydrazine (DMH) in rodents as an experimental carcinogen. This application followed studies by Lacqeur and associates who produced tumors in laboratory rats with extracts from nuts of the plant, Cycas circinalis (2). Subsequently, Druckery et al. discovered that DMH, a synthetic cycasin analog, caused a very high incidence of colon cancer in rodents (3). Since this discovery, DMH has been successfully used to induce colon tumors in rats (4,5), mice (6,7) and hamsters (8). The metabolites of DMH have also been employed to induce colon cancers in animals (9).

Epidemiological studies show that dietary fat and protein are most frequently correlated with colon cancer incidence in man (10-14). A number of studies in laboratory animals suggest that dietary fat enhances colon tumor incidence (15) although others have failed to show such enhancement (16). Summarized in this communication are animal experiments conducted by our laboratory to examine the effects of dietary protein on DMH induced carcinogenesis, mutagenesis, and toxicity.

Protein Concentration and DMH Carcinogenesis in Rats (17)

One of our early studies examined colon carcinogenesis in male Sprague-Dawley rats, ad libitum fed one of three purified diets containing 7.5, 15.0, 22.5% protein as casein. Each animal was injected intraperitoneally, once weekly for 24 weeks, with 15 mg/kg body weight of DMH. The study was terminated at 32 weeks after the initial DMH injection when all survivors were killed and necropsied.

The animals fed 7.5% protein gained less during the first six weeks of feeding than those that consumed 15 or 22.5% of total protein (Table I). The weight gain was greater between the 6th

0097–6156/85/0277–0293$06.00/0

and 26th weeks for the 7.5% protein fed rats because of catch-up
growth.

Table I. Weight gain for rats fed 7.5%, 15% and
          22.5% protein

Treatment	Wt. gain 0-6 wks	Wt. gain 6-26 wks	Weight 26 wks
7.5% protein	184	178	418
15% protein	242	156	453
22.5% protein	255	158	468

Initial average body weight 56 g.

The tumors in the colon and small intestine were principally
polypoid adenocarcinomas with histological and other characteristics of tumors induced by alkylhydrazines and their derivatives
(18). Although the percentage of rats with small intestinal or
colon tumors was not influenced by diet, the number of tumors per
rat in the small intestine and colon was significantly greater with
15.0 or 22.5% protein compared to 7.5% protein (Table II). Ear
tumors, observed first during the 21st week of the experiment

Table II. Incidence and total number of tumors in the small
           and large intestine and in the inner ear of rats
           fed different levels of protein

	% of rats with tumors			Ave. no. tumors/rat	
	Small Intestine	Large Intestine	Inner Ear	Small Intestine	Large Intestine
7.5% protein	31	84	47	0.37	1.03
15% protein	65	87	58	0.74	1.68
22.5% protein	52	91	78	0.78	1.67

32, 31, and 33 rats for 7.5, 15, 22.5% protein, respectively.

appeared as swellings on the side of the head which grew progressively and became ulcerated. These inner ear keratin-producing
papillomas of the sebacceous gland developed earlier and with a
greater incidence as the percent of protein in the diet was increased. Whether fewer tumors with 7.5% protein were due to sub-
optimal protein intake during the rapid body growth phase cannot be
answered from this study. Since all diets for practical purposes
were isoenergetic, and consumed in approximately equal amounts, the
incidence or growth of tumors cannot be ascribed to significant differences of energy, fat, minerals or vitamin consumption. All of
the evidence argues that the number of tumors in the small intestine, colon, and ear was increased by the dietary protein intake.
    The mechanism whereby dietary protein influences DMH carcino-
genesis is unknown. An attractive hypothesis concerning the effects of dietary protein on DMH metabolism is discussed later in
this manuscript. Another factor which may contribute to tumor
growth promotion in the intestine is a doubling of fecal crude
lipid excretion which we observed in mice as dietary protein was
increased from 10 to 40% of the diet (19). The association between

fecal lipids, fecal steroid excretion and colon cancer has been a
topic of extensive investigation (11,15).

Animal Versus Vegetable Protein and DMH-Induced
Colon Carcinogenesis in Rats (20)

Intake of animal protein is frequently cited as showing a strong
correlation with human colon cancer (11). It has also been hypothesized that the processing or cooking of meat may produce substances
which influence carcinogenesis. For example, benzo(a)pyrene and
other carcinogenic polycyclic aromatic hydrocarbons (PAH) are found
in meats broiled over charcoal (21). Polycyclic aromatic hydrocarbons have been shown to cause mutagenesis in bacteria (22), malignant transformation in mammalian cell culture (23), and cancer in
experimental animals (24) and man (25). Purified PAH administered
simultaneously with other carcinogens, both at low-effect levels,
have been shown to act synergistically (26,27). An attempt to test
some of these hypotheses in our laboratory compared DMH-induced
tumorigenesis in rats fed beef versus soybean protein. Charcoal-
broiled beef was also included as a variable to determine if PAH or
other factors produced during cooking would modify the carcinogenic
response (20).
    Weanling male Sprague-Dawley rats were ad libitum fed one of
the three semi-purified diets containing raw beef, charcoal-broiled
beef or soybean protein. Lean beef and beef fat were obtained from
the University of Illinois Meat Science Laboratory. Uniform 100 g
ground beef patties were prepared on an automated device. Half of
the beef was cooked by charcoal broiling on an open-topped outdoor
grill using charcoal briquets. The temperature at the surface of
the grill was approximately 230 to 290°C. Patties were turned and
cooked to a well-done state and an internal temperature of 75°C.
The cooked patties , raw beef and the beef tallow were frozen at
-20°C, lyophilized, ground to a fine powder and analyzed for fat
and protein. The beef incorporated into the diets provided 20%
protein and the fat content was adjusted to 20% with beef tallow.
Tallow from the same carcass was also used to equalize lipid content in the soybean-based diet. Each rat was given DMH intraperitoneally at 12.5 mg/kg during weeks 5 through 23 of feeding and the
study was concluded after 32 weeks. There was no evidence that
source of protein or its preparation influenced the incidence of
small intestinal or colon tumors (Table III). The results of this
study and the previous experiment suggest that the concentration
rather than the source of protein played a dominant role in determining the number of tumors.

Dietary Protein and DMH Metabolism and
Mutagenesis in Mice (28)

The next series of experiments were by Kari et al. (28) who examined the effect of dietary protein upon the activation of DMH to
its mutagenic and, presumably, carcinogenic metabolites in mice. A
combination of in vivo and in vitro assays were employed to assess
the influence of dietary protein concentration on the production of
mutagenic products from DMH, azoxymethane (AOM), and methylazoxymethanol (MAM) (Figure 1).

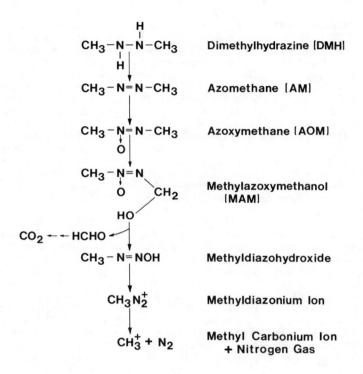

Figure 1. Postulated pathway from DMH to its proximal mutagen (carbonium ion) (Reproduced with permission from Ref. 28. Copyright 1983, Cancer Research, Inc.).

Table III.   Dimethylhydrazine-induced tumors in rats fed lyophilized
charcoal broiled beef, raw beef or soybean protein

Protein Source (20% protein)	Small Intestinal Tumors		Colon Tumors	
	% with tumors	Tumors/tumor-bearing rat	% with tumors	Tumors/tumor-bearing rat
Charcoal broiled beef	28	1.1	41	1.4
Raw beef	40	1.3	43	1.4
Soybean	32	1.1	39	1.3

In Vitro Mutagenicity of DMH, AOM, and MAM. Over the years, additions of DMH to cultures of histidine requiring Salmonella organisms have repeatedly failed to show significant mutagenesis in the
assay described by Ames (29). Our initial in vitro studies examined the mutagenic potency of DMH, AOM, and MAM, assayed with and
without activation by S-9 fractions from livers of male weanling
mice. Both DMH and AOM failed to significantly increase bacterial
mutation frequency in vitro with or without the S-9 protein fraction. In contrast, the response to MAM was positively correlated
with dosage ($p < 0.01$), and the slope of the regression line appeared to be slightly greater when the S-9 fraction was added.

Host-Mediated Assay of DMH, AOM, and MAM. We completed several
experiments employing the host-mediated bacterial assay for detection of mutagenic activity developed by Gabridge and Legator (30)
and adapted by Moriya et al. (31) for DMH. The host-mediated assay
was conducted by injecting test bacteria into the peritoneal cavity
of mice followed immediately by subcutaneous injection of the test
carcinogen. At appropriate times thereafter the mice were killed
by cervical dislocation, sterile saline was injected intraperitoneally and the abdomens were vigorously massaged. Then the peritoneal fluid was aspirated and applied to agar plates for viable
bacterial counts and mutation frequency (reversions).

       When DMH and some of its metabolites were tested. AOM pro-
duced 2 to 3 times as many mutations as DMH, and MAM was 1.5 to
10.5 as potent as AOM.

Dietary Protein and Host-Mediated Mutagenesis by DMH, AOM, and
MAM. Two experiments were conducted to compare the influence of
protein deficiency and excess on DMH, AOM and MAM mutagenesis.
Dietary protein intake produced changes in mutation frequency which
were dependent upon the mutagen tested (Table IV). For AOM, dietary protein concentration and bacterial mutation frequency were
positively correlated ($p < 0.01$).

Distribution of [^{14}C]-DMH Metabolites In Vivo as a Function of
Dietary Protein. The distribution of metabolites was studied in
mice given subcutaneous injections of [^{14}C] DMH. Most of the
radioactivity exhaled as azomethane (AM) was collected within 1 hr,
and production of this metabolite was completed by 3 hr (Figure
2). In contrast, the expiration of $^{14}CO_2$ was negligible during the
first hour and ceased after the fifth hour.
       The dietary treatments changed the quantitative relationships

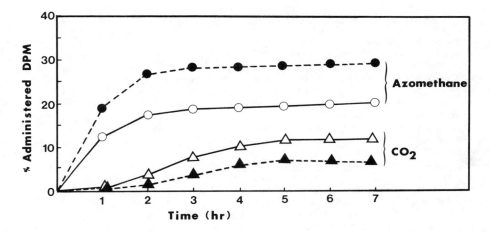

Figure 2. Effect of dietary protein concentration on cumulative
expiration of $[^{14}C]AM$ (○ , ●) and $^{14}CO_2$ (△ , ▲). Eight male
weanling mice adapted for 3 days to the control diet were randomly divided into 2 groups: Group 1, fed 2.5% casein (---);
and Group 2, 40% casein (——). Food and water were supplied ad
libitum, and feed intakes and body weights were determined for
14 days. At 9:00 on Day 14, animals were given s.c. injections
of $[^{14}C]DMH$ (0.66 mmol/kg of body weight; 120 μCi/mmol) and
placed into air-tight metabolic chambers. Solutions in the
trapping vessels were collected and replaced by fresh solutions
every hr for 7 hr, a procedure requiring about 5 min. Air flow
through each cage was individually regulated, and sampling did
not disrupt other experimental units. At the end of 7 hr, the
animals were killed, and aliquots of scrubber solutions were
assayed for radioactivity (Reproduced with permission from Ref.
28. Copyright 1983, Cancer Research, Inc.).

Table IV.   Effect of dietary protein concentration on host mediated mutagenicity of dimethylhydrazine (DMH), azoxymethane (AOM) and methylazoxymethanol (MAM) in C57BL/6
x C3HF1 male mice

Dietary protein, %	Mean revertants/10^8 survivors		
	DMH	AOM	MAM
Experiment 1			
2.5	36 ± 7	101 ± 10	--
5	62 ± 9	126 ± 28	--
10	64 ± 17	146 ± 18	--
20	60 ± 7	180 ± 22	--
40	50 ± 5	193 ± 18	--
Experiment 2.			
2.5	--	92 ± 66	814 ± 196
5	--	102 ± 14	767 ± 204
10	--	140 ± 85	898 ± 117
20	--	170 ± 35	831 ± 132
40	--	272 ± 49	866 ± 172

of the gaseous metabolites but not their time of appearance. Over
a 7 hr period after labeled DMH administration, the combined recovery of radioactivity in the expired gases, excreta and carcasses
averaged about 98%. Under these conditions the animals fed 2.5%
protein exhaled 60% of the radioactivity in AM and less than 3% in
$^{14}CO_2$ compared to 40 and 6.5% for animals fed 10% protein, respectively (Table V). The body burden of retained metabolites was 26%
for animals on the 2.5% protein diet compared to about 40% for the
animals fed 10 or 40% protein.

In summary, DMH and AOM failed to increase in vitro mutagenic
frequency with or without liver extracts. However, MAM caused a
dose-dependent increase in reversion frequency without hepatic enzymes as expected since MAM decomposes heterolytically to methyldiazonium and formaldehyde (32). Methyldiazonium ions yield nitrogen and methylcarbonium, a powerful alkylating agent. Formaldehyde
is oxidized to CO_2. In contrast to in vitro conditions, the host-
mediated assay showed that intact animals converted DMH and AOM to
mutagenic products.

It is of interest that the in vivo mutagenesis was abolished
by hepatectomy. Precursor product relationships of DMH and AOM and
MAM (Figure 1) suggest that the mutagenic activity of their metabolites should be greater as their metabolism approaches methylcarbonium ion formation. This is confirmed by our results. Since the
yield of mutagens was not the same from the administered compounds
as they were converted to methylcarbonium ion and the number of
revertants from AOM was 30% greater after an equal molar dose of
DMH, the difference had to be due to the expiration of AM, the
metabolite between DMH and AOM. The expiration of AM, therefore,
represents a loss of potentially biologically active material and
should explain the discrepancies between the mutagenic potency of
DMH and AOM on a molar basis.

The protein restricted mice also expired less $^{14}CO_2$ from
labeled DMH than their counterparts fed 40% protein. Using expired
$^{14}CO_2$ as an index of potential genetic toxicity, the burden of

Table V. Effect of dietary protein concentration distribution of [^{14}C] DMH metabolites of mice fed different intakes of protein. Measurements at 7 hours after injection

Protein %	Expired AM[1]	Expired CO	Other Expired Metabolites	Urine, feces cage rinse	Carcass	Total
2.5	60.8	2.9	6.6	2.6	26.1	99.0
10	39.4	6.6	6.8	3.4	43.4	99.6
40	45.0	9.1	3.4	1.9	38.0	97.4

[1]Azoxymethane

retained metabolites by the 10 and 40% protein groups was 2 and 3 times that for the 2.5% protein fed animals, respectively. The relationship between dietary protein concentration and DMH-induced host-mediated mutagenesis tended to parallel these findings. The loss of AM by expiration being greater on a low protein diet versus a high protein diet also represents a possible mechanism for explaining quantitative differences in the carcinogenic effects of DMH showing that 7.5% protein fed rats developed 40% fewer colon tumors than those fed 15 or 22.5%. Despite the differences in species and experimental protocol the data agree remarkably with one-third more AM and two-thirds less CO_2 expired by protein deficient mice compared to controls. This corroborates a dietary protein influence on DMH carcinogenesis and a lower body burden of proximal mutagen-carcinogen in protein restricted animals because of greater expiration of AM.

The Effects of Dietary Protein Concentration on Dietary DMH Toxicity in Mice

Our most recent studies examined the effects of dietary protein on the chronic toxicity resulting from feeding DMH in the diet. After a series of preliminary studies, $B_6C_3F_1$ male mice were fed DMH for 5 months at the following dietary concentrations: .015, .030, and .045 mg/kg of diet. The diets were based upon the AIN-76 recommendations and contained soybean protein at 10 or 40% by weight. Five to 8 week old males were used. There were 25 mice per group. The data presented are preliminary and a complete description of these studies will appear elsewhere (Visek et al., to be published).

Table VI summarizes the feed intake, organ weights and organ to body weight ratios for all of the dietary treatments. These showed a highly significant DMH dose response with several dose by protein interactions. With 0.015 g DMH/kg diet, small or moderate reductions in food consumption, body weights, heart weights and heart/body weight ratios were seen only in 10% protein fed animals. A mild decrease in liver weight, and increases in lung and testes weights relative to body weights were seen at both protein levels. However, at 0.03 g/kg reductions in food consumption and body weight were twice as great with 10% protein versus 40% protein fed animals. The absolute weights of kidneys for 10% protein fed

Table VI. Mean body weight, total food consumption, organ weights and organ/body weights of mice in five month study, by dietary protein and DMH concentrations, with standard errors of group means (25 male mice per group)

	SE of Each Group Mean	10% Protein				40% Protein			
		Controls	DMH g/kg diet			Controls	DMH g/kg diet		
			.015	.030	.045		.015	.030	.045
Weight and Food Consumption (g)									
Initial body weight[1]	0.41	25.22	24.76	24.24	25.03	24.64	24.13	24.42	25.30
Total food consumption	5	605	571	505	454	517	515	485	436
Final body weight	0.47	38.92	35.49	27.81	22.68	30.75	30.17	26.07	21.73
Organ Weights (mg) and Organ/Body Weights (x10^4)									
Liver weight	22	1335	984	763	655	1132	1021	847	684
Liver weight/body weight	6	338	279	278	284	372	344	328	309
Kidney weight	13	680	634	324	233	625	615	494	371
Kidney weight/body weight	2	173	179	117	103	205	207	191	168
Heart weight	3	160	138	116	106	146	138	105	100
Heart weight/body weight	1	41	39	43	47	48	47	41	45
Lungs weight	4	169	174	156	140	162	170	154	139
Lung weight/body weight	1	43	49	57	61	53	57	60	63
Testes weight	5	238	232	179	98	214	230	206	120
Testes weight/body weight	1	61	65	66	43	70	78	80	55

Organ weight and initial body weight data reported as observed means of each group, with standard error of group mean obtained by pooling variation in the eight groups. Organ/body weight data reported as adjusted means from an analysis of variance of the entire four carcinogen five-month study, using a model incorporating adjustment for housing positions of mice and allowing for protein level by carcinogen interactions. The standard error of a group mean is derived from this analysis. Total food consumption and final body weight were treated similarly to these, with additional covariance adjustment for initial body weight.

[1] Includes all mice. Other variables omit two mice dying early, and rare outliers.

animals dropped 50% as DMH was increased from 0.015 to 0.03 g/kg.
The drop in kidney weights was less with 40% protein. With DMH
raised to 0.045 g/kg of diet further substantial declines in feed
consumption, organ and body weight occurred at both protein levels.
Liver and kidney weight declined further, commensurate with declines in body weights.
     The liver seemed to be the organ most sensitive to DMH. At
the lowest DMH dosage a subtle but definite lesion which was designated "pre-reactive hepatitis" was seen in virtually all mice. The
lesion consisted of focal centrilobular hepatocellular necrosis,
often taking the form of eosinophilic body formation and intracellular and extracellular hemosiderin deposition. Only occasional
control mice had similar lesions. Mice consuming higher intakes of
DMH displayed a more severe "reactive hepatitis." Lobular disor-
ganization and hypertrophic hepatocytes with bizzare nuclei and
eosinophilic inclusions were seen. Centrilobular necrosis some-
times became confluent. Mice receiving 0.045 and some receiving
0.03 g DMH/kg diet also developed portal fibrosis and bile duct
hyperplasia which in some animals was so extensive that it approached an adenomatous appearance. This lesion was designated
"reactive hepatitis with triaditis". Table VII summarizes the results in relation to dosage which were highly statistically significant (P < .001). Mice fed 10% protein diet had more severe lesions
(p < .001) which is most evident at the .030 and .045 DMH dose.

Table VII. Percent mice with liver lesions by dietary
            protein and DMH dose

| Liver Status | 10% Protein | | | | 40% Protein | | | |
| | DMH g/kg diet | | | | DMH g/kg diet | | | |
	Control	.015	.030	.045	Control	.015	.030	.045
Normal	96	4	--	--	96	--	4	--
Pre-reactive hepatitis	4	96	4	--	4	100	24	--
Reactive hepatitis	--	--	84	4	--	--	68	72
Reactive hepatitis with triaditis	--	--	12	96	--	--	4	28

Twenty-five mice in each group but 10% protein and 0.045 g/kg DMH
with 24.

The low protein diet was also mildly lipogenic with moderate fatty
change present in both controls and DMH-treated mice.
     The kidneys (Table VIII) appeared less sensitive to DMH
toxicity than liver. Renal lesions consisted of focal, usually
subscapular fibrosis with atrophy and hyperplasia of tubular epithelium and variable inflammatory infiltrates. This lesion was
designated "interstitial nephritis" or "pyelonephritis" when the
renal pelvis was involved. There was no statistical basis for dif-
ferentiating the lesion with involvement of the pelvic from that
without, and therefore the two designations have been pooled for

evaluating statistical significance. As with the liver the kidney
lesions were strongly positively associated with DMH dose (p <
0.001) and were more severe with low dietary protein (p < 0.001).

Table VIII.   Percent mice with kidney lesions by dietary
protein and DMH dose

Kidney Status	10% Protein DMH g/kg diet				40% Protein DMH g/kg diet			
	Control	.015	.030	.045	Control	.015	.030	.045
Normal	96	92	0	8	100	100	60	4
Interstitial Nephritis Diagnosis A	4	4	64	46	--	--	24	48
Pyelone- phritis Diagnosis B	--	4	36	46	--	--	16	48

Twenty-five mice in each group but 10% - .015 and .045, with 24.

The lesions of the adrenal gland consisted of hyperplasia of
cortical cells with atypical nuclei and focal pigment deposition
frequently seen at 0.03 and 0.045 g/kg of diet (Table IX). This
lesion showed a strong dose response correlation (P < 0.001) and a
negative association with dietary protein level (P < 0.001).

Table IX.   Percent mice with and without adrenal hyperplasia
by dietary protein, DMH dose and severity grade

Adrenal Status	10% Protein DMH g/kg diet				40% Protein DMH g/kg diet			
	Con- trol	.015	.030	.045	Con- trol	.015	.030	.045
Normal	90	95	22	9	92	95	58	--
Hyperplasia								
0 (trace)	10	5	48	--	4	5	25	--
1 (mild)	--	--	26	9	--	--	17	41
2 (moderate)	--	--	4	59	4	--	--	50
3 (severe)	--	--	--	23	--	--	--	9

Twenty-one to 24 mice in each treatment group, due to missing
adrenals in sectioning.

Heart lesions consisting of focal myocytolysis with or without fibrosis and/or calcification were consistently observed in
mice receiving the highest dosage of DMH and also in one-third of
those receiving the intermediate dose (Table X). The dose response
relation is relatively strong (P < .001) but no evidence was found
that pathology in the heart was affected by dietary protein.
A hierarchy of pathologic lesions observed in mice fed DMH
is summarized in Figure 3. Renal damage virtually never occurred
without accompanying liver pathology, and adrenals virtually never
showed changes unless there was accompanying liver and kidney pathology. Focal myocytolysis did not fit within the same organ hierarchy as the liver, kidney and adrenal findings.

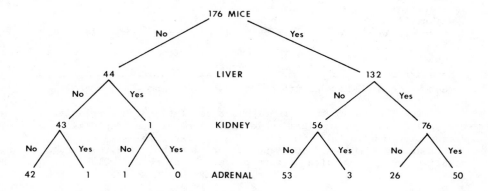

Figure 3. Sequence of developing pathologic lesions in 176 $B_6C_3F_1$ mice fed DMH.

Table X. Percent mice with and without cardiac focal
          myochytolysis

Myocardial Status	10% Protein DMH g/kg diet				40% Protein DMH g/kg diet			
	Control	.015	.030	.045	Control	.015	.030	.045
Normal	96	96	68	21	92	88	64	24
Focal myocytolysis								
0 (trace)	4	4	8	12	8	12	28	24
1 (mild)	--	--	20	46	--	--	4	48
2 (moderate) or 3 (severe)	--	--	4	21	--	--	4	4

Twenty-five mice in each group but 10% - .015 and .045, with 24.

General Discussion

The amount of dietary protein influenced the carcinogenicity of DMH
in rats and its conversion to mutagenic metabolites and toxicity in
mice. Raising protein intake in rats raised the incidence of
tumors of the inner ear and in the small and large intestines (17).
The source of protein (vegetable or animal) had no effect on DMH
intestinal carcinogenesis (20).
     Increasing dietary protein intake increased the quantities
of DMH metabolites retained by mice fed high compared to low protein diets and this is consistent with the greater yield of tumors
in rats as their protein intake was increased (28). The data argue
that lowering dietary protein reduced the capacity of liver to
metabolize DMH and increased the expiration of its volatile metabolite AM. Consequently, less DMH was converted to promutagens and
carcinogenic products. By using the host-mediated assay it was
possible to show that DMH produced mutations in histidine dependent
salmonella organisms. The essential role of the liver in making
these conversions was shown with hepatectomy studies. The fact
that mutagenesis had not been demonstrated earlier with the conventional Ames assay in which the S9 fraction was applied to an agar
plate shows that the metabolites that were necessary to cause
mutagenesis were undoubtedly lost by volatilization from the in
vitro system.
     In complete contrast with tumorigenesis in rats, higher pro-
tein intakes appear to decrease toxic effects of chronic, low dose
feeding of DMH. The 5 month toxicity study indicates that carcinogenesis observed after injection of DMH involves a different set of
metabolic processes compared to exposure after oral intake, which
is a common route of exposure to carcinogens by humans. This also
suggests that the target tissues may differ when carcinogens are
consumed in the food compared to parenteral injection which is
often used in studies with animals.

Acknowledgments

The research on DMH mutagenesis and toxicity was supported in part
by Toxicology Training Grant USPHS-ES-070001-17 and Contract US NIH

NCI CP75899. The authors acknowledge the contributions of J.
Alster, P. B. Imrey, N. S. Nandkumar, D. R. Thursh and C. R. Truex
in the studies on DMH toxicity.

Literature Cited

1. Toth, B. Cancer Res. 1975, 35, 3696-7.
2. Laqueur, G. L.; Michaelsen, O.; Whiting, M. G.; Kurland, L. T.
    J. Nat. Cancer Inst. 1963, 31, 919-33.
3. Druckrey, H.; Preussman, R.; Matzkies, F.; Ivankovic, S.
    Naturwissenchaften 1967, 54, 285-6.
4. Rogers, A. E.; Herndon, B. J.; Newberne, P. M. Cancer Res.
    1973, 33, 1003-9.
5. Reddy, B. S.; Narisawa, T.; Wright, P.; Vukusich, D.; Weis-
    burger, J. H.; Wynder, E. L. Cancer Res. 1975, 35, 287-90.
6. Wiebecke, B; Lohrs, U.; Gimmy, J.; Eder, M. Z. Ges. Exp. Med.
    1969, 149, 277-86.
7. Thurnherr, N.; Deschner, E. E.; Stonehill, E.; Lipkin, M.
    Cancer Res. 1973, 33, 940-5.
8. Osswald, H.; Kruger, F. W. Arzneimittelforschung 1969, 19,
    1891-6.
9. Pozharisski, K. M.; Likhachev, A. J.; Klimashevski, V. F.;
    Shaposhnikor, J. D. Cancer Res. 1979, 30, 165-237.
10. Doll, R. Br. J. Cancer 1969, 23, 1-8.
11. Hill, M. J. In "Dietary Fats and Health"; Perkins, E. G.;
    Visek, W. J., Eds.; American Oil Chemist's Society:
    Champaign, IL, 1983; pp. 868-80.
12. Armstrong, B.; Doll, R. Int. J. Cancer 1975, 15, 617.
13. Drasar, B. S.; Irving, D. Br. J. Cancer 1973, 27, 167.
14. Gregor, O; Toman, R.; Prusova, F. Gut 1969, 10, 1031.
15. Reddy, B. S. In "Dietary Fats and Health"; Perkins, E. G.;
    Visek, W. J., Eds.; American Oil Chemist's Society:
    Champaign, IL, 1983; pp.
16. Nauss, K.; Locniskar, M.; Newberne, P. Cancer Res.   , 43,
    4083-90.
17. Topping, D. C.; Visek, W. J. J. Nutr. 1976, 106, 1583-90.
18. Ward, J. M. Lab. Invest. 1974, 30, 505-13.
19. Hevia, P.; Truex, C. R.; Imrey, P. B.; Clinton, S. K.;
    Mangian, H. J.: Visek, W. J. J. Nutr. 1984, 114, 555-564.
20. Clinton, S. K.; Destree, R. J.; Anderson, D. B.; Truex, C. R.;
    Imrey, P. B.; Visek. Nutr. Repts. Inter. 1979, 10, 335-42.
21. Lijinsky, W.; Shubik, P. Science 1964, 145, 53-5.
22. McCann, J.; Spingarm, N.; Kobori, J.; Ames, B. Proc. Soc.
    Natl. Acad. Sci. (USA) 1975, 72, 979.
23. Diamond, L.; Sardet, C.; Rothblat, G. Int. J. Cancer 1968, 3,
    838-49.
24. Haddow, A. Perspect. Biol. Med. 1974, 17, 543-89.
25. "Evaluation of Carcinogenic Risk of Chemicals to Man, Vol. 3";
    International Agency for Research on Cancer, World Health
    Organization, Lyon, France, 1973.
26. Montesano, R.; Saffiotti, U.; Ferrero, A.; Kaufman, D. J.
    Natl. Cancer Inst. 1974, 53, 1395-7.
27. Nieman, J. Eur. J. Cancer 1968, 4, 537-43.
28. Kari, F. W.; Johnston, J. B.; Truex, C. R.; Visek, W. J.
    Cancer Res. 1983, 43, 3674-9.

29. Ames, B. N.; Lee, F. D.; Durston, W. E. Proc. Natl. Acad. Sci. U.S.A. 1973, 70, 782-6.
30. Gabridge, M. G.; Legator, M. S. Proc. Soc. Exp. Biol. Med. 1969, 130, 831-4.
31. Moriya, M.; Ohta, T.; Watanabe, K; Shirasu, Y. J. Natl. Cancer Inst. 1978, 61, 457-60.
32. Nagasawa, H. T.; Shirota, N. Nature (Lond.) 1972, 236, 234-5.

RECEIVED August 28, 1984

Nutrition and Experimental Breast Cancer: The Effects of Dietary Fat and Protein

STEVEN K. CLINTON and WILLARD J. VISEK

University of Illinois College of Medicine at Urbana-Champaign, Urbana, IL 61801

Laboratory studies examining the effects of diet on carcinogenesis began soon after animal models for cancer were developed. However, the concept that diet and nutrition may have an important role in the genesis, prevention, or treatment of human cancers has only recently become widely appreciated by the biomedical community. As the evidence accumulates from epidemiologic and laboratory studies there is increasing pressure upon the scientific community to formulate health policy guidelines. The National Research Council of the National Academy of Sciences has facilitated this process by conducting a comprehensive evaluation of the literature on diet, nutrition, and cancer (1). Based upon their findings, a series of guidelines were proposed which "are both consistent with good nutritional practices and likely to reduce the risk of cancer" (1). One of their recommendations was to reduce the consumption of both saturated and unsaturated fats from its present level of over 40% of calories to 30% of calories.

Diet and cancer relationships are an area of scientific investigation where the evidence is often vigorously debated, and extrapolation to public policy guidelines elicits much controversy. It is clear that we have not yet obtained incontrovertible evidence to define the benefits and risks which may be derived from specific changes in the fat content of our diet. However many suggest that with respect to cancer prevention, the current state of knowledge, inconclusive as it may be, is sufficient to develop recommendations which may produce significant reductions in the future incidence of certain cancers.

Women in the United States develop cancer of the breast more frequently than at any other anatomic site (2). The dietary goal suggesting a lowering of fat in the diet is aimed primarily at decreasing the incidence of breast cancer. The present communication will briefly review the epidemiological data and focus upon experimental evidence which relates total fat consumption with breast cancer incidence. The roles of dietary protein and total calories, both highly correlated with fat consumption, will also be discussed. In addition, we will review our knowledge of the mechanisms whereby dietary fat and protein may influence mammary carcinogenesis in rodents.

0097–6156/85/0277–0309$06.00/0

Epidemiologic Studies

Breast cancer has a multifactorial etiology involving numerous
genetic, metabolic, and cultural variables. Table I presents a
summary of many epidemiological studies designed to identify risk
factors for breast cancer (2-8).

Table I. Risk Factors for Breast Cancer

Factor	High-Risk Group	Low-Risk Group	Approximate Increase in Risk
Sex	female	male	99 to 1
Age	>40 yrs old	<40 yrs old	6 to 1
Family history	positive	negative	3 to 1
Mother and sister with disease; bilateral and premenopausal	positive	negative	9 to 1
Previous benign breast disease	positive	negative	3 to 1
Previous cancer in one breast	positive	negative	5 to 1
Parity	nulliparous	parous	3 to 1
Age at first birth	>35 yrs old	<20 yrs old	3 to 1
Premenopausal ovariectomy	negative	positive	3 to 1
Menarche	<12 yrs old	>12 yrs old	1.3 to 1
Menopause	>50 yrs old	<50 yrs old	1.5 to 1

The variability in breast cancer incidence between countries
has directed research toward specific environmental factors which
are characteristic of high risk populations. Based upon evidence
from 46 countries, the age-adjusted death rate from breast cancer
varies at least 6- to 10-fold among nations where accurate statistics are available (2). Countries with high incidence are typically
those with a "Western" culture such as northern Europe and North
America, whereas many developing and some industrialized nations
such as Japan show a low incidence. Studies of populations migrat-
ing from low to high incidence areas have provided additional evidence implicating lifestyle, especially diet. Investigations of
Japanese (9) and Polish (10) migrants to the United States show an
upward displacement of breast cancer risk toward the average US rate
as succeeding generations adopt American cultural habits.
        Interest in dietary components which explain differences in
breast cancer rates comes from strong correlations between nutrient
supply within nations and their age-adjusted rates for breast cancer
(11). The most frequently cited dietary components related to
higher risk of breast cancer are: total fat, total protein, calories, animal fat, animal protein, and a lack of fiber. Overall it
has not been possible to identify the specific dietary constituents
responsible for the observed incidence since the intakes of many
dietary factors such as protein, fat, and calories are strongly
intercorrelated. Other studies of nutrient intake and breast

cancer rates within countries, or between cases and controls have
provided inconclusive results (12-18).

Experimental Studies

The use of animal models for breast cancer allows control of single
dietary variables. In such studies, diets high in fat have increased the incidence of spontaneous (19-22), chemically induced (23-
26), and radiation-induced mammary tumors (27), and enhanced the
growth of transplantable breast tumors (28-31). The effects of protein on breast cancer have not been studied as extensively, and the
results have been less consistent. Several investigators have found
no effect from increasing dietary protein (32,33), whereas others
have noted a stimulation (34,35) or an inhibition of mammary tumorigenesis (36,37).

Our laboratory has completed a series of studies designed to
evaluate the simultaneous effects of dietary protein and fat on
7,12-dimethylbenz(a)anthracene (DMBA)-induced breast cancer in
rats. Sprague-Dawley female rats were assigned to nine diets in a 3
x 3 factorial arrangement with protein (casein) at 8, 16, and 32% of
kcals and fat (corn oil) at 12, 24, and 48% of kcals. As fat content was increased, all nutrients other than carbohydrate were adjusted to remain constant with respect to calories. Forty rats were
assigned to each diet for each of three experiments (Figure 1) to
examine initiation, promotion, and the combined phases of chemically-induced carcinogenesis.

For the combined phase study, all rats were maintained on
their respective dietary treatments from weaning until necropsy.
Rats fed the high protein diets showed a 5% decrease in caloric
intake and a slightly higher final body weight (Table II). Fat had
no effect on food intake or body weight. Figure 2 shows survival
curves of time to first palpated tumor. Fat consistently increased
the proportion of rats with a palpable tumors regardless of protein
intake. Table II presents the tumor number at necropsy. The effect
of dietary corn oil on the percentage of rats showing any type of
tumor was best described as a linear effect of the log of percentage
fat on the log of the odds of a rat developing a tumor. The odds of
a rat developing a tumor (probability of tumor/probability of no
tumor) increased 2.15 times for each successive doubling of dietary
corn oil. We saw no statistically significant effects of protein,
or protein by fat interactions, on the percentage of rats with
tumors. When evaluating the probability of developing multiple
tumors, we observed a significant nonlinear effect of dietary corn
oil. The odds of a second tumor was only minimally altered with an
increase in fat from 12 to 24% of kcals. However, increasing corn
oil from 24 to 48% of kcal greatly increased the risk of developing
second tumors.

Evaluation of our data by multiple logistic analyses consistently yielded statistically significant positive associations of
caloric consumption, controlled for protein and fat intake, with the
incidence of tumors. The odds of developing an adenocarcinoma, adenoma or tumor type increased by a factor of 1.10, 1.14 and 1.09, respectively, for each 1-kcal increase in intake. The effect of calories can be visualized by dividing the 351 rats into thirds

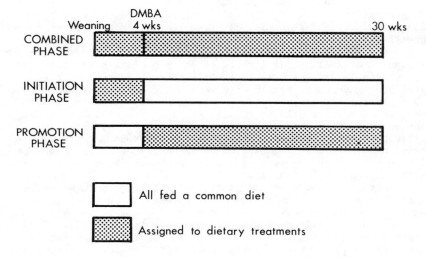

Figure 1.   Experimental design.

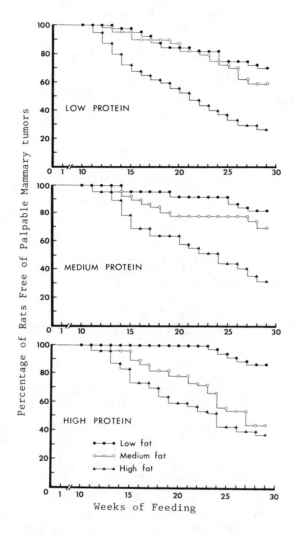

Figure 2. The interactions of dietary protein and fat on the percentage of rats free of DMBA-induced tumors. Rats were fed their respective diets from weaning for 29 weeks. DMBA was administered after 4 weeks of feeding. (Reproduced with permission from Ref. 70. Copyright 1984, American Institute of Nutrition.)

Table II. The Interactions of Dietary Protein
and Fat on Caloric Intake, Body Weight
and DMBA-Induced Breast Cancer
(Combined Phase)

Dietary Protein (% of kcals)	Dietary Fat (% of kcal)			Pooled
	12	24	48	
	Adjusted mean caloric intake, kcal/day			
8	48	49	48	48
16	47	48	48	48
32	45	45	46	45
Pooled	46	47	47	
	Adjusted mean body wt at 30 weeks, g			
8	257	261	256	258
16	264	259	255	259
32	269	267	268	268
Pooled	263	262	260	
	% of rats with any type of tumor (total no. of tumors)			
8	37 (32)	51 (29)	75 (66)	55 (127)
16	38 (18)	36 (19)	65 (45)	46 (82)
32	29 (15)	59 (33)	70 (71)	53 (119)
Pooled	35 (65)	49 (81)	70 (182)	

[1] 40 rats per diet.

according to ad libitum caloric consumption (Table III). Based on
these results, a drop of average caloric consumption by 12–13% was
associated with about a 25% reduction in the prevalence of any
tumor.

Reducing caloric intake by food restriction has consistently
reduced the incidence of tumors in a wide variety of experimental
model systems including spontaneous mammary tumors (38,39). In
contrast, our results are based upon ad libitum feed intake and
evaluated by the effects of caloric intake on tumor prevalence
using multiple logistic regression with direct rate adjustment.
Studies using dietary restriction are always associated with depressed growth rates and final body weights. In contrast, the mean
body weights in the present study for the lower or middle thirds of
caloric intake were 93 and 98% of the mean body weight recorded for
rats in the upper third of ad libitum caloric intake. This observation suggests that factors influencing the efficiency of caloric
utilization independently of their influence on body weight may
play a role in carcinogenesis.

The interactions of dietary fat and protein on the promotion
phase of breast carcinogenesis were examined by feeding weanling
rats a control diet (16% of kcal from protein and 24% of kcal from
fat) for 4 weeks and subsequent assignment to the 9 dietary treatments following DMBA administration. As in the combined phase
study we observed no protein by fat interactions or main effects of

dietary protein on tumor incidence. We did observe a significant linear effect of fat (Table IV), best described as a 1.51 increase in risk for every doubling of dietary fat concentration.

The effects of dietary fat and protein on the initiation phase of DMBA carcinogenesis were examined by feeding the 9 different diets for the 4 weeks prior to carcinogen administration. Four hours

Table III.   Prevalence and number of tumors (in parentheses) in rats divided into three equal groups based on ad libitum caloric consumption

Measure	Lower third	Middle third	Upper third
Number of rats	117	117	117
Range of kcal intake, kcal/day	29.96–46.06	46.13–48.53	48.53–55.32
Mean kcal intake, kcal/day	42.77	47.31	50.84
Weight at 4 weeks	150 ± 2	156 ± 1	154 ± 2
Weight at 30 weeks	250 ± 3	265 ± 2	269 ± 3
Percentage of rats with tumors (number of tumors)			
Any tumor	40 (88)	58 (103)	57 (137)
Adenocarcinoma	27 (62)	42 (66)	45 (84)
Adenoma	8 (12)	12 (15)	19 (25)
Fibroadenoma	8 (13)	17 (22)	14 (27)

Values with plus minus are means ± SEM.

[1] Adjusted to a uniform distribution of animals across the nine diets.

Table IV.   The main effects of dietary fat and protein on the initiation and promotion phases of DMBA-induced breast cancer in rats

Experiment	Dietary Fat (% of kcal)			Dietary Protein (% of kcal)		
	12	24	48	8	16	32
Promotion						
Incidence (%)	52	60	70	62	57	64
Total number of tumors	109	127	140	122	127	127
Initiation						
Incidence (%)	58	58	85	79	65	59
Total number of tumors	116	153	231	194	144	162

Data represents main effects of each nutrient from a 3 x 3 factorial experiment with 40 rats per diet and 120 for main effects. The rats were fed a common diet until DMBA administration at which time they were assigned among the 9 diets for an additional 28 wk. The 9 diets (3 x 3 factorial) were fed for 4 weeks, from weaning until DMBA administration. Following DMBA treatment all rats were fed a common diet.

after administration of DMBA, all rats were switched to a common
diet providing 16% of the calories from protein and 24% from fat.
There was no major increase in tumor incidence with an increase in
fat from 12 to 24% of kcal compared to an increase in risk when fat
increased from 24 to 48% kcal (Table IV). Although protein had no
significant effect on promotion we observed a decrease in tumor
incidence with increased protein fed during the period prior to
DMBA administration (initiation).

These studies showed surprisingly few interactions between
dietary fat and protein and it appears that these two macronu-
trients exert their effects independently. With regards to dietary
protein, the results agree with our previous study, which showed no
effect of protein on the promotion phase of DMBA-induced breast carcinogenesis (37) and with those of Tannenbaum and Silverstone (32)
and Ross and Bras (33) showing no effect of protein on spontaneous
breast tumors in rodents. On the other hand, Engel and Copeland
(36) observed significantly fewer 2-acetyl-aminofluorene-induced
breast cancers in rats fed diets containing 40-60% casein when
compared to 9 or 27% casein. This reduction was in part secondary
to reduced food intake caused by the diets high in protein. We
have now confirmed a previous study showing that increasing dietary
protein, during the initiation phase prior to DMBA administration,
reduced subsequent tumor incidence (37). In contrast, Shay et al.
(34) reported increased 3-methylcholanthrene-induced breast cancer
as rats were fed greater concentrations of protein. Significant
differences were reported, but their interpretation is confounded
because a standard laboratory diet was used as a control for comparison with semipurified diets containing higher levels of protein. Recently, Hawrylewicz et al. (37) also reported more breast
tumors in rats fed increasing amounts of casein. In their studies
with DMBA, the diets were fed throughout the initiation and promotion phases to offspring of dams fed graded protein diets during
mating, gestation and lactation. The above cited studies summarize
the majority of the published literature on the influence of
dietary protein on experimental mammary carcinogenesis. These
investigators have employed a variety of experimental models and
protocols, and in some instances the dietary controls have been
inappropriate. In view of these circumstances, formulation of a
unifying hypothesis concerning the effects of dietary protein on
experimental mammary cancer would be premature.

Our studies consistently showed an increased risk of breast
cancer due to higher dietary fat concentrations. The results of
the combined-phase and promotion studies are suggestive of a linear
effect of fat on tumor incidence. Although dietary fat has long
been known to influence the promotion phase we have clearly noted a
positive effect of fat during initiation. The results appear to be
in direct conflict with other studies where no effect of fat was
observed upon the initiation phase (40). One factor which may have
been responsible for these differences is the protocol followed
during DMBA administration. In all of our studies, semipurified
diets were fed. Feed was removed from the cages for 4 hr prior to
DMBA administration and replaced 4 hr later. In the studies by
Carroll, the rats were fed a chow diet for several days prior and
following DMBA dosing. Constituents of vegetable origin included

in chow diets may have influenced or blocked the effect of dietary fat on DMBA-induced carcinogenesis (41).

It is of interest to compare our results with the two classic studies from the literature using multiple levels of fat. Silverstone and Tannenbaum (42) found that the incidence of spontaneous mammary tumors in mice increased as the level of a partially hydrogenated mixture of cottonseed and soybean oil was increased from 2 to 4% of the diet up to 12 or 16% by weight. Further increments in fat intake did not significantly increase tumor incidence. Carroll and Khor (43) examined the effects of corn oil at 0.5, 5.0, 10.0 and 20.0% of the diet by weight on DMBA-induced breast cancer in rats. They observed that rats fed 0.5% or 5.0% dietary corn oil showed a slightly lower incidence and a greatly reduced total tumor number than those fed 10 or 20% corn oil. The tumor yields were not increased by the 10-fold increase from 0.5 to 5.0% or the 2-fold increase from 10 to 20% corn oil. It is of interest that both Silverstone and Tannenbaum (42) and Carroll and Khor (43) found that over 90% of their animals fed 10-12% fat developed tumors. The high tumor incidence may have masked the influence of further increases in fat intake on the percentage of rats with tumors.

It is clear that more studies are needed with various animal models, multiple levels of dietary fat, different fat sources, and differing intensities of carcinogenic stimuli if the tumor response curve to varying fat intake is to be characterized. Such data would be of value in predicting the levels and kind of fat intake that might significantly influence human breast cancer incidence.

Mechanisms: Dietary Fat and Breast Cancer

Proposed mechanisms whereby dietary fat may influence breast cancer include: (a) changes in the immune system, (b) alterations of the endocrine environment, (c) modifications of cell membrane lipids, (d) changes in the metabolism and biological activity of prostaglandins, (e) direct effects on tumor cell metabolism, (f) production of tumor promoting oxidized products from unsaturated fats, and (g) changes in the activity of carcinogen metabolizing enzymes. The present review will focus upon studies recently completed in our laboratory concerning the effects of dietary fat on estrogen and prolactin status.

Dietary Fat, Estrogen, and Breast Cancer. The presence of the ovary and its hormones clearly influences breast cancer risk in women. Metabolic epidemiologic studies showing that dietary fat influences estrogen homeostasis are suggested but unconvincing (44-49). For many years it has been known that estrogens influence breast tumor growth in rodents (50). The evidence that dietary fat influences steroid hormone concentrations in rats has been inconsistent. Chan et al. (51) noted elevated serum estrogens at metestrus-diestrus in MNU-treated Fisher rats fed 20% compared to 5% lard. Ip and Ip (52) found serum estradiol to be higher at proestrus in DMBA-treated rats fed 5 or 20% vs 0.5% corn oil. They found no difference in estradiol between rats fed 5 or 20% fat, although the percentage with tumors was 46 and 75, respectively.

However, others (53,54) have found that changes in the level or
type of fat had no effect on serum estrogen or progesterone
concentrations.

We have completed a study to determine if intact, cycling
ovaries are necessary for enhancement of breast tumor incidence by
dietary fat. Female, Sprague-Dawley rats were given DMBA at 50-55
days of age. Twenty-four hr later they were divided into 3 groups:
(1) ovariectomy and a subcutaneous estrogen implant to provide constant serum estrogen levels, (2) ovariectomy and an empty implant,
and (3) sham-ovariectomy and an empty implant. The rats were then
placed on diets containing 4 or 20% corn oil by weight. Although
estrogen status clearly influences tumor incidence, dietary fat had
a similar effect on tumor incidence in normally cycling rats and in
ovariectomized rats with constant estrogen levels maintained by im-
plants (Table V). We conclude that the effect of fat is independent of the cyclic function of the ovary. In a parallel study in
rats not given DMBA we saw no effect of dietary fat on total serum
extrogens (Table VI).

Table V. The effects of dietary fat concentration (4 or
          20% corn oil) on DMBA-induced mammary carcino-
          genesis in control, ovariectomized, and ovariec-
          tomized-estrogen treated rats

Treatment	Incidence (%)		Number of tumors	
	4% fat	20% fat	4% fat	20% fat
Controls	59	84	53	117
Ovariectomy	12	22	6	10
Ovariectomy + Estrogen	47	81	61	95

Thirty rats per group. Diets were fed during the promotion
phase.

Table VI. The effects of dietary fat concentration (4 vs. 20%
           corn oil) on serum estrogens and prolactin

Diet	Prolactin (ng/ml)		Estrogens (pg/ml)	
	Diestrus	Proestrus	Diestrus	Proestrus
4% corn oil	7 ± 2	328 ± 43	83 ± 15	149 ± 15
20% corn oil	12 ± 5	275 ± 45	76 ± 10	159 ± 12

Values represent means ± SEM after 18-20 weeks of feeding.

Dietary Fat, Prolactin, and Breast Cancer. Prolactin may also
interact with diet to influence breast cancer. Although the role
of prolactin in human breast cancer etiology is relatively obscure,
its role as a promotor in rodent mammary carcinogenesis has been
well established (55,56).

Studies in humans have suggested that serum prolactin may be
lower on vegetarian-low fat diets (57,58). As previously noted for
serum estrogen, studies in laboratory animals have shown inconsistent effects. Some studies report elevations of serum prolactin
with high fat diets (51,59,60) whereas others show no change

(53,54). We have observed no effect of fat on serum prolactin levels in three separate studies like that summarized in Table VI. There are a number of possible explanations for the inconsistency in results observed between laboratories. Those studies showing an effect of fat compared levels of 0.5% to 20.0% (51,59,60). Low fat concentrations, especially with lard or another saturated fat, do not satisfy the recommended daily allowances for essential fatty acids (61). Diets marginal or deficient in essential fatty acids may reduce serum prolactin levels or reduce apparent breast tumor incidence by reducing tumor growth rate (29,31), inhibiting mammary gland development (62,63), or reducing the number of hormone receptors (64).

Earlier studies showing an effect of fat on serum prolactin utilized ether anesthesia while obtaining blood samples (51-59). The stress of ether produces a rapid secretion of prolactin by the pituitary (64). The effect of fat noted when ether was used may have been a result of altered pituitary sensitivity to regulators of prolactin secretion. This hypothesis is reinforced by a study by Sinha et al. (66). Mice fed a semipurified diet containing 60% fat by weight showed a 25% greater response to perphenazine, a potent prolactin stimulating drug, than mice fed a non-purified, closed-formula, commercial diet. In a recent study, with carefully defined diets, we observed no effect with dietary corn oil supplying from 12 to 24 to 48% of calories on serum prolactin concentrations following perphenazine (Figure 3).

Serum hormone concentrations reflect both the rate of secretion and clearance by peripheral tissues. In parallel with our studies on prolactin secretion we have evaluated the effects of dietary fat on the metabolic clearance rate of prolactin. Rats were initially treated with ergocryptine to suppress endogenous prolactin secretion. We then measured the disappearance of immuno-reactive prolactin from the sera after a single intravenous injection of prolactin. No significant effect of dietary fat on the clearance of prolactin was observed (Figure 4).

Evidence is accumulating that the enhancement of breast tumorigenesis by dietary fat is independent of alterations in prolactin or estrogen homeostasis. It is clear that dietary fat may influence breast cancer incidence by other mechanisms which should be more vigorously pursued.

Mechanisms: Dietary Protein and Breast Cancer

We observed a protective effect of increased dietary protein on DMBA-induced breast tumor incidence when the diets varying in protein were fed prior to carcinogen administration. We have investigated the hypothesis that dietary protein may influence carcinogenesis via effects on the mixed-function oxidase (MFO) enzyme systems involved in carcinogen metabolism.

Aryl hydrocarbon hydroxylase (AHH) is a complex mixed function oxidase enzyme which converts polycyclic aromatic hydrocarbons such as DMBA to more hydrophilic and readily excretable products. During this process metabolites that are more carcinogenic than the parent compound can be produced. The distribution of MFO enzymes, their activity, and the balance between conversion of procarcinogens to active carcinogens and their detoxification is probably a

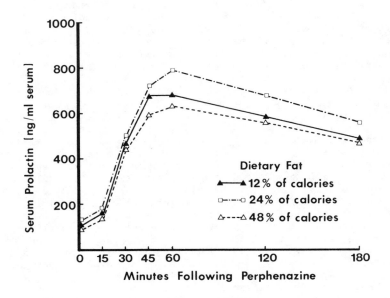

Figure 3. The effects of dietary fat on perphenazine stimulated prolactin release in female rats after 18 weeks of
feeding.

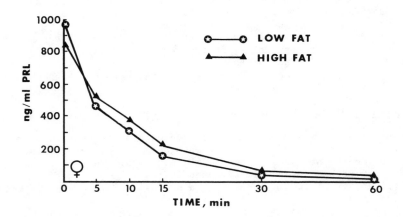

Figure 4. Metabolic clearance rate of prolactin in female rats
fed diets containing 4 (low fat) or 20% (high fat) corn oil for
18 weeks.

determining factor in carcinogenesis by DMBA. As can be seen in
Figure 5, dietary protein influences the activity of these enzymes
in growing rats significantly (66). Our evidence supports the
theory that dietary protein modifies the carcinogenic response by
enhancing hepatic metabolism of DMBA to detoxified products. The
liver has the greatest capacity to metabolize polycyclic aromatic
hydrocarbons (PAH) thereby influencing their biological activity.
Enhancing the hepatic metabolism of DMBA to inactive and readily
excretable metabolites may significantly alter the amount of potentially active carcinogen in the peripheral circulation thereby influencing the carcinogenic response. Wattenberg found that natural
inducers of hepatic AHH present in the cruciferous vegetables such
as brussels sprouts, cabbage, and cauliflower, reduces the number of
PAH-induced cancers (67). Induction of hepatic AHH by chemical antioxidants and noncarcinogenic PAH prior to exposure to DMBA also reduced the number of tumors (68). Somogyi et al. (69) found that pretreatment with steroids capable of inducing hepatic aryl hydrocarbon
hydroxylase (AHH) activity protects rats from DMBA-induced adrenal
necrosis. Our in vivo experiments and those of others show that
enhanced hepatic AHH at the time of carcinogen exposure is indicative of detoxification processes possibly responsible for lower
tumor incidence.

Summary and Prospects

Breast cancer has a multifactorial etiology, with both genetic and
environmental factors playing important roles. Among the nutritional variables which are correlated with breast cancer incidence,
dietary fat has shown consistently high correlations in epidemiological data and stimulatory effects in numerous rodent experimental
models. Despite this large body of evidence about the influence of
dietary fat on mammary tumorigenesis, our present understanding is
insufficient to predict what fraction of breast cancer in women can
be attributed to dietary fat intake. Human diets vary in content
and source of protein, fat, carbohydrate, fiber, vitamins and minerals. Many nutrients appear to have individual effects on experimental breast cancer, and undoubedly participate in significant synergistic and antagonistic interactions.
    A critical question concerns the possible value of dietary
intervention as a preventive or therapeutic measure. There is
little doubt that fat intake influences breast cancer development in
rodents at levels which are found in the human diets. However, conclusive evidence is lacking about the quantitative and qualitative
aspects of these processes and how fat in diets may be modified to
reduce human cancer incidence. It is likely that dietary intervention may prove useful initially as a preventive or therapeutic measure in isolated groups of high risk individuals. As genetic, hormonal, and immunologic risk factors became more clearly defined,
individuals at high risk and those with breast cancer may benefit
from therapeutic low-fat diets whose efficacy will require assessment in well-designed clinical studies.

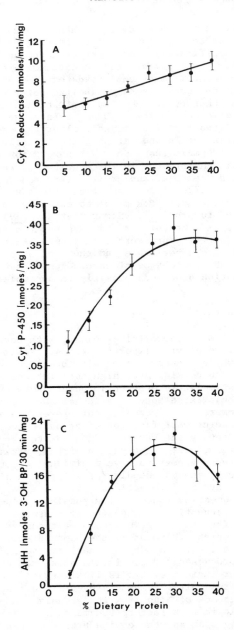

Figure 5. Dietary protein and hepatic mixed function oxidase activity (cytochrome c-reductase, cytochrome P-450, aryl hydrocarbon hydroxylase). (Reproduced with permission from Ref. 71. Copyright 1983, American Dairy Science Association.)

Acknowledgments

The authors wish to acknowledge our co-investigators Anthony L. Mulloy, Peter B. Imrey and Joan M. Alster for their contributions to the studies described.

Literature Cited

1. "Diet, Nutrition, and Cancer," Committee on Diet, Nutrition, and Cancer, National Research Council, National Academy of Sciences, 1982.
2. Silverberg, E. Ca-Cancer J. Clin. 1982, 32, 15-31.
3. Mason, T. J.; McKay, F. W.; Hoover, R.; Blot, W. J.; Frowmeni, J. F. "Atlas of Cancer Mortality for US Countries 1950 to 1969," US Dept. of Health, Education and Welfare, 1975.
4. Kelsey, J. Epid. Rev. 1979, 1, 74-109.
5. Lynch, H. T. "Genetics and Breast Cancer"; Van Nostrand Reinhold Co., 1981.
6. Staszewski, J. J. Natl. Cancer Inst. 1971, 47, 935-40.
7. Choi, N. W.; Howe, G. R.; Miller, A. B. Am. J. Epidemiol. 1978, 107, 510-21.
8. Trichopoulous, D.; MacMahon, B.; Cole, P. J. Natl. Cancer Inst. 1972, 48, 605-13.
9. Buell, P. J. Natl. Cancer Inst. 1973, 51, 1479-83.
10. Staszewski, J.; Haenszel, W. J. Natl. Cancer Inst. 1965, 35, 291-7.
11. Armstrong, B.; Doll, R. Int. J. Cancer 1975, 15, 617-31.
12. Phillips, R. L. Cancer Res., 1975, 35, 3513-22.
13. Phillips, R. L.; Garfinkel, L.; Kuzma, J. W.; Beeson, W. L.; Lotz, T.; Brin, B. J. Natl. Cancer Inst. 65, 1097-107.
14. Kinlen, L. J. Lancet 1982, 1, 946-9.
15. Bjarnason, O.; Day, N.; Snaedal, G.; Tulinius, H. Int. J. Cancer 1974, 13, 689-96.
16. Miller, A. B.; Kelly, A.; Choi, N. W.; Matthews, V.; Morgan, R. W.; Munan, L.; Burch, J. D.; Feather, J.; Howe, G. R.; Jain, M. Am. J. Epidemiol. , 107, 499-509.
17. Hirayama, T. Prev. Med. 1978, 7, 173-95.
18. Lubin, J. H.; Burns, P. E.; Blot, W. J.; Ziegler, R. G.; Lees, A. W.; Fraumeni, J. F. Int. J. Cancer 1981, 28, 685-9.
19. Tannenbaum, A. In "The Pathophysiology of Cancer"; Homberger, F., Ed.; Holber-Harper: New York, 1959; pp. 517-62.
20. Tannenbaum, A. Cancer Res. 1942, 2, 468-75.
21. Tinsley, I. J.; Schmitz, J. A.; Pierce, D. A. Cancer Res. 1981, 41, 1460-5.
22. Benson, J.; Lev, M; Grand, C. G. Cancer Res. 1956, 16, 135-7.
23. Dunning, W. F.; Curtis, M. R.; Maun, M. E. Cancer Res. 1949, 9, 354-61.
24. Engel, R. W.; Copeland, D. H. Cancer Res. 1951, 11, 180-3.
25. Gammal, E. G.; Carroll, K. K.; Plunkett, E. R. Cancer Res. 1967, 27, 1737-42.
26. Chan, P. C.; Head, J. F.; Cohen, L. A.; Wynder, E. L. J. Natl. Cancer Inst. 1977, 59, 1279-83.
27. Silverman, J.; Shellabarger, C. F.; Holtzman, S.; Stone, J. P.; Weisburger, J. H. J. Natl. Cancer Inst. 1980, 64, 631-4.

28. Giovarelli, M.; Padula, E.; Ugazio, G.; Cavallo, G. Cancer
     Res. 1980, 40, 3745-9.
29. Hillyard, L. A.; Abraham, S. Cancer Res. 1979, 39, 4430-7.
30. Hopkins, G. J.; West, C. E. J. Natl. Cancer Inst. 1977, 58,
     753-6.
31. Rao, G. A.; Abraham, S. J. Natl. Cancer Inst. 1976, 56, 431-2.
32. Tannenbaum, A.; Silverstone, H. Cancer Res. 1949, 9, 162-73.
33. Ross, M. H.; Bras, G. J. Nutr. 1973, 103, 944-63.
34. Shay, H.; Gurenstein, M; Shimkin, M. J. Natl. Cancer Inst.
     1964, 33, 243-53.
35. Hawrylewicz, E. J.; Huang, H. H., Kissane, J. Q.; Drab, E. A.
     Nutr. Rep. Int. 1982, 26, 793-806.
36. Engel, R. W.; Copeland, D. H. Cancer Res. 1952, 12, 905-8.
37. Clinton, S. K.; Truex, C. R.; Visek, W. J. J. Nutr. 1979, 109,
     55-62.
38. Tannenbaum, A. In "The Pathophysiology of Cancer"; Homberger,
     F., Ed.; Holber-Harper: New York, 1959; pp. 517-62.
39. Tannenbaum, A. Cancer Res. 1945, 5, 609-15.
40. Carroll, K. K.; Khor, H. T. Cancer Res. 1970, 30, 2260-4.
41. Wattenberg, L. W. Adv. Cancer Res. 1978, 26, 197-226.
42. Silverstone, H.; Tannenbaum, A. Cancer Res. 1950, 10, 448-53.
43. Carroll, K. K.; Khor, H. T. Lipids 1971, 6, 415-20.
44. Cole, P.; MacMahon, B. Lancet 1969, 1, 604-6.
45. MacMahon, E.; Cole, P.; Brown, J. B.; Aoki, K.; Lin, T.;
     Morgan, R.; Woo, N. Lancet 1971, 2, 900-2.
46. MacMahon, B.; Cole, P.; Brown, J. J. Natl. Cancer Inst. 1973,
     50, 21-42.
47. Hoggins, C. Science 1967, 156, 1050-4.
48. Bulbrook, R. D.; Swain, M.; Wang, D.; Hayward, J.; Kumaoka, S.;
     Takatani, O.; Abe, O.; Utsunomiya, J. Eur. J. Cancer 1967, 12,
     725-35.
49. Murray, W. S. J. Cancer Res. 1928, 12, 18-25.
50. Welsch, C. W.; Aylsworth, C. F. In "Dietary Fats and Health";
     Perkins, E. G.; Visek, W. J., Ed.; American Oil Chemist's
     Society: Champaign, IL, 1983; pp. 790-816.
51. Chan, P. C.; Head, J. F.; Cohen, L. A.; Wynder, E. L. J. Natl.
     Cancer Inst. 1977, 59, 1279-83.
52. Ip, C.; Ip, M. J. Natl. Cancer Inst. 1981, 66, 291-5.
53. Hopkins, G.; Kennedy, T.; Carroll, K. J. Natl. Cancer Inst.
     1981, 66, 517-22.
54. Wetsel, W. C.; Rogers, A. E.; Rutledge, A.; Leavitt, W. Cancer
     Res. 1984, 44, 1420-5.
55. Welsch, C. W.; Nagasawa, H. Cancer Res. 1977, 37, 951-63.
56. Meites, J. J. Natl. Cancer Inst. 1972, 48:1217-24.
57. Hill, P.; Garbaczewski, L.; Helman, P.; Huskisson, J.;
     Sporangisa, E.; Wynder, E. Am. J. Clin. Nutr. 1980, 33,
     1192-8.
58. Hill, P.; Wynder, E. Lancet 1976, 2, 806.
59. Chan, P. C.; Didato, F.; Cohen, L. A. Proc. Soc. Exp. Biol.
     Med. 1975, 149, 133-5.
60. Ip, C.; Yip, P.; Bernardis, L. L. Cancer Res. 1980, 40, 374-8.
61. "Nutrient Requirements of Laboratory Animals"; No. 10, National
     Research Council, National Academy of Sciences, 1978.
62. Kidwell, W. R.; Monaco, M. E.; Sicha, W. S.; Smith, G. S.
     Cancer Res. 1978, 38, 4091-100.

63. Wicha, M. S.; Liotta, L. A.; Kidwell, W. R. Cancer Res. 1981, 39, 426-35.
64. Neiil, J. D. Endocrin. 1970, 87, 1192-7.
65. Sinha, Y. N.; Thomas, J. W.; Salocks, C. B.; Wickes, M. A.; Vanderlaan, W. R. Horm. Metab. Res. 1977, 9, 277-82.
66. Clinton, S. K.; Truex, C. R.; Imrey, P. B.; Visek, W. J. In "Microsomes, Drug Oxidations, and Chemical Carcinogenesis"; Coon, M. J., Ed.; Academic Press: New York, 1980; pp. 1129-32.
67. Wattenberg, L. W.; Loub, W. D.; Lam, L. K.; Speier, J. L. Fed. Proc. 1976, 35, 1327-31.
68. Wattenberg, L. W. Cancer Res. 1975, 35, 3526-3531.
69. Somogyi, A.; Kovacs, K.; Kuntzman, R.; Conney, A. H. Life Sci. 1971, 10, 1261-71.
70. Clinton, S. K.; Imrey, P. B.; Alster, J. M.; Simon, J.; Truex, C. R.; Visek, W. J. J. Nutr. 1984, 114, 1213-1223..
71. Visek, W. J. J. Dairy Sci. 1984, 67, 481-498.

RECEIVED November 30, 1984

Promotion of Liver Carcinogenesis
Interactions of Barbiturates and a Choline-Deficient Diet

H. SHINOZUKA, A. J. DEMETRIS, S. L. KATYAL, and M. I. R. PERERA

Department of Pathology, University of Pittsburgh School of Medicine, Pittsburgh, PA 15261

A choline deficient (CD) diet has been shown to exert
a strong promoting effect on the emergence of foci of
enzyme altered hepatocytes and on the induction of
hepatomas in rats initiated with a carcinogen.
Earlier, we demonstrated that inclusion of barbiturates in a CD diet resulted in a synergistic enhancement of tumor promotion, but inhibited the CD diet-
induced stimulation of liver DNA synthesis and liver
cell proliferation. In the present study, we examined
how modifications of the quality of fat in a CD diet
alters the promoting effect and the diet-induced lipid
peroxidation in the liver. Feeding a CD diet for one
week induced lipid peroxidation of liver microsomal
membrane lipids as determined by diene conjugate
formation. A CD diet with corn oil as the source of
fat exerted a stronger promoting effect and induced
lipid peroxidation earlier and more intensely than did
a CD diet containing Primex and corn oil. Dietary
administration of phenobarbital in a choline supplemented diet induced no lipid peroxidation and no
evidence of enhanced lipid peroxidation was noted when
phenobarbital was added to a CD diet. Thus, a CD diet
and barbiturates exert their promoting effects through
different mechanisms and the combination results in a
synergistic enhancement.

During the past ten years, the concept of initiation and promotion
of chemical carcinogenesis, originally demonstrated in the skin of
mice and rabbits, has been extended to several other organ systems
including the liver (1,2). Thus, hepatocellular carcinomas can be
induced in experimental animals by a relatively brief initiation by
a carcinogen followed by prolonged imposition of a promoting stimulus. A number of promoters with diverse properties have been identified in liver tumor induction (1). Table I lists several known
liver tumor promoters which can be arbitrarily divided into two
broad categories; agents which are inducers of microsomal mono-

0097-6156/85/0277-0327$06.00/0

oxygenases and the ones which are not. It is evident that a large number of xenobiotics which act as primary hepatotoxicants are promoters of liver carcinogenesis. The mechanisms by which different agents or conditions exert the common effect of liver tumor promotion are not known.

TABLE I

Promoting Agents of Hepatocarcinogenesis

Enzyme[*] Inducers	Non-Inducers
Phenobarbital (other barbiturates)	Estradiol-17-phenylpropionate
	Ethinyl estradiol
Dichlorodiphenyltrichloro-ethane (DDT)	Lithocholic acid
Polychlorinated (brominated) biphenyl(s)	Choline-deficient diet
3-(3,5-dichlorophenyl)5,5'-dimethyloxazoline-1,4-dione	Methapyrilene
	Orotic acid
2,3,7,8-tetrachlorodibenzo-p-dioxin (TCDD)	
Hexachlorocyclohexane	

[*]Microsomal monoxygenases.

We have been investigating a few selected aspects of the mechanism of liver tumor promotion by a diet devoid of choline, a choline deficient (CD) diet. The diet is an effective promoter of the emergence of early presumptive preneoplastic foci of γ-glutamyltranspeptidase (GGT)-positive hepatocytes as well as of the progression of GGT-positive foci to hepatomas (3,4). A CD diet with a high fat content (14%) exerted a stronger promoting action than a CD diet with a low fat content (5%) (5). The addition of phenobarbital, another type of liver tumor promoter, to a CD diet resulted in a marked synergistic enhancement on liver tumor promotion (6). In both cases, however, the efficacy of the promotion was not directly correlated with the extent of liver cell proliferation induced by the diets (5,7). Thus, as in the case of skin tumor promotion (8,9), the stimulation of cell proliferation in target cells may be important but may not be sufficient conditions for liver tumor promotion. It has been postulated that certain promoters of carcinogenesis may act by generating oxygen radicals and resulting in lipid peroxidation (10,11). This notion stemmed from the observation that several free radical generating compounds such as benzoyl peroxide, lauryl peroxide and chloroperbenzoic acid have been shown to induce skin tumors in mice (12,13). Lipid peroxidation may lead to structural and functional perturbation of the cellular membranes and/or DNA, and such alterations may serve as an underlying mechanism of tumor promotion. Among promoters of liver tumor induction, phenobarbital, TCDD and a CD diet have been reported to induce lipid peroxidation in the liver under certain experimental conditions (14,15,16,17). In this paper, we will present some of our recent data on, modification of the CD-diet mediated promotion by changing the quality of dietary fat, generation of lipid peroxidation by a CD diet and the effects of phenobarbital on CD-diet-induced lipid peroxidation.

Quality of Fat as a Modifying Factor of Liver Tumor Promotion by a CD Diet

Experimentally, dietary fats, both quantity and quality, play important roles in the genesis of cancers of many organs (18,19). Earlier, we demonstrated that a high fat CD diet is a more efficient liver tumor promoter than the diet with a low fat content (5). The proportion of saturated and polyunsaturated fatty acids in a CD diet is an important determining factor for the severity of the diet-induced fatty liver (20,21). Saturated fatty acids containing 14 to 18 carbons in the diet appeared to increase the deposition of fat in the liver more so than unsaturated fatty acids (22). It became of considerable interest to determine whether and how changing the quality of fat in a CD diet modifies the promoting efficacy of the diet.

Male Sprague Dawley rats weighing 180-200 gm were initiated with a single dose of diethylnitrosamine (DEN) at 40 mg/KG 18 hours after partial hepatectomy. One week thereafter, groups of rats were fed a choline supplemented (CS) or CD diet in which the degree of saturation of fat was obtained by using hydrogenated vegetable oil (saturated) (Primex) and corn oil (polyunsaturated) (CO). The regular CS and CD diets contained 4% CO and 10% Primex while the CS and CD-CO diet contained 14% CO and the CS, CD-primex diets 14% Primex. After 7 weeks of promotion by the different dietary regimens, the animals were killed and enzyme altered foci (GGT) in the liver were quantitated (3). The results as shown in Table II indicate that feeding the CS diets of different fat quality showed no promoting activity. The number of GGT-positive foci developed after 7 weeks of promotion by the CD diet with predominantly CO was 2.6 times higher than that by the regular CD diet.

TABLE II

Induction of GGT(+) Foci by Various Regimens of Dietary Promotion.

Group[*]	Dietary Promotion	No. Foci/cm^2
1	CS = Regular	0.98 ± 0.3[**]
2	CS = Corn Oil	1.20 ± 0.5
3	CS = Primex	0.90 ± 0.4
4	CD = Regular	10.8 ± 1.6[***]
5	CD = Corn Oil	28.5 ± 5.0
6	CD = Primex	4.9 ± 1.0

[*]Initiation: Each animal received a single intraperitoneal
injection of diethylnitrosamine (DEN) (40 mg/KG) 18 hours
after partial hepatectomy.
[**]Each figure represents the Mean ± S.E. of 7-8 rats.
Differences between the means were evaluated statistically
by Student's t test.
[***]P < 0.02 when compared with group 5 and P < 0.05 when compared with group 6.

        The CD diet with Primex as the sole source of fat was a
less effective promoter than the regular CD diet. Therefore,
inclusion of polyunsaturated fat in the CD diet enhances the
promoting action of the CD diet. Diets high in unsaturated fat
per se appear to promote pancreatic carcinogenesis in azaserine-
treated rats (23). Studies with the 7, 12, dimethylbenz(α)-
anthracene-rat model of mammary gland carcinogenesis, unsaturated
fat promoted more mammary tumors than saturated fat (24). In the
present study, the modification of the quality of fat in a CS diet
showed no significant effects on the emergence of GGT-positive
foci in the DEN-treated rats indicating that polyunsaturated fat
per se is not a good promoter of liver carcinogenesis. Since
there is good experimental evidence that polyunsaturation of fat
in a CD diet lessens the severity of fatty liver (21), the
efficacy of the promoting action does not appear to be related to
the amount of fat accumulated in the liver.

Lipid Peroxidation in the Liver of Rats Fed a CD Diet

One of the early effects of a CD diet on the liver is metabolic
alterations of phospholipids. These include a decrease in phosphatidylcholine (25), a shift toward an increase in the content of
polyunsaturated species of phosphatidylcholine (26), and a

decrease in the hepatic phosphatidylcholine/phosphatidylethanol-amine ratio (27). These changes occur predominantly in cellular membranes, and may lead to disturbances of many membrane associated functions. Cell membranes may become vulnerable to free radical attack. Indeed, feeding a CD diet has been shown to induce lipid peroxidation in the kidney of weanling rats and in the liver of young rats (28,17). Lipid peroxidation in the kidney after feeding a CD diet has been suggested to play a pivotal role in the development of the pathological lesions, called acute hemorrhagic kidney (28).

Recently, evidence has been presented to indicate that a CD diet induces subtle cell necrosis in the liver which may trigger compensatory cell proliferation (29,30). Liver cell proliferation has been repeatedly shown to act as a good promoter of liver tumor induction in both mice and rats (30,31). However, it remains questionable that cell proliferation is solely responsible for liver tumor promotion. Phenobarbital, a prototype of liver tumor promoters is not a good stimulator of cell proliferation after repeated injections or chronic feeding (6). It is possible that the secondary effects of lipid peroxidation on cell membranes and/or DNA may serve as an underlying mechanism of certain tumor promoters (10). Accordingly, we re-examined whether feeding a CD diet results in lipid peroxidation in the liver and how the changes in the quality of fat modify such pathological lesions.

Male Sprague Dawley rats (180-200 gm) were fed CS, CD, CS-CO and CD-CO diets for for 2, 7 and 14 days. The microsomes were isolated from the liver and the total lipids extracted by the methods of Folch et al. (33). 1 mg lipid samples in 1 ml CH_3OH were scanned spectrophotometrically from 300 through 220 nm. The mean difference spectra were obtained by subtracting the mean values of the control spectra from the mean values of the experi-mental spectra (34). Diene conjugates resulting from a rearrange-ment of the double bonds in unsaturated lipids characteristically absorb at 233 nm (34).

Figure 1 shows the results obtained 2 days after feeding various diets. There is no significant difference in the absorbance patterns of microsomal lipids of rats fed a CD and CS diet. In rats fed a CD-CO diet, there is a distinct peak at 233 nm as evidenced from the profile of the difference spectrum. Feeding a CD diet for 1 week resulted in generation of diene conjugates which remained evident after 2 weeks of the dietary feeding (Figure 2). Feeding a CD-CO diet for 1 and 2 weeks induced higher levels of diene conjugates as compared to 2 days after the dietary feeding (Figure 3). At 2 weeks, the level of the difference spectrum in the CD-CO group is considerably higher than that in the CD group.

The results of the present experiments confirmed the earlier observation of Ugazio et al. (17) that feeding a CD diet induces lipid peroxidation of the microsomal membrane lipids in the liver. Similar findings were also reported recently by Ghoshal et al. (35) who demonstrated that in rats fed a CD diet lipid peroxida-tion of nuclear membrane lipids occurred much earlier than that of microsomal lipids. The significance of the early and selective effects of a CD diet on nuclear membrane is not clear. The onset

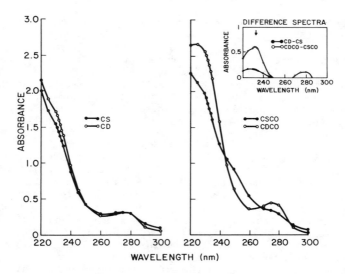

Figure 1. Conjugated diene absorption in rat liver 2 days after feeding choline-deficient (CD), choline-supplemented (CS), choline-deficient with corn oil (CDCO) or choline-supplemented with corn oil (CS-CO) diets. The difference spectrum (inset) is obtained by subtracting the mean values of the control spectra from the mean values of the experimental spectra.

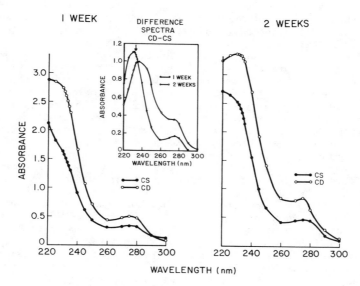

Figure 2. Conjugated diene absorption in the liver of rats fed a CD or a CS diet for 1 and 2 weeks. The inset shows the difference spectrum.

of detectable diene conjugate formation in the rats fed a CD-CO diet occurred prior to those fed a regular CD diet. The intensity of lipid peroxidation was higher in rats fed a CD-CO diet, which correlates with the efficacy of the promoting action exerted by a CD or CD-CO diet. The critical questions to be answered are whether lipid peroxidation is responsible for the induction of liver cell necrosis by the diet and subsequent stimulation of cell proliferation or whether it generates other secondary effects on other cellular macromolecules. Lipid peroxidation may further damage the structural and functional properties of the plasma membranes and/or cellular DNA, and the changes in these structures were frequently associated with certain types of tumor promoters (36). Further studies are needed to clarify the consequences of lipid peroxidation in liver cells induced by a CD diet and their relationship to the action of tumor promotion.

Effects of Phenobarbital on a CD Diet-induced Lipid Peroxidation

As indicated earlier, both phenobarbital and a CD diet are independently good promoters of liver carcinogenesis. It is not known, however, whether they share any common mechanisms. Our earlier observation (7) that when phenobarbital and a CD diet are combined, they exerted a synergistic effect, strongly suggests a different mechanism of action by each agent. Hahn et al. (14,15) earlier demonstrated that intraperitoneal injections of phenobarbital to rats on a relatively high fat diet induced lipid peroxidation in liver microsomes. Weddle et al. (37) also showed that endogenous lipid peroxidation is enhanced in liver cells from phenobarbital-treated animals. Since we observed that lipid peroxidation of rat liver microsomes was one of the early responses to feeding of a CD diet, it became of interest to determine whether the addition of phenobarbital to a CD diet modifies the extent of the diet-induced lipid peroxidation.

Groups of rats (male Sprague Dawley) were fed a CS or CD diet or the same diets containing 0.06% phenobarbital for 2 weeks. Lipid peroxidation of liver microsomes was determined by the methods described above. The results are shown in Figure 4. The distinct peak absorbance of diene conjugates was again noted in rats fed a CD diet. In both groups of rats fed either a CS or CD diet containing phenobarbital, no peaks corresponding to diene conjugates were apparent. Thus, under the present experimental conditions, the administration of phenobarbital did not induce lipid peroxidation of liver microsomes, and, rather suppressed the CD diet-induced lipid peroxidation. The demonstration of lipid peroxidation in phenobarbital treated rats reported by Hahn et al. (14,15) may be due, in part, to the use of a high fat diet in their experiments.

Our results of the effects of phenobarbital on the CD-diet-induced lipid peroxidation are analogous to the earlier findings that phenobarbital inhibited a CD diet-induced cell proliferation. Since the combination of phenobarbital and a CD diet resulted in a synergistic effect on promotion, the findings support the notion that the promoting effects of a CD diet and phenobarbital are mediated through different mechanisms. While sustained liver cell

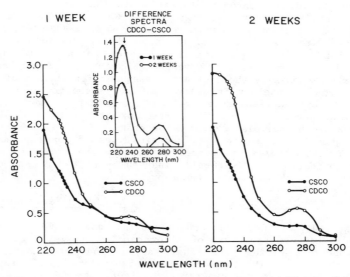

Figure 3. Conjugated diene absorption in the liver of rats fed a CD-CO or a CSCO for 1 and 2 weeks. The inset shows the difference spectrum.

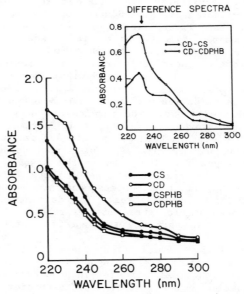

Figure 4. Conjugated diene absorption in the liver of rats fed a CS or CD diet and the same diets containing 0.06% phenobarbital (CSPHB, CDPHB) for 2 weeks. The difference spectrum is in the inset.

proliferation and/or membrane lipid peroxidation may be important underlying mechanism(s) of CD diet promotion, phenobarbital and other barbiturates may exert their effect through different, as yet unclarified mechanisms.

The finding that the combination of two promoters of different mechanistic action may act synergistically has possible practical significance in the analysis of the genesis of human cancers. As indicated in Table 1, many liver tumor promoters are xenobiotics found in environmental contaminants, and risks of exposure to these chemicals by humans are always high. A high fat diet and polyunsaturated fat have been implicated as promoters of several types of cancer, such as of the breast and pancreas. We have shown that the dietary deficiency of certain nutritional components exert a strong promoting stimulus to liver tumor development. It is likely that the combination of the diet-mediated tumor promotion and exposure to promoting chemicals may result in a greater risk of developing cancers. Further elucidation of the mechanisms by which different tumor promoters exert their action is critically important to understand the significance of the interactions of two or more types of promoters in mutually enhancing their actions.

Acknowledgments

The authors wish to thank Ms. L.A. Witkowski for her technical assistance and Mrs. D. Pronio for typing of the manuscript. The work was supported by grants awarded by the National Cancer Institute, Department of Health and Human Service (CA-26556) and by the Samuel Emma Winters Foundation.

Literature Cited

1. Farber, E. Biochim. Biophys. Acta 1980, 605, 149–66.
2. Pitot, H.C.; Sirica, A.E. Biochim. Biophys. Acta 1980, 605, 191–215.
3. Sells, M.A.; Katyal, S.L.; Sell, S.; Shinozuka, H.; Lombardi, B. Brit. J. Cancer 1979, 40, 274–83.
4. Takahashi, S.; Lombardi, B.; Shinozuka, H. Int. J. Cancer 1982, 29, 445–50.
5. Shinozuka, H.; Takahashi, S.; Lombardi, B.; Abanobi, S.E. Cancer Letters 1982, 16–43–50.
6. Abanobi, S.E.; Lombardi, B; Shinozuka, H. Cancer Res. 1982, 42, 412–15.
7. Shinozuka, H.; Lombardi, B. Cancer Res. 1980, 40, 3846–9.
8. Boutwell, R.D. Prog. Exp. Tumor Res. 1964, 4, 207–50.
9. Colburn, N.H.; Wendel, E.J.; Abruzzo, G. Proc. Nat. Acad. Sci. 1981, 78, 6912–16.
10. Ames, B.N. Science 1983, 221, 1256–64.
11. Copeland, E.S. Cancer Res. 1983, 43, 5631–7.
12. Slaga, T.J.; Klein-Szanto, A.J.P.; Triplett, L.L.; Yotti, L.P.; Trosko, J.E. Science 1981, 213, 1023–25.
13. Logani, M.K.; Solanki, V.; Slaga, J.J. Carcinogenesis 1982, 3, 1303–6.
14. Hahn, H.K.J.; Tuma, D.J.; Barak, A.J.; Sorrell, M.F. Biochem. Pharmacol. 1976, 25, 769–72.

15. Hahn, H.K.J.; Barak, A.J.; Tuma, D.J.; Sorrell, M.F. Biochem Pharmacol. 1977, 26, 164-5.
16. Stohs, S.J.; Hassan, M.Q.; Murray, W.J. Biochem. Biophys. Res. Commu. 1983, 111, 854-9.
17. Ugazio, G.; Gabriel, L.; Burdino, E. Lo Sperimentale 1967, 117, 1-17.
18. Clayson, D.B. Cancer Res. 1975, 35, 3292-300.
19. Rogers, A.E. Cancer Res. 1983, 43, 2477s-84s.
20. Channon, H.J.; Hanson, S.W.F.; Loizides, P.A. Biochem. J. 1942, 36, 214-20.
21. Carroll, C.; Williams, L. J. Nutr. 1977, 107, 1263-8.
22. Benton, D.A.; Harper, A.E.; Elvehjen, C.A. J. Biol. Chem. 1956, 218, 693-700.
23. Roebuck, B.D.; ;Yager, J.D. Jr.; Longnecker, D.S.; Wilpone, S.A. Cancer Res. 1981, 41, 3961-6.
24. Carroll, K.K., Khor, H.T. Lipids 1971, 415-20.
25. Chen, S.H.; Estes, L.W.; Lombardi, B. Exp. Mol. Path. 1972, 176-86.
26. Lombardi, B.; Pani, P.; Schlunk, F.F.; Chen, S.H. Lipids 1969, 67-75.
27. Chalvardjian, A. Canad. J. Biochem. 1970, 48, 1234-40.
28. Monserrat, A.J.; Ghoshal, A.K.; Hartroft, W.S.; Porta, E.A. Am. J. Path. 1969, 55, 163-90.
29. Ghoshal, A.K.; Ahluwali, M.; Farber, E. Am. J. Path. 1983, 113, 309-14.
30. Giambarressi, L.I.; Katyal, S.L.; Lombardi, B. Br. J. Cancer 1982, 46, 825-9.
31. Cole, L.J.; Nowell, P.C. Science 1965, 150, 1782-6.
32. Pound, A.W.; McGuire, L.J. Br. J. Cancer 1978, 37, 585-94.
33. Folch, J.; Lees, M.; Sloane Stanley, G.H. J. Biol. Chem. 1957, 226, 497-509.
34. Recknagel, R.O.; Glende, E.A. Jr.; Waller, R.L.; Lowrey, K. In Toxicology of the Liver 1982, Ed. Plaa, G.L.; Hewitt, W.R., Raven Press, p. 213-241.
35. Ghoshal, A.K.; Rushmore, T.H.; Lim, Y.P.; Farber, E. Proc. Am. Assoc. Cancer Res. 1984, 25, 94.
36. Emerit, I.; Cerutti, P.A. Proc. Nat. Acad. Sci. 1982, 79, 7509.
37. Weddle, C.C.; Hornbrook, K.K.; McCay, P.B. J. Biol. Chem. 1976, 251, 4973,8.

RECEIVED November 30, 1984

Modulation of Chemical Mutagenesis in a *Salmonella*/Mammalian Tissue Bioassay by Vitamin A and Other Retinoids

MALCOLM B. BAIRD

Masonic Medical Research Laboratory, Utica, NY 13504

Mutagenesis induced in Salmonella typhimurium by 2-fluorenamine and other chemical carcinogens was inhibited by low levels of retinol and other retinoids when carcinogen activation was carried out by rat liver microsomes. In contrast, low levels of retinoids enhanced mutagenesis when carcinogen activation was mediated by whole liver homogenates. There was no effect of the provitamin β-carotene in this test system. The enhancement factor was shown to be localized to the post-microsomal soluble fraction, was heat labile, has a molecular weight between 50,000 and 100,000 daltons, and was not precipitable by $(NH_4)_2 SO_4$ in the range from 1.0 to 2.0 M. The results parallel those observed in whole animal studies, which generally show that high levels of vitamin A inhibit, while low levels enhance tumorigenesis. Thus, these studies demonstrate the utility of in vitro short term bioassays in gaining a more thorough understanding of the role of nutritional and other factors on the metabolism of xenobiotics.

Vitamin A and its derivatives, the so-called retinoids (1), exert anti-tumor activity at a variety of organ sites in various animal model systems (2-8). Recent studies suggest that high serum levels of vitamin A (retinol) are related to a reduced tumor incidence in human populations (9-10), and that a high dietary intake of foods rich in vitamin A reduces tumor yield (11-14). Thus, there is considerable interest, and effort made in elucidating the mechanism by which vitamin A and retinoids exert anti-tumor activity.

It is widely accepted that retinoids inhibit tumor growth and development, or the promotional phase of tumorigenesis (15) since it is well known that vitamin A plays a marked, as yet ill-defined, role in controlling the growth and differentiation of epidermis and epidermally-derived structures (16-18). Experimental evidence for this hypothesis rests primarily on the observation that conditions of hypervitaminosis A significantly inhibit tumor production even when initiated after application of the carcinogenic insult. Thus, 13-cis-retinoic acid inhibits the induction of transitional cell

0097-6156/85/0277-0337$06.00/0

tumors in rodent bladder by N-butyl-N(4-hydroxybutyl) nitrosamine
(7), and squamous cell tumors induced in the same organ by N-methyl-
N-nitrosourea (8), even when the retinoid is applied at some time
interval following carcinogen treatment. Therefore, retinoids appear
to modulate the promotional phase of tumorigenesis in rat bladder
epithelium when tumors are induced by direct-acting carcinogens.
    However, it seemed to us that suggesting a single role for
retinoids vis-á-vis tumor formation seemed overly conservative,
especially when other experimental observations were considered.
Georgieff (19) demonstrated that a number of compounds, including
the provitamin β-carotene, were effective at trapping active forms of
oxygen. Hill and Shih (20) showed that fourteen different forms of
vitamin A effectively altered the metabolism of polycyclic aromatic
hydrocarbons (PAHs), including 3,4-benzo[a]pyrene. A vast number,
if not the majority, of chemical carcinogens including 3,4-benzo[a]
pyrene require metabolic activation to the ultimate carcinogenic form
(21). Furthermore, this transformation is mediated by tissue mixed-
function oxidases which utilize an active form of oxygen (22). Thus,
we hypothesized that retinoids inhibit chemically-induced tumorigenesis by modulating the activation of these compounds (23), thereby
affecting the initiation phase of tumor formation (15).
    We chose to test our hypothesis using a Salmonella/mammalian
microsome test system, since we could utilize this system to isolate
the effects of retinoids in modulating the metabolic activation of
chemical carcinogens to forms which can covalently interact with
bacterial DNA. We also wished to examine, and possibly establish,
the limits of usefulness of the widely used Salmonella bioassay in
examining the modulation of xenobiotic metabolism by nutritional and
other factors.

Methods of Procedure

The Salmonella plate bioassay was used in these studies as described
in detail by Ames and his co-workers (24-26), unless otherwise
indicated. Details for obtaining rat liver preparations, and of the
assay itself, have been described previously (23). All determinations were carried out in triplicate, and all experiments were
repeated at least three times. Experiments were rigidly controlled
by taking into consideration the recommendations of de Serres and
Shelby (27). All other pertinent experimental details appear in the
appropriate figure headings, table legends or in the text.

Modulation of Mutagenesis by Retinoids

Enhancement of Mutagenicity by Retinol or Retinyl Acetate. We
initially examined the effect of vitamin A alcohol (retinol) on 2-
fluorenamine-induced mutagenesis in S. typhimurium (TA98) (23).
These studies clearly demonstrated that high levels of retinol
totally inhibited mutagenicity when carcinogen activation was
carried out by S9 (9,000xg supernatant of whole liver homogenate) or
by microsomes sedimented from S9 by centrifugation at 105,000xg for
one hour. Control studies have eliminated the likelihood that the
effect of retinol was a result of one of several possible artifacts
in the standard plate test. One such artifact was the plate test
itself. Therefore, the modulation of mutagenicity induced by

2-fluorenamine by retinol was determined in a liquid assay. Salmonella typhimurium (TA98) was grown overnight in a nutrient bath.
Aliquots of the bacterial suspension were centrifuged at 2,800 rpm
for five minutes, and the bacteria resuspended in sterile 0.155 M KCl
to a concentration of $\approx$ 2-3x10^9 bacteria/ml. 0.1 ml of bacterial
suspension, 0.5 ml of S9 mix, 1.0 µg 2-fluorenamine and varying concentrations of retinol were incubated with gentle shaking at 37°C,
for one hour, following which the tube contents were mixed with 2 ml
of molten top agar and poured onto petri dishes containing Vogel-
Bonner minimal medium E agar. The results of this study are shown
in Table I, which yielded results virtually identical to those
obtained in the plate test.

Table I. Dependence upon carcinogen activator source of
2-FA-induced mutagenesis in S. typhimurium
(TA98) in liquid culture by retinol

additions to culture medium[a]	his[+] revertants per plate	
	S9	microsomes
bacteria	16	23
bacteria + 2-FA	243	210
bacteria + 2-FA + retinol:		
5 µg	268	188
10 µg	385	162
25 µg	280	123
50 µg	122	19
100 µg	70	9

[a] 1.0 µg 2-FA and the retinol were added to the incubation medium in
10 µl dimethyl sulfoxide.

Polychlorinated biphenyls (PCBs) are routinely used to induce rodent
hepatic mixed-function oxidases in tissues used in the Ames test.
The presence of PCBs in the tissue preparations themselves, or an
effect of PCBs in vivo could be responsible for the retinol effect
on mutagenicity induced by 2-fluorenamine. This possibility was
eliminated by preparing S9 and microsomes from male rats not treated
with PCBs. Utilizing these preparations in the plate test yielded
results identical to those obtained in the standard assay (Table II).

Table II. Modification of 2-FA-induced mutagenesis in S. typhimurium TA98 by retinol utilizing carcinogen activation
sources prepared from rats not treated with polychlorinated biphenyls

additions to plate[a]	his[+] revertants per plate	
	S9	microsomes
bacteria	4	8
bacteria + 2-FA	380	39
bacteria + 2-FA + retinol	432	15

[a] 1.0 µg 2-FA and 5.0 µg retinol were added to the top agar in 10 µl
dimethyl sulfoxide.

We had previously eliminated the possibility that retinol affected
bacterial viability in this assay. The likelihood of a non-specific
inhibitory effect of retinol was also eliminated, since there was no
effect of vitamin A alcohol on mutagenicity induced by adriamycin, a
direct-acting mutagen in Salmonella (23). Thus, these findings
demonstrated that retinol inhibited the metabolism of 2-fluorenamine
by rat liver tissue preparations to forms capable of producing mutations in S. typhimurium.

      These conclusions were subsequently confirmed by other workers.
Busk and Ahlborg (28) have shown that retinol inhibits the mutagenicity of aflatoxin B_1, an hepatic carcinogen which requires metabolic activation for mutagenicity in Salmonella, while having no
effect on mutagenicity induced by the direct-acting carcinogen
diepoxybutane. More recently Rocchi et al. (29) have shown that
vitamin A palmitate inhibits the mutagenicity of three different
polycyclic aromatic hydrocarbons (PAHs) in EUE cells, a human epi-
thelial-like cell line. The inhibition of mutagenicity by vitamin A
palmitate correlated directly with a decrease in covalent binding of
metabolites of radioactively labelled PAHs to cellular DNA. Thus,
naturally occurring retinoids inhibit the mutagenicity of PAHs,
aflatoxin B_1 and aromatic amines, procarcinogens which require metabolic biotransformation to active forms of Salmonella or in human
cell short term assays.

Enhancement of Mutagenicity by Retinol and Retinyl Acetate. We
originally reported that low concentrations of retinol often enhance
mutagenicity when carcinogen activation was mediated by S9, but
not when activated by microsomes (23). This effect is illustrated
for retinyl acetate in Figure 1, which demonstrates that low concentrations of retinyl acetate actually enhance mutagenicity when
activated by S9, while high concentrations inhibit mutagenicity.
No such enhancement by retinyl acetate was observed when 2-fluoren-
amine activation was carried out by rat liver microsomes prepared
from S9 (Figure 2).

      We have begun to characterize the retinoid enhancement factor.
Reconstitution studies clearly show that the factor is present in
the post-microsomal soluble fraction (Table III) in rat liver (there
is a factor(s) present in the 17,000xg pellet which normally inhibits
this factor (Table III)). The retinoid enhancing factor is heat
sensitive, since its activity in the presence of retinol is lost
when supernatant is incubated for 15 minutes at 45°C (Figure 3).
Similar results were obtained by incubating the supernatant at 50°C
for five minutes.

      The postmicrosomal supernatant was filtered through Amicon
membrane filters of varying pore size, and assayed for its effectiveness in the presence of retinol. These results are summarized in
Table IV which shows that the enhancing factor has a molecular weight
between 50,000 and 100,000 daltons. Finally, this factor is not
precipitated from the soluble fraction by $(NH_4)_2SO_4$ in the range
from 1.0 to 2.0 M.

      Retinoid enhancement activity appears to be distinct from the
enhancement activity reported to result from the addition of post-

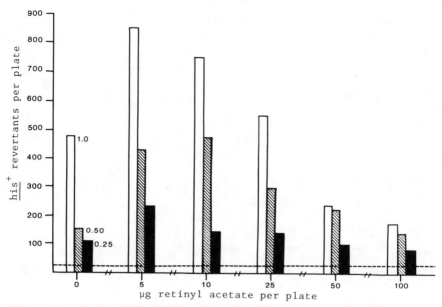

Figure 1. Modulation of S9-mediated 2-fluorenamine (2-FA)-induced metagenesis in S. typhimurium (TA98) by retinyl acetate. Horizontal dashed line shows average number of spontaneous his[+] revertants per plate Open bars - 1.0µg 2-FA/plate; cross-hatched bars - 0.5µg 2-FA/plate; solid bars - 0.25µg 2-FA/plate.

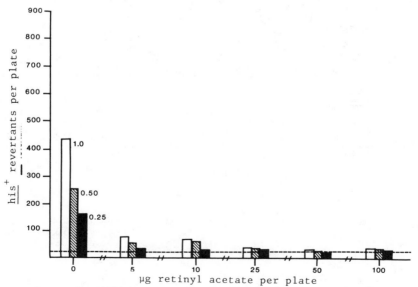

Figure 2. Inhibition of microsome-mediated 2-fluorenamine (2-FA)-induced mutagenesis in S. typhimurium (TA98) by retinyl acetate. Horizontal dashed line shows average number of spontaneous his[+] revertants per plate. Open bars - 1.0µg 2-FA/plate; cross-hatched bars - 0.5µg 2-FA/plate; solid bars - 0.25µg 2-FA/plate.

Table III. Complete reconstitution of the enhancement of 2-FA-
           induced mutagenesis in S. typhimurium (TA98) by retinol

additions to plate[a]	his[+] revertants per plate
bacteria	12
bacteria + S9	32
bacteria + microsomes	26
bacteria + supt. + microsomes	24
bacteria + supt. + microsomes + 17,000g pellet	31
bacteria + S9 + 2-FA	115
bacteria + microsomes + 2-FA	131
bacteria + supt. + microsomes + 2-FA	124
bacteria + supt. + microsomes + 17,000g pellet + 2-FA	84
bacteria + S9 + 2-FA retinol	269
bacteria + microsomes + 2-FA + retinol	29
bacteria + supt. + microsomes + 2-FA + retinol	400
bacteria + supt. + microsomes + 17,000g pellet + 2-FA retinol	133

[a]2-fluorenamine (0.5μg per plate) and retinol (10μg) were added in 10μl
 dimethyl sulfoxide.

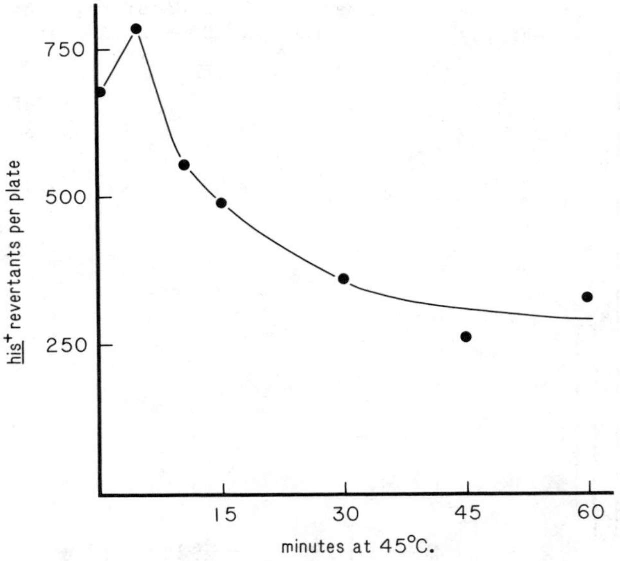

Figure 3. Thermal inactivation of the 105,000xg cytosolic
retinoid enhancement activity of 2-fluorenamine-induced mutagenesis in S. typhimurium (TA98).

Table IV. Membrane filtration of the soluble factor which effects
enhancement by retinol of 2–FA–induced mutagenesis in S.
typhimurium (TA98)

experiment #	additions to plate[a]	his[+] revertants per plate
	bacteria	17
	bacteria + S9	33
	bacteria + S9 + 2–FA	541
1	bacteria + microsomes	31
	bacteria + microsomes + 2–FA	437
	bacteria + microsomes + supt. + 2–FA + retinol	715
	bacteria + microsomes + 2–FA + retinol + filtrate:	
	300,000 mw	549
	100,000 mw	420
	bacteria	36
	bacteria + microsomes	50
2	bacteria + microsomes + 2–FA	198
	bacteria + microsomes + supt. + 2–FA + retinol	718
	bacteria + microsomes + 2–FA + retinol + filtrate:	
	50,000 mw	64
	20,000 mw	51
	1,000 mw	66

[a]2-fluorenamine (2–FA, 0.5µg per plate) and retinol (50µg per plate)
were added to the top agar in 10µl dimethyl sulfoxide.

105,000xg supernatant to purified and washed microsomes (30-32),
since retinoid enhancement activity is present in S9 preparations.
The greater-than-expected enhancement of 2-FA mutagenesis when S9 is
reconstituted by mixing purified microsomes and post 105,000xg supernatant, in the presence of retinol may reflect the summation of two
(or more) enhancement activities.

Modulation of Mutagenesis by β-carotene and 13-cis-Retinoic Acid. The
provitamin β-carotene, and a synthetic derivative of vitamin A, 13-
cis-retinoic acid, were examined with respect to their capacity to
modulate 2-fluorenamine-induced mutagenicity in Salmonella. These
studies were carried out since dietary and serum levels of β-carotene
vary widely among humans. Also, there is considerable interest in
the anti-tumor activity of 13-cis-retinoic acid and other synthetic
retinoids.
      When carcinogen activation was mediated by S9, high concentra-
tions of 13-cis-retinoic acid were slightly inhibitory toward mutagenicity in Salmonella (Table V), while 13-cis-retinoic acid was
extremely inhibitory to mutagenesis induced by 2-fluorenamine when
carcinogen activation was carried out by microsomes (Table VI).

Table V.   Effect of retinol, 13-cis-retinoic acid and β-carotene on
           2-FA-induced mutagenesis in S. typhimurium (TA98) mediated
           by S9

additions to plate[1]	his^+ revertants per plate
bacteria	24
bacteria + S9	31
bacteria + S9 + 2-FA	366
bacteria + S9 + 2-FA + 13-cis- RA:	
50 µg	297
100 µg	235
bacteria + S9 + 2-FA + β-carotene:	
50 µg	342
100 µg	339
200 µg	367
bacteria + S9 + 2-FA + retinol	84

Carcinogen activation carried out by 5µl S9 per plate.

[1] 2-fluorenamine (2-FA, 0.5µg per plate), 13-cis-retinoic acid (13-cis
RA), β-carotene, and retinol (50µg per plate) were added to top agar
in 10µl dimethyl sulfoxide.

In no instance did the synthetic retinoid possess as great an inhibitory capacity as do retinol or retinyl acetate. In addition, the
provitamin β-carotene had no effect on mutagenicity of 2-fluorenamine
in Salmonella regardless of the carcinogen activation system (Tables
III and IV). Thus, β-carotene would apparently require enzymatic
cleavage to vitamin A in order to have an effect in this in vitro
bioassay and exerts no role by itself in modulating the metabolism of
chemical carcinogens in the model system.

Table VI. Effect of retinol, 13-<u>cis</u>-retinoic acid and β-carotene on
          2-FA-induced mutagenesis in <u>S</u>. <u>typhimurium</u> (TA98) mediated
          by purified microsomes

additions to plate [1]	<u>his</u>[+] revertants per plate
bacteria	10
bacteria + microsomes	35
bacteria + microsomes + 2-FA	318
bacteria + microsomes + 2-FA + 13-<u>cis</u>-RA:	
50µg	198
100µg	168
200µg	99
bacteria + microsomes + 2-FA + β-carotene:	
50µg	314
100µg	256
200µg	273
bacteria + microsomes + 2-FA + retinol	34

Carcinogen activation carried out by 5µl purified microsomes per
plate.

[1] 2-fluorenamine (2-FA, 0.5µg per plate), 13-<u>cis</u>-retinoic acid
(13-<u>cis</u>-RA), β-carotene and retinol (50µg per plate) were added in
10µl dimethyl sulfoxide.

<u>Modulation of Mutagenicity by the Intestinal Carcinogen 3,2'-Dimethyl-
4-Aminobiphenyl</u>. We wished to examine the effect of retinol, β-
carotene and 13-<u>cis</u>-retinoic acid on yet another aromatic amine,
3,2'-dimethyl-4-aminobiphenyl (DMAB), which is an intestinal carcinogen in rats (<u>33,34</u>). When the carcinogen was activated by S9, 13-
<u>cis</u>-retinoic acid slightly enhanced mutagenicity in <u>Salmonella</u>
(Table VII), but was extremely inhibitory toward mutagenicity when
the carcinogen was activated by purified microsomes (Table VIII).
Retinol in high concentrations inhibited DMAB mutagenicity in
<u>Salmonella</u> regardless of the activation system (Tables VII and VIII).
There was no effect of β-carotene upon the mutagenicity of DMAB in
<u>Salmonella</u>.

Conclusions and Significance

The following conclusions may be drawn from these studies:
1) High levels of retinol or retinyl acetate inhibit mutagenicity
induced by aromatic amines in a <u>Salmonella</u>/mammalian microsome assay
when carcinogen activation is carried out by S9 or purified microsomes.
2) Low levels of retinol or retinyl acetate enhance mutagenicity
induced by 2-fluorenamine in <u>Salmonella</u> <u>typhimurium</u> when activation
is carried out by S9, while inhibiting mutagenicity when activation
is mediated by microsomes.
3) There is no effect of retinoids on mutagenicity induced in
<u>Salmonella</u> by direct-acting carcinogens.

Table VII. Effect of retinol, 13-cis-retinoic acid and β-carotene on
            DMAB-induced mutagenesis in S. typhimurium (TA98) mediated
            by S9

additions to plate[1]	his+ revertants per plate
bacteria	13
bacteria + S9	32
bacteria + S9 + DMAB	309
bacteria + S9 + DMAB + 13-cis-RA:	
50µg	500
100µg	440
200µg	501
bacteria + S9 + DMAB + β-carotene:	
50µg	275
100µg	303
200µg	312
bacteria + S9 + DMAB + retinol	399

Carcinogen activation carried out by 5µl S9 per plate.

[1] 3,2'-dimethyl-4-amino-biphenyl (DMAB, 5.0µg per plate), 13-cis-
retinoic acid (13-cis-RA), β-carotene and retinol (50µg) were added
to top agar in 10µl dimethyl sulfoxide.

Table VIII. Effect of 13-cis-retinoic acid, β-carotene and retinol on
             2-FA-induced mutagenesis in S. typhimurium (TA98) mediated
             by purified microsomes

additions to plate[1]	his+ revertants per plate
bacteria	11
bacteria + microsomes	35
bacteria + microsomes + DMAB	152
bacteria + microsomes + DMAB + 13-cis-RA:	
50µg	87
100µg	48
200µg	46
bacteria + microsomes + DMAB + β-carotene:	
50µg	164
100µg	149
200µg	129
bacteria + microsomes + DMAB + retinol	28

Carcinogen activation carried out by 5µl purified microsomes per
plate.

[1] 3,2'-dimethyl-4-amino-biphenyl (DMAB, 5.0µg per plate), 13-cis-
retinoic acid (13-cis-RA), β-carotene and retinol (50µg per plate)
were added in 10µl dimethyl sulfoxide.

4) The modulation of mutagenicity of aromatic amines in Salmonella is not a result of (a) PCB treatment of rats, or the presence of residual PCB's in liver preparations, (b) vagaries of the Salmonella plate test, or (c) the effect of retinoids upon bacterial viability.
5) Similar effects were observed with the synthetic retinoid 13-cis-retinoic acid, while β-carotene was without effect in modulating the mutagenicity of aromatic amines in Salmonella.
6) The retinol enhancing factor is thermosensitive, localized in the soluble liver fraction, not precipitated by $(NH_4)_2SO_4$ in the range from 1.0 to 2.0 M, and has a molecular weight between 50,000 and 100,000 daltons.

The results of our studies, as well as those from other laboratories, clearly indicate that the Salmonella/mammalian microsome assay and other short term bioassays have been useful specifically in elucidating the mechanism by which retinoids modulate mutagenesis by modulating the activation of chemical carcinogens which are mutagenic in these assays. We obviously recognize that extrapolation from in vitro assays to phenomena which occur in intact animals is fraught with inherent unpredictability. However, it has been clearly shown that vitamin A inhibits the initiation phase of tumorgenesis in the rat mammary gland by 7,12-dimethylbenzanthracene (33,36) since the greatest inhibitory effect is manifest when vitamin A is present during the period of the time of carcinogen application. In addition, vitamin A deficiency decreases the covalent binding of metabolites of chemical carcinogens to hamster trachea in an in vitro organ culture (37). Finally, both naturally-occurring and synthetic retinoids inhibit the changes produced on mouse prostate in organ culture by the polycyclic aromatic hydrocarbon 3-methylcholanthrene (38). Thus, there is ample evidence to suggest that retinoids inhibit carcinogen metabolism both within intact animals and in organ culture, therefore decreasing the concentration of ultimate carcinogen capable of interacting with target biological molecules. Furthermore, the results presented here suggest that this process may be isolated from other processes by application of short term tests in examining the modulation of the metabolism not only of chemical carcinogens, but of other xenobiotics present in the environment.

Acknowledgments

The author acknowledges the expert technical assistance of George Sfeir, Mary Jones and Cathleen Slade. The Salmonella strains were kindly provided by Professor Bruce Ames. Aroclor 1254 was generously provided by Montsanto Co., and 3,2'-dimethyl-4-amino-biphenyl was generously supplied by the National Cancer Institute.

Literature Cited

1. Sporn, M.B.; Dunlop, N.M.; Newton, D.L.; Smith, J.M.   Federation Proc. 1976, 35, 1332.
2. Chu, E.W.; Malmgren, R.A.   Cancer Res. 1965, 25, 884.
3. Shamberger, R.J.   J. Natl. Cancer Inst. 1971, 47, 667.
4. Bollag, W.   European J. Cancer, 1972, 8, 689.
5. Cone, M.V.; Nettsheim, P.   J. Natl. Cancer Inst. 1973, 50, 1599.
6. Bollag, W.   European J. Cancer 1975, 11, 721.

7. Grubbs, C.J.; Moon, R.C.; Squire, R.A.; Farrow, G.M.; Stinson,
    S.F.; Goodman, D.G.; Brown, G.B.; Sporn, M.B. Science (U.S.)
    1977, 198, 743.
8. Sporn, M.B.; Squire, R.A.; Brown, C.C.; Smith, J.M.; Wenk, M.L.;
    Springer, S. Science (U.S.) 1977, 195, 487.
9. Vark, J.D.; Smith, A.H.; Switzer, R.R.; Hames, G.C. J. Natl.
    Cancer Inst. 1981, 66, 7.
10. Wald, N.; Idle, M.; Bareham, J.; Bailey, A. Lancet 1980, 2, 813.
11. Bjelke, E. International J. Cancer 1975, 15, 561.
12. Mettlin, C.; Graham, S. Amer. J. Epidemiol. 1979, 110, 255.
13. Mettlin, C.; Graham, S., Swanson, J. J. Natl. Cancer Inst. 1979,
    62, 1435.
14. Shekeller, R.B.; Lepper, M.; Liv, S. et al. Lancet 1981, 2, 1185.
15. Berenblum, I. In "Cancer: A Comprehensive Treatise"; Becker,
    F.F., Ed.; Plenum: New York, 1975, Vol. I, p. 323.
16. Mori, S. Johns Hopkins Hosp. Bull. 1922, 33, 357.
17. Wolbach, S.D.; Howe, P.R. J. Exp. Med. 1925, 42, 753.
18. DeLuca, L.M.; Shapiro, S.S. "Modulation of cellular interactions
    by vitamin A and derivatives (retinoids). ANNALS OF THE NEW
    YORK ACADEMY OF SCIENCES, Vol. 359, New York, 1981.
19. Georgieff, K.K. Science (U.S.) 1971, 173, 537.
20. Hill, D.L.; Shih, T.W. Cancer Res. 1974, 34, 564.
21. Heidelberger, C. Annual Rev. Biochem. 1975, 44, 79.
22. Strobel, H.R.; Coon, M.J. J. Biol. Chem. 1971, 246, 7826.
23. Baird, M.B.; Birnbaum, L.S. J. Natl. Cancer Inst. 1979, 63,
    1093.
24. Ames, B.N. In "Chemical Mutagens: Principles and Methods for
    Their Detection"; Hollander, A., Ed.; Plenum: New York, 1971,
    Vol. I, p. 267.
25. Ames, B.N.; Durston, W.E.; Yamasaki, F.; Lee, F.D. Proc. Natl.
    Acad. Sci. (U.S.) 1973, 70, 2281.
26. McCann, J.; Choi, E.; Yamasaki, E.; Ames, B.N. Proc. Natl.
    Acad. Sci. (U.S.) 1975, 72, 5135.
27. DeSerres, F.J.; Shelby, M.D. Science (U.S.) 1979, 203, 563.
28. Busk, L.; Ahlborg, U.G. Toxicol. Letters 1980, 6, 243.
29. Rocchi, P.; Arfellini, G.; Capucci, A.; Grilli, M.P.; Prodi, G.
    Carcinogenesis 1983, 4, 245.
30. Forster, R.; Green, M.H.L.; Priestly, A. Carcinogenesis 1981,
    2, 1081.
31. Prival, M.J.; Mitchell, V.D. Cancer Res. 1981, 41, 4361.
32. Saccone, G.T.P.; DasGupta, B.R.; Pariza, M.W. Cancer Res. 1981,
    41, 4600.
33. Spjut, H.J. Cancer 1970, 28, 29.
34. Spjut, H.J.; Noall, M.W. In "Carcinoma of the Colon and Antece-
    dent Epithelium"; Burdette , W.J., Ed.; Thomas: Springfield,
    1970, p. 280.
35. McCormick, D.L.; Burns, F.J.; Albert, R.E. Cancer Res. 1980, 40,
    1140.
36. Moon, R.C.; McCormick, D.L.; Mehta, R.G. Cancer Res. (suppl.)
    1983, 43, 2469 .
37. Genta, V.M.; Kaufman, D.G.; Harris, C.C.; Smith, J.M.; Sporn,
    M.B.; Saffioti, U. Nature (London) 1974, 247, 48.
38. Lasnitzki, I.; Goodman, D.S. Cancer Res. 1974, 34, 1564.

RECEIVED August 17, 1984

Effects of Hormone and Diet on Hepatic Enzymes

OLGA GREENGARD

Departments of Pediatrics and Pharmacology, Mount Sinai School of Medicine of The City University of New York, New York, NY 10029

Enzymes subserving hepatotypic functions are acquired in three major clusters at critical stages of normal development. It has been possible to evoke the precocious synthesis of specific groups of enzymes with injection of appropriate hormones, and to show that the normal time schedule is regulated primarily by sequential changes in the circulatory level of glucocorticoids, thyroid hormones and glucagon. The results provide insights into defective hepatic functions frequently noted in apparently healthy newborn infants, and point to means for circumventing them. The process of biochemical differentiation, though normally unidirectional, suffers partial reversal in the cancer-free liver of tumor-bearing rats: the regulatory properties of enzymes and, more importantly, their overall quantitative pattern changes towards that in normal fetal liver. This immature hepatic enzyme composition, seen also in the histologically normal liver samples of human subjects of extrahepatic cancers, contributes to the metabolic deterioration and eventual cachexia of the host organism.

This account deals with pathological or physiological variations in hepatic functions which, occuring in the face of an intact genome, involve quantitative alterations in qualitatively normal gene products. Studies on the liver of adult rats treated with hormonal or nutritional factors(1) were the first to demonstrate that alterations in the concentrations of appropriate enzymes play a primary role in metabolic regulations by several hormones or nutritional conditions. Adult animals were also used for the initial demonstration that stimulated mRNA synthesis, or in some cases increased rate of translation, underlies the induction of mammalian enzymes(2,3). It has then become apparent that viewing this phenomenon from the vantage point of differentiation, provides further insights into the underlying mechanisms, and aids the interpretations of disease-associated hepatic enzyme patterns not only in the immature but also in the adult organism.

The impetus for the developmental studies came not from embryology but from clinical observations on the postnatal organism, on metabolic problems frequently seen in newborn children. They occurred in the absence of genetic or morphological abnormalities, were often transient, indicated defects in hepatic functions, and had a higher incidence in premature than in term infants. For these reasons, Dawkins(4) suggested that several important hepatic enzymes are acquired only shortly before or after term, so that the newborn is not immediately ready to take over functions which, like detoxifixations, had been carried out by the maternal liver.

TABLE I - Enzyme concentration in developing human liver

Enzyme	AQ	
	Midgestation	Term
Phenylalanine hydroxylase	0.59	0.51
Arginase	0.46	0.46
Aspartate aminotranferase	0.28	0.62
Cystathionine synthetase	0.21	0.53
Phenylalanine pyruvate amino-transferase	0.59	0.51
Cystathionase	0.00	0.0-0.6
Tyrosine aminotransferase	0.07	--
Alanine aminotransferase	0.04	0.04
UPD-glucuronyl transferase	0.10	0.1
Phosphoenolypyruvate carboxy-kinase	0.08	0.11* 0.42+

To obtain activity Quotients (AQ), enzyme activities (units per g liver) were divided by those in normal, adult liver. For further details see reference 5.

*7 months of gestation.

+3 days after birth.

Subsequent studies have shown (e.g. 5,6, Table I) that the liver of newborns is indeed deficient in enzymes needed not only for drug metabolism but also for the elimination of natural products. For example, because of the lack of UDP-glucuronyl transferase resulting in the inability to dispose of bilirubin, the newborn is at risk for brain damage by kernicterus. That PEP carboxykinase, the key catalyst of gluconeogenesis de novo is absent at 7 months and still at low titers 3 days after birth (Table I), probably contributes to the fact that transient hypoglycemia (which can also cause brain damage) represents a hazard to full term as well as premature infants. The immaturity of the hepatic enzyme composition imposes limitations on the choice of nutrients used to supplement or replace the natural diet. For example, in connection with the species difference in the amino acid composition of milk proteins, the lack of cystathionase and half the adult levels of other enzymes in amino acid metabolism (Table I) become a problem, in that they seem to underlie the potentially harmful, low methionine and abnormally high phenylalanine levels in infants fed on protein-enriched formulae (7).

The more extensive information available for rats(8) showed that the capacity for hepatotypic functions is acquired in three major steps, with the sudden, simultaneous upsurge of a dozen or more enzymes at each of three critical stages of development. Fig. 1, which lists some representatives of each cluster, illustrates that the time schedule "makes sense" in terms of the changing functional requirements of the organism. For example, owing to the late fetal emergence of enzymes necessary for glycogen deposition, an energy source is available by the time the continuous maternal glucose supply is cut, and a few hours after birth, by which time the hepatic glycogen store is used up, the liver can begin to engage in gluconeogenesis from amino acids or lactate. That malic enzyme emerges only with the late suckling cluster is in accord with the need for fatty acid synthesis when changing from milk to the relatively high carbohydrate-containing solid diet.

The process of biochemical differentiation is not an unresolvable succession of predestined events. In rat liver several individual enzymes or specific groups of enzymes which have been caused to be formed "out of step" a few hours after the administration of the appropriate stimulus, can attain levels normally associated with a more mature morphology and overall enzyme profile. To mention a few examples, rats given a prenatal injection of thyroxin are born with more cytochrome c reducatase than untreated ones, and only 24 hours later does the control animal attain the same level of this component of the microcomal drug metabolising system (Figure 2). Additional enzymes undergoing such a precocious rise in reponse to thyroxine are those of the urea cycle, while prenatal cortisol injection, stimulating the formation of glycogen synthetase, results in rats born with more extensive hepatic glycogen deposits. The fact that in the normal rat fetus glucocorticoid and thyroid hormone secretions begin at about the same time (the 16th day)(10), explains the sudden, simultaneous upsurge of the different enzymes of the late fetal cluster. On the other hand, the secretion of glucagon (rising after birth in the human as well as rat circulation) is a natural trigger for the synthesis of the neonatal cluster of enzymes, since the prenatal formation of several of these was evoked by an injection of glucagon(11,12).

The general conclusion would thus be that the timing of the appearence of different groups of enzymes is attributable to the sequential appearance of different endocrine factors in the circulation. However, the emergence of the last, the late suckling cluster of enzymes, cannot be attributed to a new hormone, but to the secondary quantitative increase (following an early postnatal ebb) in glucocorticoid and thyroid hormone secretion(13,14). Why did these enzymes fail to respond to the first, prenatal and much more impressive rise in these secretions that occurred prenatally?

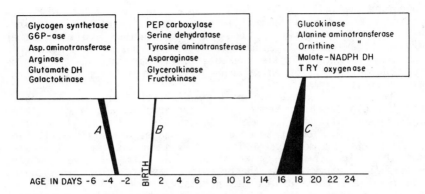

Figure 1. The sequential emergence of enzyme clusters in developing liver.

For additional members of the late fetal (A), neonatal (B), and late suckling (C) cluster of enzymes see ref. 8. G6P-ase, glucose-6-phosphatase; glutamate DH, glutamate dehydrogenase; malate-NADP DH, malic enzyme; TRY Oxygenase, tryptophan oxygenase.

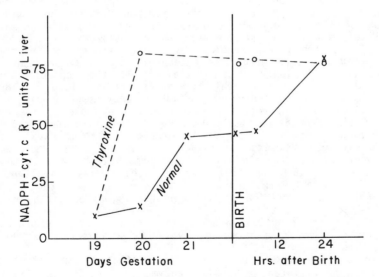

Figure 2. Precociously induced enzyme formation in developing rat liver.

Half of the fetuses in each pregnant rat on the 19th gestational day were injected with 3 micrograms thyroxine (circles) and the other half with saline (crosses). They were killed at the difference pre- or postnatal times indicated by the abscissa, and cytochrome c reductase (ordinate) was quantified.

And why is it that, while we could evoke these enzymes by cortisol (e.g. alanine aminotransferase) or thyroxine (malic enzyme) in neonatal life, we could not do so prenatally? The explanation can clearly cannot lie in receptor availability since the same hormones do induce alternative enzymes at the same fetal stage.

It was not unexpected to come up against such puzzles, since one of them had already become apparent in connection with the first evidence for the feasibility of precocious enzyme inductions. Throughout postnatal life, tyrosine aminotransferase is exquisitely sensitive to glucocorticoid, and yet an injection of glucagon or cAMP (which are not effective inducers in adulthood) is what caused it to rise in fetal liver from undetectable to adult levels(15). Both cortisol and glucagon act on transcription, but as shown recently(16), in fetal liver in vivo only glucagon (or cAMP) can stimulate the synthesis of messenger RNA specific for tyrosine aminotransferase. Thus, the same gene can respond to different inducers at different stages of development. The event of birth per se is not necessarily the crucial factor since, after a prenatal injection of glucagon, cortisol can also induce the synthesis of tyrosine aminotransferase in fetal liver(17). It appears, that once exposed to the developmental stimulus, the synthetic system becomes competent to respond to new regulators. The sensitivity of

Table II

Changes with age in the inducibility of arginase in vivo

Increase of Hepatic Arginase:

Hormone injected 24 hr before assay:	Fetal	9 days	28 days	35 days	adult rats
Thyroxine, 2.5µg/g	52%				N.S.
Hydrocortisone, 2.5 µg/g	N.S.[+]	360%	20%	N.S.*	N.S.
Glucagon, 5 mg/g	N.S.		61%	N.S.*	N.S.

*from Brebnor et al (25).

[+]N.S., no significant change.

tyrosine aminotransferase to its new regulator (glucocorticoid) persists, whereas (as explified in Table II and also in Table V) the inducibility of many other enzymes continues to vary with postnatal age and metabolic state. This changing competence is of immediate practical importance to designing hormone treatments for correcting developmental delays or disease associated enzyme deficiencies. Also, study of the as yet obscure molecular mechanisms involved should greatly advance current thinking about mechanisms of gene expression. Another puzzle brought up by the developmental studies will be postponed until after discussing a disease syndrome in adulthood, namely, the multiplicity of enzymic lesions in the liver caused by anatomically distant, cancerous growth in the organism.

In early studies of the cancer-free liver of animals carrying various subcutaneous neoplasms, a variety of enzymes were reported to exhibit decreased or increased levels, or changes in isozyme pattern. To examine this phenomenon more systematically, we turned to the above-described classification of enzymes according to their developmental behavior, and assayed the liver of mammary carcinoma-bearing rats for some two dozen enzymes, representing each of the 3 clusters emerging at critical stages of ontogeny and also a hitherto unmentioned cluster, one whose members undergo a decrease during postembryonic differentiation. The many enzymes thus found

Table III

The tumor-induced undifferentiation of the enzymic composition in the cancer-free liver

	Enzyme units per g liver		Developmental
Rats:	Tumor-bearing adult	Normal fetal	emergence
Enzymes	(normal adult=1.0)		
Alanine aminotransferase	0.53±0.10	0.1	3rd postnatal
Ornithine amino-transferase	0.30±0.15	0.1	week
Malic enzyme	0.50±0.16	0.1	"
Glucokinase	0.41±0.15	0.1	"
Glutamine synthetase	0.60±0.07	0.2	"
Serine dehydratase	0.64	0.10	neonatal
Arginase	0.85±0.13	0.10	late fetal
Cytochrome c reductase	0.66±0.1	0.12	"
Hexokinase	1.66±0.09	1.1	embryonic
-glutamyl trans-peptidase	3.20±0.6	9.4	"
Phosphofructokinase	3.1	2.8	"

Further information on tumor-bearing and fetal rats are in reference 8 and 18, respectively.

to be sensitive to tumor implantation (a portion of the results is shown in Table III), were quite heterogenous with respect to metabolic functions, subcellular location or regulatory properties. The only common denominator behind this diversity was that "adult" enzymes (i.e. clusters emerging at late stages of ontogeny) were the only ones at diminished titers in the host's liver, and that those responding positively were all enzymes at higher levels in normal fetal than in more mature liver(18). Thus, while the adult host's liver showed no histological loss of differentiation, its overall quantitative pattern of enzymes shifted towards that of immature liver. Since the cluster which is the last to emerge in the course of normal development showed the most striking response to tumor-bearing (in terms of the number of enzymes involved and the extent to which they decreased) it appeared as if we were dealing with an almost orderly reversal of the process of enzymic differentiation. Qualitatively similar patterns of change were then found in rats with transplanted renal, hepatic, muscle or salivary gland tumors, and also in the histologically normal liver samples of human subjects of extrahepatic cancers(19,20).

The biochemical undifferentiation of the liver was found to begin long before the onset of ill-health: losses of enzymes, detectable 4-6 days after transplantation when the tumor is not yet palpable,(18,19) are clearly not a consequence of malnutrition or other side-effects. On the contrary, they must be among the causes of the metabolic deterioration seen at later stages of the disease. It is worth illustrating, therefore, that a relatively small, quantitative change in the amount of an enzyme ascertained by assay under unnatural, in vitro conditions (i.e. at saturating substrate and cofactor concentrations) is associated with significant functional changes in vivo. Figure 3 shows that in tumor-bearing rats with an only 30% reduction of hepatic cytochrome c reductase the duration of hexobarbital hypnosis was appreciably longer than normal, and that the further loss of enzyme (with increasing tumor size) was paralelled by a progressive increase in sleeping time. Each responsive hepatic enzyme, including cytochrome c reductase, was found to revert to normal levels a few days after surgical eradication of the tumor(21). Correspondingly, sleeping time became normalized (see dark triangles, as opposed to open ones for sham-operated animals in inset of Fig. 3), except in those few rats whose autopsy revealed tumor regrowth (see half dark triangels). Thus, the length of the sleeping time provides indication as to whether surgery was successful or whether it failed to remove all the cancer cells.

Such simple, non-invasive tests are not yet available for determining the physiological consequences of tumor-induced changes in the many other catalysts (e.g. Table III). It stands to reason, however, that a hepatic enzyme pattern akin to that of immature liver would put the adult organism at a disadvantage. It would contribute to aspects of the cancer patient's morbidity that often cannot be explained by anorexia or by the thermodynamic cost of synthesizing tumor constituents. That weight-loss bears no necessary correlation to food intake or to tumor burden(22) indicates that the problem lies not merely in the availability, but in the utilization of nutrients. Glucokinase and malic enzyme may be implicated in anomalies shown by cancer patients in carbohydrate utilization and its appropriate adaptation to changing food intake. In tumor-bearing animals (Table IV) their basal levels are low, show an excessive loss upon starvation, and no recovery is seen

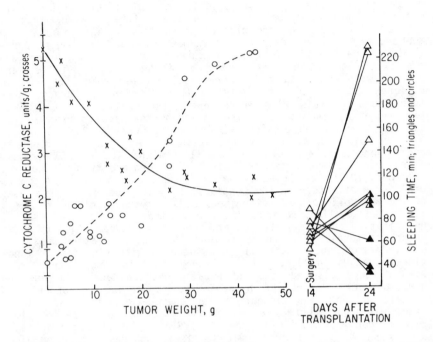

Figure 3. Changes of hepatic cytochrome c reductase content and hexobarbital sleeping time with fibrosarcoma growth.

Tumors (approximately 10^6 cells) were implanted subcutaneously into one of the flanks of adult male KX rats. Left side: points refer to individual rats without tumors (abscissa = 0) or 4-30 days after transplantation. Cytochrome c reductase activity (μmoles/ min/g of liver, crosses) and hexobarbital sleeping time (open circles, right ordinate) are plotted against tumor weight. Right side: each line connects the sleeping time of one rat measured twice: a few hours before surgery (when tumors were 5-9 g) and 10 days later. Autopsy examination detected no tumor (▲) or 0.2 to 4.5 g regrowth (▲) of the apparently totally resected tumors. In the three sham-operated animals (△) at 30 days, the tumors weighed 30-50 g.

after 48 hours of refeeding (whereas in tumor-free amimals the partial loss of glucokinase and malic enzyme is completely restored within two days of refeeding).

Table IV

Effects of fasting and refeeding on adult normal
and tumor-bearing rats

| | | Enzyme units/g liver | | |
		Control	Fasted, 48 hr.	Refed, 48 hr.
Glucokinase	Normal	1.42 ± 0.75	0.60 ± 0.26	1.24 ± 0.08
	Tumor-bearing	0.58 ± 0.10	0.03	0.03
Malic Enzyme	Normal	1.0 ± 0.15	0.65 ± 0.22	1.07 ± 0.15
	Tumor-bearing	0.60 ± 0.16	0.32 ± 0.02	0.33 ± 0.14

Adult male Fischer rats without and with transplanted mammary carcinoma 5a were deprived of food for 48 hr and were analyzed at this time (fasted) or after a 48-hr period of refeeding the normal diet. The results are means (± SD) of determinations on 3 or more rats.

Several lines of evidence indicate that macromolecules of as yet unidentified chemical nature, produced by cancers and released into the systemic circulation, are responsible for the biochemical alterations in the liver and other host organs. In view of the diverse regulatory properties of the many different enzymes that increase or decrease towards their immature level (see Table III), a deficiency or excess in any given endocrine or dietary factor can clearly not explain the phenomenon. Nor has it been possible to implicate reductions in the efficacy of these factors. Subnormal concentration of the nuclear thyroid hormone receptor has been noted in the liver of tumor-bearing animals(24); however, since losses in the T3-inducible catalysts of the same liver occurred at much earlier stages of tumor-bearing,(24) the subnormal receptor concentration could clearly not be the cause of these losses but was probably another, and rather late, reflection of the process of biochemical undifferentiation.

In recent studies(23,26) attempts were made to normalize the tumor-induced abnormalities in the levels of hepatic enzymes. It is known that catalysts of the urea cycle are induced by high protein diet, while high carbohydrate intake, decreasing the levels of alanine aminotransferase, increases those of malic enzyme and pyruvate kinase. In each case, the same percent change was seen in tumor-bearing and normal adult animals (Table V), so that the tumor-induced defiency of such enzymes seen in rats on a normal diet was also apparent on these altered diets. Hormone treatments,

Table V

The effect of tumor bearing on enzyme inductions

	Adult rats		Immature rats
	Normal	Tumor-bearing	(5-28 day old)
	% change		
Argininosuccinate synthase			
βmethasone	N.S.	100	+
glucagon	N.S.	113	+
DcAMP	N.S.	117	+
high protein diet	43	30	
Arginase			
βmethasone	N.S.	28	+
glucagon	N.S.	25	+
DcAMP	N.S.	35	+
high protein diet	27	29	
Alanine aminotransferase			
cortisol	N.S.	90	+
high carbohydrate	-28	-30	-
Malic enzyme			
thyroxine	373	600	+
high carbohydate	530	700	+
Pyruvate kinase			
thyroxine	N.S.	63	+
high carbohydrate	238	258	+

The results on the first two enzymes, and on the others, are from Brebnor et al.(26), and from Greengard and Cayanis(23), respectively. For increases and decreases (plus and minus signs) under "Immature rats" see refs 8 and 25. DcAMP, dibutyryl cyclic AMP; N.S., no significant change.

on the other hand, did abolish or minimize some of the enzymic differences. In normal adult rats, as opposed to immature ones (see Table II and positive signs in Table V), the level of urea cycle enzymes failed to respond to an injection of glucocorticoid (hydrocortisone or βmethasone), glucagon or cAMP. After tumor implantation, however, all three agents became effective again; the results by Brebnor et al.(26) on argininosuccinate synthase, the rate limiting enzyme in urea synthesis, illustrate this most strikingly (Table V). Our studies on enzymes of the late suckling cluster yielded similar results. An injection of cortisol which triggers the developmental formation of alanine aminotransferase, had no effect on this enzyme in normal adult liver, but caused a 90 percent increase in tumor-bearing animals. Glucocorticoids play no role in the development of the last two enzymes in Table V; thyroid hormones were found to enhance their early postnatal formation(13). It may be seen that the responsiveness of malic enzyme, which is not entirely lost with age, was smaller in normal than in tumor bearing adult animals. The results on pyruvate kinase are somewhat more striking, in that the response to thyroid hormone is entirely lost with age, but becomes significant again after tumor implantation. The general picture emerging from these studies is that in tumor-bearing animals not only the basal levels of hepatic enzymes, but their responsiveness to appropriate hormonal stimuli, reverts to that characteristic for normal, immature liver. It is possible that, as in the case of alterations in basal levels, so the increasing inducibility of enzymes is attributable to the direct action of factors that tumors elaborate and release to the systemic circulation. The only evidence for this at present is the recently reported(26) experiment with plasma from tumor hosts: its administration to normal mature rats not only reduced the basal level of urea cycle enzymes but also made them responsive again to glucagon.

Despite this accumulating information, the molecular mechanism of the cancer-induced undifferentiation of the liver is still a mystery. This is not too surprising since, as will be illustrated with another puzzle brought up by the developmental studies, we do not even understand the mechanism whereby the differentiated functional state of the liver is normally maintained.

It has been noted in the case of several enzymes that their artificial prococious induction is reversible in that, unless the injection of the appropriate hormone is repeated, the enzyme disappears again. Why is it then that after its natural appearance at the scheduled time, the persistence of the enzyme does not hinge on the continued action of that hormone? For example, glucocorticoid is undoubtedly the essential developmental stimulus for the hepatic ornithine aminotransferase(14), a member of the late suckling cluster. Its normal emergence on day 12 can be prevented by prior adrenalectomy, its precocious synthesis (5-10 days before schedule) can be evoked by an injection of cortisol, and yet no loss at all is incurred by adrenalectomy performed at or after the time at which ornithine aminotransferase has attained near adult or adult values (i.e. on day 20 or later).

Other enzymes with an absolute dependence on glucocorticoid or thyroid hormone for their development, may show a small quantitative decrease upon depreviation of these hormones in maturity, but in no case is this extirpation of the corresponding gland followed by the disappearance of the appropriate enzyme. An explanation we proposed was that with maturation new, positive regulators come into play(8). Alternatively, one may postulate that the continued expression of these genes is made possible by the disappearance with age of "negative regulators" which, present at earlier stages, were responsible for the evanescence of enzymes induced precociously (and also for our inability, mentioned earlier, to induce some of these enzymes before birth). Although such repressive factors have been shown to be present in the embryonic environment, the attractive hypothesis that analogous factors elaborated by cancer cells are responsible for the biochemical undifferentiation of the hosts' liver, lacks factual support. It is clear, however, that study of tumor-bearing animals may provide insights into mechanisms which normally preserve the functional potentials acquired by the liver during development. In fact, unless we learn to explain the mechanisms underlying the immature enzyme pattern in the histologically normal liver of cancer hosts, we cannot claim to have a good understanding of the normal process of biochemical differentiation.

Acknowledgments

These studies were supported by NIH Research Grants CA 25005 and HD 17636.

Literature Cited

1.   Knox, W.E.; Auerbach, V.H.; Lin, E.C.C. Physiol. Rev. 1956, 36, 164.

2.   Schutz, G.; Killewich, L.; Feigelson, P. Natl. Acad. Sci. 1975, 72, 1017-1020.

3.   Schimke, R.T.; Sweeney, E.W.; Berlin, C.M. J. Biol. Chem. 1965, 240,322-331.

4.   Dawkins, M.J.R. Br. Med. Bull. 1966, 22, 27-33.

5.   Greengard, O. Pediat. Res. 1977, 11, 669-676.

6.   Raiha, N.C.R.; Lindros, K.O. Ann. Med. Exp. Biol. Fenn. 1969, 47, 146-

7.   Gaull, G.E.; Rassin, D.K.; Raiha, N.C.R.; Heinonen, K. J. Pediat. 1977, 90, 348-355.

8.   Greengard, O. Essays Biochem. 1971, 7, 159-205.

9.   Greengard, O. Science 1969, 163, 891-895.

10. Jost, A. Recent Prog. Hormone Res. 1966, 22, 541-569.

11. Greengard, O.; Dewey, H.K. J. Biol. Chem. 1967, 242, 2986-2991.

12. Yeung, D.; Oliver, I.T. Biochem. J. 1968, 108, 325-331.

13. Greengard, O.; Jamdar, S.C. Biochim. Biophys. Acta 1971, 237, 476-483.

14. Herzfeld, A.; Greengard, O. J. Biol. Chem. 1969, 244, 4894-4898.

15. Greengard, O. Biochem. J. 1969, 115, 19-24.

16. Ruiz-Bravo, N.; Ernest, M.J. <u>Proc. Nat. Acad. Sci. U.S. - Biol. Sci</u> 1982, 79, 365-368.

17. Greengard, O. In "Perinatal Pharmacology: Problems and Priorities"; Dancis J.; Hwang, J.C.; Eds.; Raven Press Publishers, New York, 1974, pp. 15-26.

18. Herzfeld, A.; Greengard, O. <u>Cancer Res.</u> 1972, 32, 1826-1832.

19. Herzfeld, A.; Greengard, O. <u>Cancer Res.</u> 1977, 37, 231-

20. Herzfeld, A.; Greengard, O.; McDermott, W.V. <u>Cancer</u> 1980, 45, 2383-2388.

21. Greengard, O. <u>Biochem. Pharmacol.</u> 1979, 28, 2569-2572.

22. Costa, G.; Donaldson, S.S. <u>N. Engl. J. Med.</u> 1979, 300, 1471-1474.

23. Greengard, O.; Cayanis, E. <u>Cancer Res.</u> 1983, 43, 1575-1580.

24. Grajower, M.M.; Surks, M.I. <u>Endo.</u> 1979, 104, 697-703.

25. Brebnor, L.; Phillips, E.; Balinsky, J.B. <u>Enzyme</u> 1981, 26, 265-270.

26. Brebnor, L.D.; Grimm, J.; Balinsky, J.B. <u>Cancer Res.</u> 1981, 41, 2692-2699.

RECEIVED September 5, 1984

INDEXES

Author Index

Subject Index

A

Arachidonic acid (AA) metabolism,
    enzymatically regulated lipid
    peroxidation, 255
Aryl hydrocarbon hydroxylase (AHH)
  detoxification of xenobiotics, 4
  effect of cigarette smoke, 235
  effect of dietary fat on
      activity, 141t
  protective effect of dietary protein
      on DMBA-induced breast
      tumor, 319
  and xenobiotic metabolism, 151
Ascitic tumors, inhibition by
    selenium, 275
Ascorbic acid
  inhibition of in vitro formation of
      N-nitroso compounds, 114
  plasma level, effect of cigarette
      smoke, 232
Atherosclerosis
  free radical involvement, 78t,79
  and lipid peroxidation, 255
Autoxidation
  inhibited, linoleic acid, 8
  kinetics of inhibited, linoleic
      acid, 89
  linoleic acid, quantitative
      study, 84-92
  and lipid hydroperoxide
      production, 82
  styrene, 90
  unsaturated lipids, cigarette smoke
      extract, 229
Azo dye metabolites, HPLC, 98
Azo dye oxidation, lipid peroxide
    catalyzed, 98
Azofluorene formation, effect of
    DNA, 103
Azoxymethane (AOM)
  effect of dietary protein on
      mutagenic products, 295
  fiber effects on experimental colon
      carcinogenesis, 56
  induced colon cancer, effect of
      fiber, 58t

B

Bacteria, cecal, effect of dietary
    fiber, 41,43t
Bacterial assay, host-mediated, DMH,
    AOM, and MAM, 297
Barbiturates, interaction with dietary
    choline deficiency in promoting
    liver cancer, 327-35
Bay region dihydrodiol epoxide of
    DMBA, DNA-reactive
    metabolites, 190

Beef, charcoal broiled, effect on
    human drug metabolism, 62
Beef fat, effect of type and amount of
    dietary fat on colon tumors, 124t
Beef protein, cooked, effect on DHM
    induced colon cancer, 295
Benzoflavone, inhibition of DMBA-DNA
    binding, 203
Benzo(a)pyrene (BaP) metabolism,
    effect of dietary sulfur amino
    acids, 151-60
Benzo(a)pyrene (BaP) metabolite
  effects of phenolic antioxidants on
      DNA adducts, 241-48
  typical fluorescence
      chromatogram, 155
Bile acids
  and colon tumor promotion, 126
  excretion, effect of dietary fat and
      fiber, 125
  related to dietary fat and fiber and
      colon cancer, 169
Binding
  DNA, during aminofluorene catalyzed
      oxidation by peroxide, 101
  DNA-carcinogen, monitor for elec-
      trophilic metabolites, 187-206
Biochemical transformation of drugs,
    effect of foods, 222
Biosynthesis, hepatic ascorbic acid,
    stimulation, 232
Bood cell concentrations, rats exposed
    to cigarette smoke, 231
Bowman-Birk inhibition, possible
    sites, 289
Bowman-Birk protease inhibitor,
    soybean flour, 285
Bowman-Birk type protease inhibitors,
    anticarcinogens, 284
Bran
  effect on induced colon cancer, 56
  influence on dimethylhydrazine-
      induced colon cancer, 58t
Breast cancer
  BHT protection, 142
  DMBA-induced, 136f
  effect of dietary fat and hormone
      level, 319
  effect of fat, 178,317,330
  effect of fat and
      antioxidants, 131-47
  effect of fat and protein, 309-21
  effect of
      selenium, 110,269t,271,272t
  effect of various antioxidants, 137
  human, Bowman-Birk soybean trypsin
      and chymotrypsin inhibitor, 289
  mechanism of inhibition
    dietary fat, 317

Production by Anne Riesberg
Indexing by Susan Robinson
Jacket design by Pamela Lewis

Elements typeset by Hot Type Ltd., Washington, D.C.
Printed and bound by Maple Press Co., York, Pa.